NURSING EDUCATION

NURSING EDUCATION

PLANNING AND DELIVERING THE CURRICULUM

Jennifer Boore
and Pat Deeny

SAGE

Los Angeles | London | New Delhi
Singapore | Washington DC

SAGE

Los Angeles | London | New Delhi
Singapore | Washington DC

SAGE Publications Ltd
1 Oliver's Yard
55 City Road
London EC1Y 1SP

SAGE Publications Inc.
2455 Teller Road
Thousand Oaks, California 91320

SAGE Publications India Pvt Ltd
B 1/I 1 Mohan Cooperative Industrial Area
Mathura Road
New Delhi 110 044

SAGE Publications Asia-Pacific Pte Ltd
3 Church Street
#10-04 Samsung Hub
Singapore 049483

First published 2012

Editor: Susan Worsey
Assistant editor: Emma Milman
Production editor: Katie Forsythe
Copyeditor: Helen Fairlie
Proofreader: Elisabeth Rees Evans
Marketing manager: Tamara Navarathnam
Cover design: Lisa Harper
Typeset by: C&M Digitals (P) Ltd, Chennai, India
Printed and bound by: the MPG Books Group

Library of Congress Control Number: 201194313

British Library Cataloguing in Publication data

A catalogue record for this book is available from the British Library

MIX
Paper from responsible sources
FSC www.fsc.org FSC® C013604

ISBN 978-0-85702-743-6
ISBN 978-0-85702-744-3 (pbk)

This book is dedicated to the late Gordon Rae, Emeritus Professor of Psychology and Jenny's husband, whose encouragement and advice on education and statistics helped to make this book possible.

Table of Contents

List of Figures, Tables and Boxes

Figures

Tables

Boxes

About the Authors

The authors have worked together for many years in nursing education at the University of Ulster, and have developed considerable expertise in curriculum development and nursing education in general. Their involvement in curriculum innovations have included the first examples of a community nursing programme integrating the four branches of nursing, an international online masters degree in disaster relief nursing, and a professional Doctorate in Nursing. They have contributed to the nationally and internationally recognised research profile of the School.

Pat Deeny is a Senior Lecturer and Course Director for Specialist Nursing Practice programmes. As external examiner and nursing education consultant, he has provided support to curriculum teams in universities in Ireland, United Kingdom, Finland, United States and South Korea on critical care nursing, pre-hospital care, disaster relief nursing and emergency preparedness. He and his wife Kate live on a farm in the North Sperrins in Northern Ireland with their three daughters Aoife, Bronagh and Dearbhla.

In 1984 Jennifer Boore became the first Professor of Nursing in the island of Ireland when appointed as Head of Department at the University of Ulster. She now lives in Portstewart, Northern Ireland and holds the title of Emeritus Professor of Nursing. During her career she has seen nursing education move from the apprenticeship system through Project 2000 diploma programmes to degree qualifications for entry to the profession. She has substantial experience of teaching and examining pre and post-registration nursing education programmes and research degrees. She is a Fellow of the Royal College of Nursing in the UK, holds an OBE and is still actively involved in review of papers for publication in both nursing and higher education journals and in pre-doctoral education in South Africa.

Acknowledgements

The authors wish to acknowledge the valuable help of the large number of people who have contributed in various ways:

Numerous colleagues in the University of Ulster, including nursing academics, technical and senior administrative staff, particularly those responsible for academic affairs, quality management and student services and the students' union.

Nursing academic colleagues elsewhere in the UK, in Finland, Australia and the USA.

Staff at the numerous organisations consulted particularly the NMC, and QAA.

The staff at SAGE Publications who have been a delight to work with (and who have been so kind during Jenny's recent and sudden bereavement).

List of Abbreviations

AEI	Approved Education Institutions (term used by NMC)
APL	Accreditation of Prior Learning: 'a process for accessing and, as appropriate, recognising prior experiential learning or prior certificated learning for academic purposes'.
CATS	Credit Accumulation and Transfer
CBL	Case Based Learning
CPD	Continuing Professional Development
CQC	Care Quality Commission
CST	Communication Skills Teaching
ECTS	European Credit Transfer and Accumulation System
EHEA	European Higher Education Area
FHEQ	Framework for Higher Education Qualifications for England, Wales and Northern Ireland
FQ-EHEA	Framework for Qualifications of the European Higher Education Area
GCSE	General Certificate of Secondary Education, normally taken at age 16
HE	Higher Education; third level or university level education
HEFCE	Higher Education Funding Council for England
HEI	Higher Education Institution (NMC refers to AEIs or Approved Education Institutions)
ICN	International Council of Nurses
IELTS	International English Language Testing System. Consists of 4 sections: listening, reading, writing and speaking.
IPE	Interprofessional Education
NGO	Non-Governmental Organisation
NHS Trust	Organisation which provides health care within UK National Health Service
NICATS	Northern Ireland Credit Accumulation and Transfer System

NIPEC	Northern Ireland Practice and Education Council for Nursing and Midwifery
NLN	National League for Nursing, USA
NMC	Nursing and Midwifery Council; the Statutory Body for Nursing in the UK
NSL	Nursing Skills Laboratory
OBE	Outcomes-Based Education
OSCE	Objective structured clinical examination
PBL/EBL/TBL	Problem-Based Learning/Enquiry-Based Learning/Task-Based Learning
PCN	Person-Centred Care
QAA	Quality Assurance Agency for Higher Education
RCN	Royal College of Nursing; the major professional organisation and one of the trade unions for Nurses in the UK
REF (RAE)	Research Excellence Framework (replacing the Research Assessment Exercise) a regular audit of research quality in the UK
SCQF	Scottish Credit and Qualifications Framework
UCAS	University and College Admission System

1 ORIENTATION TO BOOK

INTRODUCTION

Nursing education is about preparing the next generation of nurses and, thus, must be done well to ensure that patients continue to receive high quality care. This book hopes to make a contribution to this through helping those involved in the preparation of nurses. This chapter aims to provide an orientation to the book as a whole and considers how it might be used by the wide range of staff who contribute to nursing education.

VALUES UNDERPINNING THIS BOOK

A book about education has the potential to become very focused on education itself, with the subject of the education becoming secondary. However, we consider that the professional practice of nursing has characteristics which mean that the subject area should strongly influence the educational approaches and is as important as the educational knowledge and skills. The key is the appropriate merging of the two and the clarification of the values underpinning nursing education.

As authors of this book, we declare that we are coming from a perspective of nursing as caring – caring which requires a high level of knowledge and skill applied with compassion and empathy within an ethical framework. Chapter 2 examines nursing in rather more detail; later chapters consider the different aspects of the educational enterprise and endeavour to integrate both nursing and educational knowledge and approaches.

THE READERSHIP

This is a book originating within the UK and, of necessity, is founded on the nursing education system in this country in which programmes are required by the Nursing and Midwifery Council to be offered in partnership between Higher Education (HE) and the health services (NMC, 2010a). Education involves staff working in different institutions with a range of differing responsibilities, as discussed in greater detail in later chapters.

In the UK, a number of key educational roles are identified by the Nursing and Midwifery Council (NMC, 2008a):

- the teacher, who holds an appointment in HE or a joint appointment between HE and service;
- the practice teacher employed in service whose educational role focuses mainly on the practice-based preparation of nurse specialists or community public health nurses;
- the service employed mentor who in addition to providing patient care plays an important role in the practice-based education of pre-registration nursing students.

In addition, there are other organizational and educational posts within service whose holders interact with HE in the management of practice learning for nursing.

This book aims to provide a broad view of nursing education and to help all those involved to understand the structures and process. In particular, teachers need to understand the total picture including the social context of education in order to integrate all parts into a coherent whole. Newly appointed teaching staff are moving from an environment where they are confident in their abilities and understand the structures, processes and roles within the organisation. This book will provide information about HEIs (HE Institutes) and how they work, and offer guidance for new teachers that will help them with some aspects of their new role. In time they will develop into an 'expert nurse academic' within the new context. Some chapters will be more relevant to those in specific roles. In addition, other healthcare professionals may find some of the content of this book useful for their own programmes.

Nursing is developing in different ways in different countries of the world. Nurses have varying priorities depending on the needs of their own communities, and will be prepared in different ways. However, it is hoped that this book will be valuable to those involved in nursing education in many parts of the world.

MAJOR AIMS OF THE BOOK

This book examines all aspects of pre-registration nursing education, although some parts of it are equally applicable to post-registration programmes. It focuses on the planning and provision of nursing education, aiming to stimulate creativity and to empower those involved in education in the academic institution and the clinical environment. Creativity and empowerment are prerequisites for undertaking research and will encourage development of the educational research role of those who are primarily educators and clinicians. This book does not examine methodologies for educational research as that information can be found in any good research text (for example, Parahoo, 2006). However, it does endeavour to indicate the evidence base for educational practice in nursing, including some findings which do not always correspond with our expectations.

An examination of education has the potential to become a theoretical discourse with debate about philosophical issues of considerable value to academics (for example, Billings and Halstead (2009) cover this aspect in detail). While we consider that some of this content is useful for all those involved in teaching, the major focus here is realism tempered with idealism. This book aims to be of practical use both to nursing academics and to the clinical practitioners who make a vital contribution to the education of nurses. We also hope it will motivate all those involved in nursing education to work to achieve the highest possible quality of care from their graduates. It is concerned with a variety of different approaches and methods in learning, teaching and assessment, with some information about theoretical underpinnings to nursing education and its application. It includes practical guidance through discussing ideas for teaching methods and provides examples of good practice. The final chapter specifically focuses on quality management although the whole book aims to facilitate the provision of high quality education. This concept frequently receives relatively little attention in curriculum development, often largely consisting of quotations from the HEI's own documentation, but a thorough understanding of what quality is and how it can be achieved is essential. Of particular importance is recognition of the roles of both main partners, the HEI and the clinical service provider, and how these must be integrated in ensuring the quality of the overall programme of nursing education.

Perhaps the most important point to make is that this is not a recipe book, rather it aims to stimulate thought. It also endeavours to enable nursing professionals to identify risks associated with their teaching in relation to care provided to patients by nursing students, and to develop systems for teaching and practice learning to manage such risks.

It aims to facilitate **academic** staff involved in curriculum planning and delivery in making appropriate choices about approaches and methods of delivery. These choices start with identifying their client base (that is, what is their student population) and planning a programme that will enable the recruits to become skilled, compassionate, professional nurses.

Overall this book aims to be precise and to the point, providing useful guidance primarily to those becoming newly involved in this exciting activity, although it may also be useful for more experienced educators.

HOW TO USE THIS BOOK

Different people will use the book in different ways. It is probably most useful for those who are in the early stages of their educational career. Many newly appointed lecturers have moved from being experienced practitioners in practice into being novice academics and need readily available guidance. Many will have been mentors but have not yet completed preparation and recording of their qualification as a teacher on the NMC Register. They are expected to complete this programme within a few years of appointment but, in the meantime, need some guidance on educational issues. However, even in the early stages of a career in nursing education, lecturers may well become involved in curriculum development, contributing their clinical expertise and, perhaps, research competence.

It is easy for experienced teachers to become settled into the routine of teaching and assessment and this book can be valuable in reviving interest and creativity. In many areas of education new writings introduce developments and some of these are discussed here. Experienced staff members are likely to be referring to other publications as well. We consider that Chapters 2 and 3 are essential reading for all those designing a new curriculum.

Some teachers have moved from hospital-based Schools of Nursing or from other educational institutions, such as Colleges of Further Education, into HE. They will need to understand how HEIs work and the principles underpinning some of their practice. One major example of important content is the Bologna Process. Discussion of this in Chapter 4 helps to clarify how it is incorporated into the work of the UK Quality Assurance Agency (QAA) within the European context. This is important with the increasing emphasis on nursing as an international activity, and with students having increasing opportunities to spend some time abroad.

Mentors and practice teachers will gain an understanding of how their roles fit into the total picture of nursing education, and also of the importance of their roles in the development of clinical competence in nursing. Some guidance is provided on approaches to this within the team involved in supporting practice learning. Again, there are publications which focus specifically on these aspects of nursing education (for example, Gopee, 2010; Hinchliff, 2009; Gopee, 2008; The Practice Education Group, 2006).

Some of those appointed to education management roles within health service organisations will not hold a teacher's qualification recorded with the NMC. This book will help them to achieve an adequate understanding of how nursing education is organised and functions, and enable them to work effectively within their collaborating role with HE. Chapter 3 provides useful ideas on how this may be achieved.

NURSING IN HIGHER EDUCATION

As in the UK, most nursing education worldwide now takes place within the Higher Education sector of education (in universities or colleges of higher education), or is moving in that direction. This book is aimed at all those providing that education, or preparing to do so, including those working primarily in the academic institution and those within the practice setting where students gain the essential clinical experience.

University Schools of Nursing are involved in much more than education. Some staff working in such a context are primarily educators or researchers, although many are expected to be both and, however arranged, the integration of the two roles is paramount for enhancing patient care and the development of the nursing profession. However, in addition, staff may be contributing to practice development, dissemination of knowledge, nursing and health policy development, educational and research developments within the institution, regionally, nationally and internationally. While this book focuses on nursing education, it is important that all members of the School see themselves as contributing through the work of the School to the development of nursing and enhancing patient care, and are working from a common set of values.

2 DEFINING THE PROGRAMME

INTRODUCTION

In this book the term 'curriculum' means the totality of the **programme** offered, including the theoretical content, clinical experience, approaches to academic and practice teaching, learning and assessment, student support and maintaining quality. This chapter examines the different dimensions which determine the structure of the curriculum.

Developing a curriculum is a creative process that has potential to empower teaching staff who contribute to it. It should result in a sense of ownership which will enhance creativity in the future delivery of the programme. The process should be founded upon the principles and philosophies of nursing and education, as well as the statutory requirements (NMC, 2010a). This chapter provides a map of the complexity of curriculum development, arriving at a structure that will guide future development of content. This chapter deals with issues which curriculum development teams often find difficult. However, defining the programme is an essential stage in the process, and the time and effort expended on this will make the later stages of curriculum planning easier and more satisfying.

This chapter examines theoretical and philosophical issues in relation to developing nursing education programmes. At the outset it is important to be clear about what we mean by nursing and to be able to specify the characteristics of the students exiting the programme, and the approaches to education that will achieve the desired ends.

In preparing and providing an educational programme in nursing there are a number of key considerations and choices to be made about the application of theory. A number of issues are presented in this chapter from which the team can select those which fit their own orientation. The important concern is that the choices made should be appropriate and useful in helping to achieve the goal of a caring professional nurse working within society. Some consideration of philosophy and theory can help in this enterprise.

There are three major areas for consideration for effective curriculum development:

- *Nursing*: Philosophy, definitions and other issues to help to define the outcome of the programme in terms of the sort of nurse we want to prepare, that is an autonomous practitioner holding appropriate values.
- *Education*: What can we learn from the study of education that will be of value in the education of nurses? What do we need to know about the models and philosophies used in the broader education domain, and how might these contribute to the delivery of the nursing programme which will prepare an autonomous learner who will become an autonomous practitioner?
- *Nursing and Midwifery Council (NMC) Standards and QAA Benchmarks*: What does the NMC (the statutory body for the regulation of nursing in the UK) say about what the programme being planned must achieve? What do the QAA benchmarks for nursing tell us about the expectations for courses at specified academic levels?

Although it must be recognised that these cannot be dealt with in great depth here, they can be explored through further examination of the literature.

PHILOSOPHY FOR NURSING EDUCATION

What is Philosophy?

Philosophy is about the quest to understand fundamental issues about '*knowledge, truth, reason, reality, meaning, mind and value*' through systematic inquiry and reflection. Originally the study of philosophy encompassed '*all aspects of the world and humankind*' but as knowledge has been divided into separate areas of study (for example, history, physics, psychology), philosophy itself has been subdivided into numerous areas (Grayling: 1995: 1–6).

The word itself is derived from the Greek for 'love of wisdom' and The Concise Oxford English Dictionary (OED, 2006) has defined it as:

- The study of the fundamental nature of knowledge, reality, and existence; a set of theories of a particular philosopher; the study of the theoretical basis of a branch of knowledge or experience.
- A theory or attitude that guides one's behaviour.

In nursing the word philosophy tends to be used as a combination of these two sets of definitions above, particularly *'the study of the theoretical basis of a branch of knowledge or experience'* and *'a theory or attitude that guides one's behaviour'*. In the context of this discussion the second of the two is particularly applicable as nursing is essentially a profession which is demonstrated through behaviour. Many of the facets of philosophy are relevant to nursing (Drummond and Standish, 2007), but two in particular are important in relation to nursing education: ethics and epistemology.

Ethics

Ethics has been described as '*enquiry into the nature of value*' (Drummond and Standish, 2007: 5) and it underpins all aspects of nursing practice – clinical, management, education, research, policy development. Ethics relates to what we think nursing is, what sort of nurse we want to prepare and what we expect the nurses to be able to do. The section below on values and beliefs builds on this understanding.

Epistemology

This is the branch of philosophy dealing with the nature of knowledge – clearly highly relevant for nursing, the practice of which is based on knowledge. Rodgers (2005) discusses the philosophical bases for the development of nursing knowledge from the classical period onwards and emphasises the role of the university-based nursing lecturer in the continuing development of knowledge through research, thus influencing education and practice.

Defining nursing knowledge is crucial to the appropriate selection of content in the development of curricula. Fawcett (2005) has identified five levels of contemporary nursing knowledge: metaparadigm at the highest level of abstraction; philosophies; conceptual models; theories; and empirical indicators being the most concrete level. She discusses each of these in some detail and some are considered later in this chapter.

Writing a Philosophy

Supported by theories from social psychology it is evident that values and beliefs influence human motivation and guide human behaviours. Designing a curriculum, like any social activity, will be influenced by values and beliefs which when articulated, normally in writing, are commonly known as a 'philosophy'. Many nurses are already familiar with the idea of writing a '*philosophy of care*' which should articulate the values of the organisation or team and provide a valuable strategic approach. The term '*mission statement*' may also be used to provide a strategic focus. Such statements provide direction for the delivery of the service or production of a quality product, but mission statements normally do not articulate values and beliefs about specific aspects of the service or processes associated with the delivery, hence the need for a philosophy.

It is important therefore that at the beginning of curriculum development, the first stage in educational provision, there is agreement about what nursing is and what values and beliefs underpin nursing practice and nursing education. This enables clarification about the attributes of the nurses the team are aiming to prepare. It is important to articulate these value-belief systems early in the design process so that everyone is aware of such influences and the end product reflects the values and beliefs underpinning the curriculum. As these are articulated they can also help stimulate ideas related to content; for example, values and beliefs that promote a philosophy of nursing that highlights the importance of person-centredness will have themes that reflect this throughout the curriculum.

A philosophy that will underpin a nursing curriculum is slightly different from those that underpin curricula in other disciplines. Clearly, for a nursing curriculum the philosophy must take account of values and beliefs about nursing practice often inherent in nursing codes of practice and nursing theories, as well as values and beliefs and theoretical frameworks which influence the nature and practice of teaching and learning in nursing. In particular the values pertaining to teaching, learning and assessment of competence, a concept which reflects the fundamental basis of nursing practice and professional accountability, are very important. While the national or international codes of practice contribute to a philosophy for nursing, values about other specific aspects of nursing and nursing knowledge must also be considered such as person, environment, nursing and health. Other ideas influencing the nature of nursing and the concept of care, including cultural context and public health, need to be addressed as well as wider social, economic and political perspectives.

Fundamentally the philosophy should provide the reader (who eventually will be the students, teachers and mentors who experience the programme) with a clear idea of the values and beliefs that underpin the curriculum. Writing a philosophy to underpin a nursing curriculum is an in-depth process and requires the team to articulate value and belief statements on nursing practice, nursing knowledge and nursing education. What are the values and beliefs that guide the practice of nursing (and thus equate to a philosophy as discussed above), and what do we expect nurses to be able to do?

Values and Beliefs: Personal and Professional

The profession of nursing is founded on moral values and beliefs about those issues directly relevant to nursing practice. An agreed understanding of these is needed to underpin the whole of the educational enterprise – or even all the work – of the School of Nursing. One approach to achieving such an agreed statement is shown in Box 2.1.

Box 2.1 Agreeing Concepts, Values and Beliefs about Nursing

Issue: New staff join a School of Nursing and it is important to reach agreement on concepts, values and beliefs about nursing as the focus for the work of the newly extended School.

Resolution: During an away-day the four items of the nursing metaparadigm (person, health, environment and nursing) were used as a starting point. Working groups of about 10–12 staff members were allocated one of the four metaparadigm factors each and endeavoured to reach agreement on their beliefs and values in relation to that topic. This was shared with other groups working on the same topic, reconsidered and perhaps modified.

At the end of the day all the statements were ordered for further review. These statements were sent to all those in the School, and in further (shorter) sessions were reviewed; staff were also given the opportunity to send in comments. Statements were added, subtracted, merged and divided. They were then reorganised under different topic areas, and additional areas included.

Eventually a two-page statement of concepts, values and beliefs held by nursing staff was achieved. The agreed statement is intended to underpin all aspects of the School and is included at the beginning of course documents. It is reviewed at intervals.

Box 2.2 shows an example of the concepts, values and beliefs about nursing which may be developed by a School and will represent the fundamental foundation for their work, including education. Although dense, it summarises the complexity of nursing as practice and a profession.

Box 2.2 Example of Statement of Concepts, Values and Beliefs

Person: *Patients/clients, the family, community, population, students or colleagues*

Each person is unique with biological, psychological, social, cultural and spiritual dimensions, and merits respect and to be treated with dignity. Individuals are presumed autonomous and responsible for their own actions; when they cannot be fully responsible their potential in these respects must be maximised. They participate in decisions affecting their own lives, such as lifestyle, care and treatment. Individuals have a right to have an informed professional speak for them as an advocate if necessary. In some cultures, the wellbeing of the group or community supersedes the wellbeing of the individual.

Health: *Personal health of individuals, community health of groups, public health of populations*

Based on the dynamic interaction of biological, psychological and social determinants of health embedded in cultural, socio-economic, political and spiritual influences. Support and empowerment of individuals, families and communities should begin at birth and continue throughout the lifespan to promote health including wellbeing.

Environment: *Physical, psychological and social environment to promote health and facilitate independence*

Settings where people exist and influence the lifestyle and wellbeing of individuals and their community. People should have living conditions and social and health care for a satisfactory state of health and wellbeing. Healthcare professionals should act as advocates for the promotion of a safe, healthy environment incorporating the individual's subjective view of what their living environment should be like. Within the political and economic environment healthcare professionals have a responsibility to participate in policy decisions, locally, nationally and internationally to influence the health status of the population.

Nursing: *Enhancement of health and wellbeing based on shared values and ethical understanding*

Nursing is a person-centred activity. It is about 'being with people', showing compassion, promoting and maintaining health, minimising the effect of illness and caring for individuals across their lifespan. It is about working in partnership with individuals, families, communities and populations, to enable, empower and promote attainment of full potential within their cultural context. It is a reflective and empathetic process based on aesthetic, personal, empirical and ethical knowledge from nursing, psychology, physiology, communication,

(Continued)

(Continued)

ethics, sociology etc. applied in a holistic approach. Therapeutic relationships at levels within communities and across the lifespan of individuals demand creativity and sensitivity to changing human needs, goals and aspirations. Nurses provide high quality, cost-effective care and support based on the best available evidence, promoting innovation and facilitating change as necessary in unidisciplinary, multidisciplinary and multisectoral contexts.

Professionals: *With attributes, rights, and duties conferred by professional education*

They have a duty to maintain and improve their own knowledge and competence through lifelong learning. Through leadership and management they ensure the continuing development of their profession. They have a responsibility to develop the theoretical and scientific knowledge base for practice through research and inquiry. They should generate a culture in which new ideas can be fostered and new and changing areas of practice identified, developed and shared. They have a duty to facilitate the learning of students and colleagues.

Education: *Promoting learning of knowledge, skills and attitudes for professional practice*

Nursing education is based on humanism, demonstrated through genuineness, acceptance and empathic understanding of students and colleagues. Nursing education is based on Knowles' focus on andragogy, that is, the principles of teaching adults. It aims to develop independent learners for lifelong learning through using students' previous experiences in collaborative working. Education programmes are designed so that new content builds on previous learning with an appropriate balance between different modes of learning and methods of teaching. Appropriate experience with reflection is used to promote learning from clinical practice.

The beginning of curriculum development, the first stage in educational provision, needs to be about achieving agreement on what nursing is, what values underpin nursing practice and the attributes of the nurses to be prepared. The educational team, including the partners in education (see Chapter 3), may begin by reviewing, clarifying and perhaps modifying the School statement of values, beliefs and core concepts about nursing (see Box 2.2). Through a process of discussion, negotiation and compromise the different members of the team reach agreement on the values accepted by all as underpinning the programme. The achievement of agreement between those starting with different views takes time, effort and an understanding that consensus is needed. These concepts, values and beliefs demonstrate an agreed philosophical stance of the team. The staff involved in nursing education need to work in a person-centred way in terms of the values they propose relating to the practice of nursing, and by demonstrating these values through the way in which they interact with, teach and support their students.

The concepts, values and beliefs agreed by the team arise mainly from the backgrounds of the different individuals involved. The different members of the team will bring with them their own professional values and conceptual understanding derived from their clinical experience and previous learning about professional issues and models of nursing. Their individual personal values will also influence discussion and will be modified by their own life experiences and family values. In turn, these will be influenced by their cultural background; for example, in Western countries individual personal views and rights are paramount, but in Chinese culture societal rights take precedence, and obedience and compliance are the norm (Leininger and McFarland, 2002). The student's own values and beliefs need to be compatible with those underpinning the practice of nursing.

Having achieved consensus about these concepts, values and beliefs should be the key elements which form the foundation for the programme and are regularly visited. They are applied through a holistic approach to the programme emphasising the integration of theory and practice; the evidence base and global nature of nursing; and expectations of patients and the public – set within current healthcare policies and structures. Following discussion and, perhaps, adaptation with partners in education, this statement (Box 2.2) provides the total underpinning for the curriculum. It is important to recognise that the standards implied by these statements may be difficult to achieve with student intake numbers in the hundreds. However, as beliefs and values have a strong influence on behaviour and practice it is imperative that we do our utmost to achieve them.

Where do Models and Theories in Nursing Fit?

The term 'theory' is often used broadly to encompass different ways of describing nursing knowledge. However, Dickoff and James defined it more precisely as '*a conceptual system or framework invented to some purpose; and as the purpose varies so too must vary the structure and complexity of the system*' (1968: 198); and, of the levels of theory identified, '*situation-producing theory*' (1968: 201) was the most relevant for nursing practice. This level identifies the situation and action required by the practitioner to achieve the anticipated goals.

Nursing has been described in various ways through a number of conceptual models produced by nursing theorists. The knowledge of these held by those involved in developing the statement of concepts, values and beliefs will contribute to achieving the agreed understanding of nursing and the structure and content of the programme. Models of nursing explain nursing in different ways, for example the biologically-based Roy's Adaptation Model, Orem's Self-Care Deficit Model, Neuman's Systems Model (all discussed in Fawcett, 2005) or the Activities of Living Model (Roper et al., 2002) used in the UK. The author of each model describes in relatively abstract terms how the different concepts relevant to nursing are to be interpreted in the context of that model and each model provides a unique perspective on nursing.

Theories are more concrete descriptions of the relationships between concepts described in conceptual models and are more limited in scope than models. Theories applied in nursing may be developed directly from nursing, such as Peplau's Theory of Interpersonal Relations (discussed in Fawcett, 2005), or derived from other sciences, for example the theory of stress from biology or locus of control from psychology.

In the past some Schools of Nursing used a single nursing model as the framework for the whole curriculum, often within the School where the author was a member of staff. However, this approach is now considered outdated as none of the current nursing models provide an explanation of nursing in all contexts and cannot, therefore, adequately be used as the framework for a complete pre-registration curriculum. Models and theories play a valuable role in helping to structure care in particular situations and some of these will be referred to in more detail later in this book, at points where they are relevant to specific content.

Although the different models present some very different perspectives on nursing, there is general agreement by all nurse theoreticians on the four key themes of person, health, environment and nursing as proposed by Fawcett (2005) as the metaparadigm for nursing, which acts as a framework which underpins the art and science of nursing. As discussed in Box 2.1, these four concepts can be used to develop your own agreed view (or philosophy) of nursing which will provide the anchor points for the curriculum.

Definitions of Nursing

Also influencing the statements of values and beliefs and, thus, the structure and content of the curriculum is the way in which nursing has been defined. Nursing has been described in numerous ways by different national and international nursing organisations. The International Council of

Nurses (ICN, 2010) has now defined nursing simply as follows:

> Nursing encompasses autonomous and collaborative care of individuals of all ages, families, groups and communities, sick or well and in all settings. Nursing includes the promotion of health, prevention of illness, and the care of ill, disabled and dying people. Advocacy, promotion of a safe environment, research, participation in shaping health policy and in patient and health systems management, and education are also key nursing roles.

This incorporates the key concepts proposed by Fawcett (2005) and identifies the major roles in which nurses should be active.

The Royal College of Nursing of the UK has drawn on worldwide expertise in developing a more complex but very useful document, *Defining Nursing*. The definition they have published is in two major parts. Firstly it states that:

> Nursing is the use of clinical judgement in the provision of care to enable people to improve, maintain, or recover health, to cope with health problems, and to achieve the best possible quality of life, whatever their disease or disability, until death (RCN, 2003: 3).

They then specify defining characteristics of nursing under the six headings shown in Box 2.3 which help to clarify the context and focus of nursing. The definition developed by the RCN includes all the concepts of Fawcett's (2005) metaparadigm and additionally incorporates many of the other concepts considered in different conceptual models. This definition gives a good indication of aspects of the curriculum to be covered.

Box 2.3 The Defining Characteristics of Nursing Are ...

1 ***A particular purpose***: The purpose of nursing is to promote health, healing, growth and development, and to prevent disease, illness, injury, and disability. When people become ill or disabled, the purpose of nursing is, in addition, to minimise distress and suffering, and to enable people to understand and cope with their disease or disability, its treatment and its consequences. When death is inevitable, the purpose of nursing is to maintain the best possible quality of life until its end.

2 ***A particular mode of intervention***: Nursing interventions are concerned with empowering people, and helping them to achieve, maintain or recover

(Continued)

(Continued)

independence. Nursing is an intellectual, physical, emotional and moral process which includes the identification of nursing needs; therapeutic interventions and personal care; information, education, advice and advocacy; and physical, emotional and spiritual support. In addition to direct patient care, nursing practice includes management, teaching, and policy and knowledge development.

3 ***A particular domain***: The specific domain of nursing is people's unique responses to and experience of health, illness, frailty, disability and health-related life events in whatever environment or circumstances they find themselves. People's responses may be physiological, psychological, social, cultural or spiritual, and are often a combination of all of these. The term 'people' includes individuals of all ages, families and communities, throughout the entire lifespan.

4 ***A particular focus***: The focus of nursing is the whole person and the human response rather than a particular aspect of the person or a particular pathological condition.

5 ***A particular value base***: Nursing is based on ethical values which respect the dignity, autonomy and uniqueness of human beings, the privileged nurse–patient relationship, and the acceptance of personal accountability for decisions and actions. These values are expressed in written codes of ethics, and supported by a system of professional regulation.

6 ***A commitment to partnership***: Nurses work in partnership with patients, their relatives and other carers, and in collaboration with others as members of a multi-disciplinary team. Where appropriate they will lead the team, prescribing, delegating and supervising the work of others; at other times they will participate under the leadership of others. At all times, however, they remain personally and professionally accountable for their own decisions and actions.

THEORIES AND PHILOSOPHIES OF EDUCATION

The next major area to consider is how to deliver the curriculum to achieve the desired outcome. As for nursing, philosophical approaches and models used in education need to be considered for application in nursing programmes. Some models have been derived from philosophy, psychology, sociology and applied in education, while others have been developed from the practice of education itself. In Figure 2.1 some of the key theoretical and philosophical ideas relevant to nursing education are indicated, with some emphasised and selected for discussion here. Other concepts and principles from education are applicable in the context of teaching, learning and assessment within the nursing curriculum, and are considered in later chapters. These include

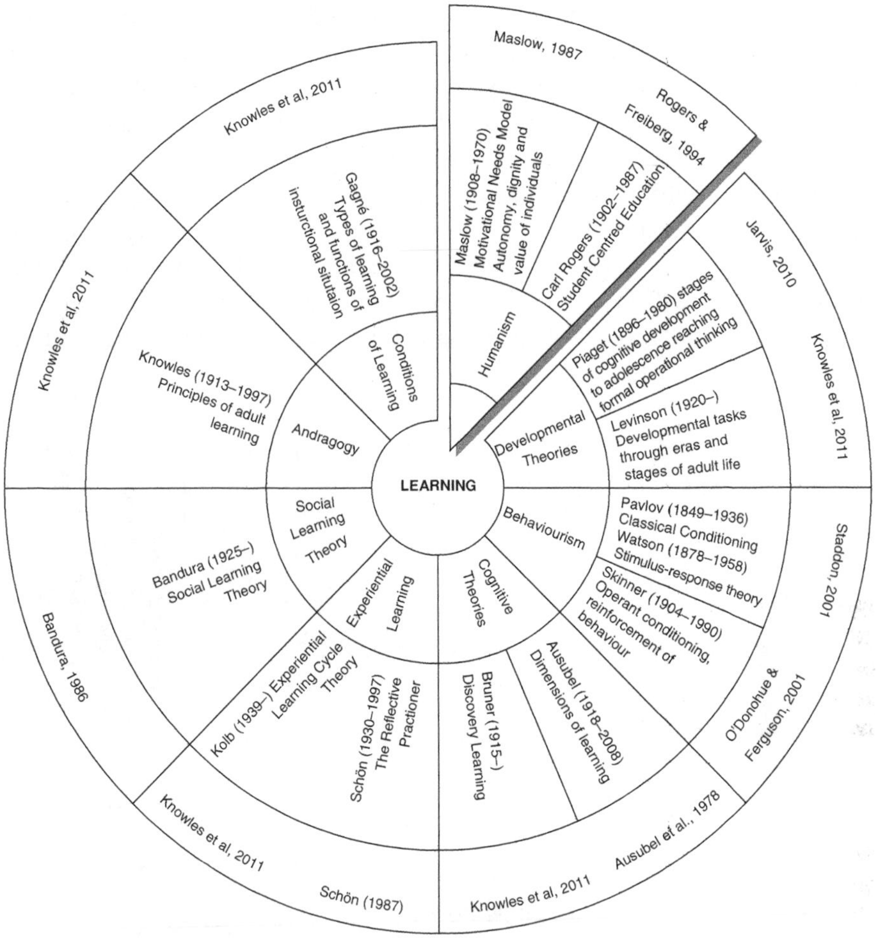

FIGURE 2.1 *Educational Philosophies and Models of Learning*

reflection on and in experience and adult learning theories and models – both of which are essential aspects of a nursing programme.

Humanism Underpinning Nursing Education

Derived from psychology, humanism is based on beliefs about the autonomy, dignity and value of individual human beings and, in the context of education, supports student-centred programmes which aim to help students to 'learn to learn' and to develop their independence and creativity. The values of humanism are congruent with those of nursing and this is an appropriate foundation for nursing education.

Some Schools of Nursing are clear about basing their curricula on the principles of humanism, using Maslow (1987) and Carl Rogers (Rogers and Freiberg, 1994) as the major exemplars. Maslow is well known in nursing for his theory of human motivation and hierarchy of needs but we also need to consider this in the context of education. Figure 2.2 indicates the aspects of this hierarchy which are dealt with through the content of the curriculum and those needs of students that are (hopefully) met through the educational processes in presenting the curriculum. It is also hoped that **academic staff** will strive to achieve self-actualisation through creativity and imagination in the activity of curriculum development and nursing education.

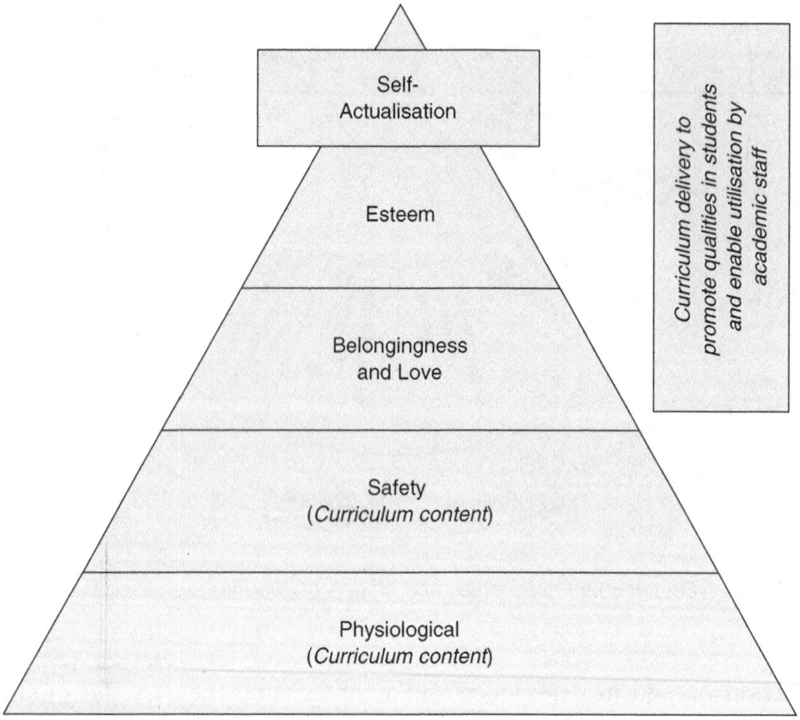

FIGURE 2.2 *Maslow's Hierarchy of Needs in Nursing Education*

Carl Rogers is the other humanist whose ideas are important in nursing education as well as in the context of counselling where he began. He focuses on the importance of the interpersonal relationship in education, as in nursing, and emphasises the role of the educator as being a facilitator of learning, rather than as a teacher. He identifies three attributes which he considers essential for the educator to be an effective facilitator. These are:

- *genuineness:* in which the educator develops an honest relationship with each student, rather than playing a role as a teacher;

- *acceptance:* in which the educator values the student as an individual with feelings and opinions which are prized;
- *empathy or empathic understanding:* when the educator is sensitive to the students' reactions and is able to understand their position.

These are comparable to the attributes we wish to see nursing students demonstrate in their interactions with patients. When academic staff use such an educational approach students will have a role model for their own professional practice where similar attributes are important. Approaches should be used to facilitate learning in which valuing students, students taking responsibility and personal autonomy are paramount.

Domains of the Curriculum

Barnett and Coate (2005) identified a framework for curricula consisting of three domains, with curriculum in the centre, which can be applied to different professional disciplines, including nursing (Figure 2.3). The three domains of knowing, acting and being are intended to be used as the focus for determining the content and structure of the curriculum and are of varying importance in different academic disciplines. Our earlier discussion

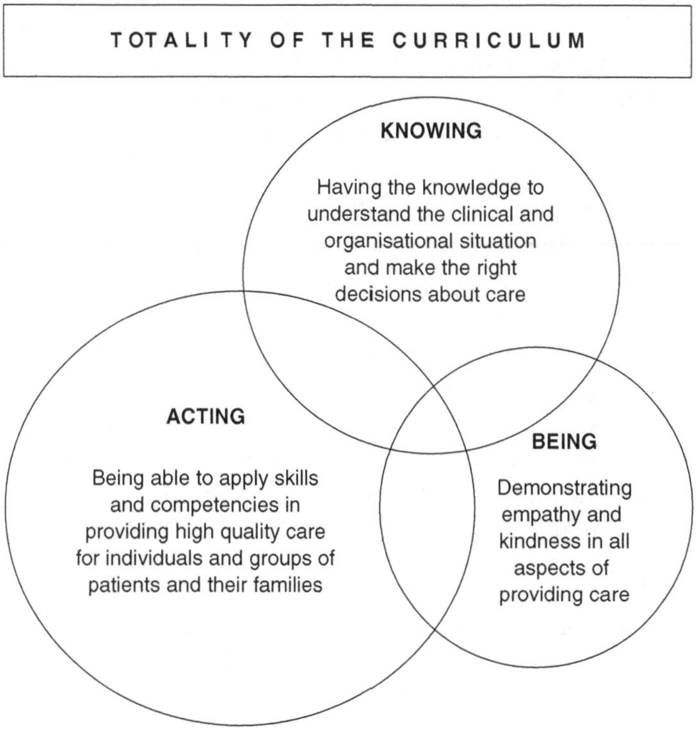

FIGURE 2.3 *Domains of the Curriculum in Professional Subjects*

Source: Barnett and Coate (2005) *Engaging the Curriculum in Higher Education* © Reproduced with the kind permission of Open University Press. All rights reserved.

has demonstrated the importance of 'knowing', but the practice of nursing is essentially 'acting' (based on knowledge) and a crucial focus for the curriculum is preparation for selection and implementation of appropriate action. However, the 'being' of the nurse is absolutely essential in providing humanistic, ethical person-centred care.

STATUTORY BODY STANDARDS AND QAA BENCHMARKS

NMC Standards for Pre-Registration Outcomes

In many countries the Statutory Body for Nursing, or a State Board, specifies the content and outcomes of a programme leading to registered nurse status, or for a higher level of nursing qualification. In the UK, the mandatory NMC (2010a) *Standards for Pre-Registration Nursing Education* provide detailed instructions on the competencies to be achieved and the structure of the programme, ensuring that the requirements of society are met. However, in some countries a legal framework for nursing does not yet exist and those responsible for training nurses have to determine the competencies to be achieved and the knowledge and skills needed to demonstrate these.

Although the standards may appear to be the most appropriate place to start curriculum planning, we suggest that it is important to remember that these standards apply to the outcomes to be achieved and the steps on the way to that end. The interpretation and implementation of these standards should be built on the values and philosophies about nursing and education held by the staff (academic and clinical). When staff understand and apply the agreed values and philosophies about nursing and education, the students will absorb and use them in their own practice. These values and philosophies will strongly influence the quality of the student experience and the humanity of the nurse produced. In addition, as nursing is an academic discipline it is expected that we are able to explain the underpinning philosophy of the subject. While each country will have their own directives, all nurse curriculum planners need to begin with philosophy of nursing and philosophies and models of education to set the groundwork for detailed curriculum planning.

In the UK the Nursing and Midwifery Council (NMC) was established in law to regulate the profession

> The principal functions of the Council shall be to establish from time to time standards of education, training, conduct and performance for nurses and midwives and to ensure the maintenance of those standards (UK Statutory Instrument, 2002:4).

The NMC in the UK regularly updates the standards for practice, for pre-registration training and for post-registration education programmes. For example, the 2010 standards replaced the 2004 version for pre-registration education and were completed following consultation with the profession and others. They are presented in considerable detail on the NMC website (NMC, 2010a). Figure 2.4 shows an outline of the different components of these standards. From the left hand side, for each of the four fields of practice, four domains of practice are identified within which the essential skills clusters can be incorporated. Within each of these domains for each field of practice competencies are specified, some generic to all fields and some field specific. The right hand side of the figure identifies the key progression points in the programme.

The UK is unusual in preparing pre-registration nursing students for one of four fields of practice: Adult Nursing, Mental Health Nursing, Learning Disability Nursing and Children's Nursing. During the consultation period for these new standards the possibility of moving towards preparation of a generic nurse, with specialisation post-qualification, was considered. However, it became clear that nurses working within mental health and learning disability in particular believed strongly that the quality of care could not be maintained with the proposed move away from pre-registration specialisation. One of the key areas of concern was recruitment as currently a considerable number of those entering these fields have personal experience of people, often family members, with such health difficulties and these recruits may not wish to spend three years training to become a generic nurse.

The NMC Standards include the detailed competencies to be achieved before registration within the four domains of: professional values; communication and interpersonal skills; nursing practice and decision-making; and leadership, management and team working. In addition to the competencies within these domains, the five essential skills clusters are separately presented. These were developed through consultation with service users and thus relate to issues of concern to the general public. These clusters are: care, compassion, and communication; organisational aspects of care; infection prevention and control; nutrition and fluid management; and medicines management. These can be fitted within the four domains previously identified. The NMC standards for pre-registration education also now specify the skills and professional values which must be achieved at specified progression points at the ends (normally) of years one and two, as well as at the end of the programme (NMC, 2010a).

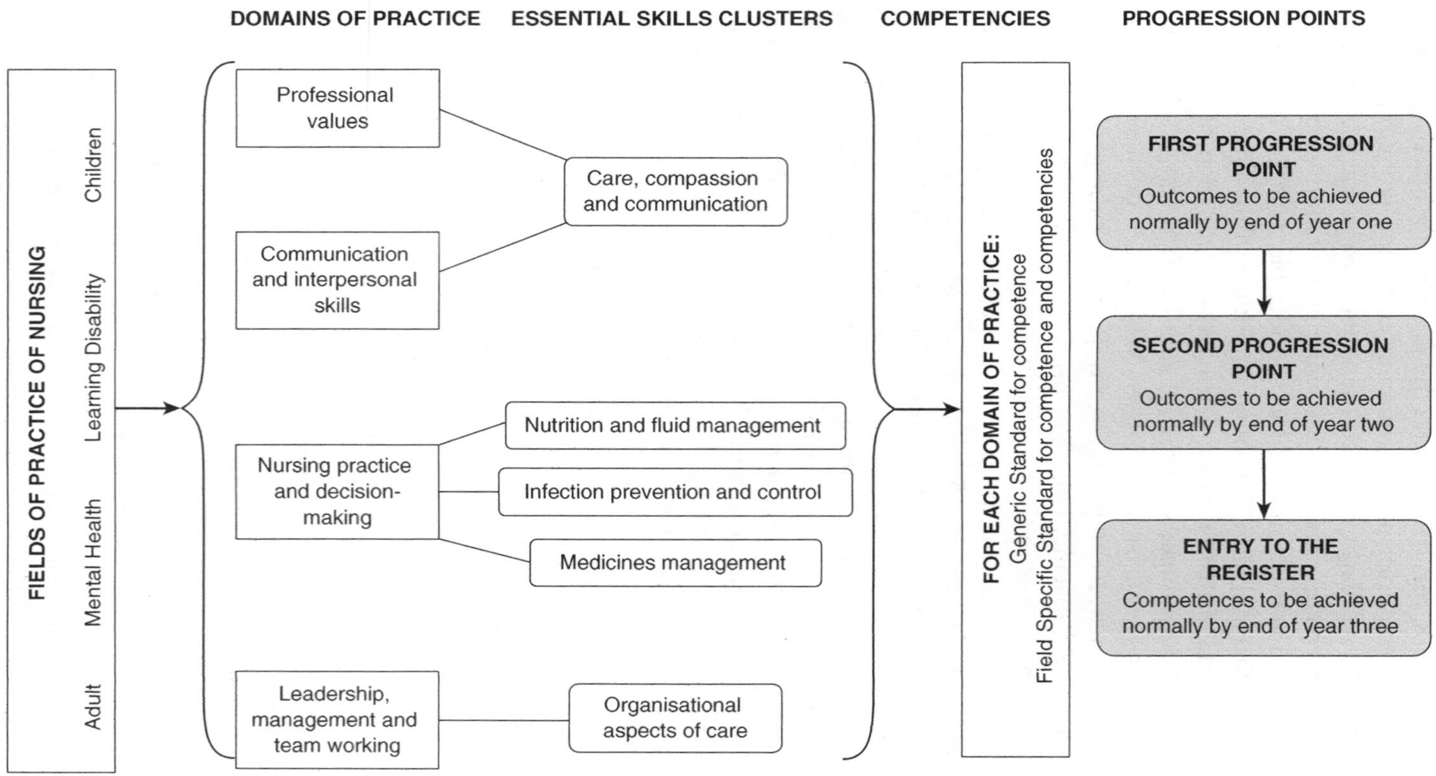

FIGURE 2.4 *Outline of NMC Standards*

NMC Standards for Education

Standards that must be met by the educational institution for the provision of courses are also specified. These state the requirements in relation to a number of issues which aim to ensure that suitable individuals undergo a well-organised programme of theory and practice to achieve the specified outcomes. Students are supported by well-prepared educators who have adequate resources for teaching and assessment, and who maintain a well-managed system of quality assurance. These standards are also obligatory and, in curriculum development, these must be achieved even if they are incompatible with some of the HE institutional standards. Incorporated within the NMC standards are the requirements specified in the European Union Directive 2005/36/EC of the European Parliament and of the Council of 7 September 2005 (EU, 2005) on the recognition of professional qualifications. This specifies the requirements for recognition of general nurses across the EU which member states are required to meet, with new members working to achieve the necessary level.

All the standards specified by the NMC (2010a) will be interpreted and incorporated within the curriculum as moderated through the values held by the School.

QAA Benchmark Statements

The benchmarks for healthcare subjects are prepared by working groups of academics, practitioners and representatives of professional and statutory bodies. These statements act as a frame of reference when planning and reviewing educational programmes and allow judgements to be made about standards. However, they do not specify the curriculum.

The benchmarks for nursing were developed in collaboration with other healthcare professionals and begin with the framework for the healthcare professions. The nursing benchmarks follow. Table 2.1 shows the outline of these statements, which can be seen in detail on the QAA website (QAA, 2001).

The value of these statements is that they enable differentiation between the expectations at the different academic levels, which the NMC Standards do not. However, the current nursing benchmarks were published in 2001 and include Standards for both Diploma of Higher Education (the threshold standard for registration to be superseded by non-honours degrees in new courses commencing after September 2011) and **Honours degree**. Nevertheless, the benchmarks for the Honours degree are useful as the only statement available for expectations at this level in nursing.

TABLE 2.1 *Outline of Nursing Subject Benchmarks*

Health Professions Framework			
A	Expectations of the health professional in providing patient/client services	A1	Professional autonomy and accountability
		A2	Professional relationships
		A3	Personal and professional skills
		A4	Profession and employer context
B	The application of practice in securing, maintaining or improving health and well-being	B1	Identification and assessment of health and social needs
		B2	Formulation of plans and strategies for meeting health and social care needs
		B3	Practice
		B4	Evaluation
C	Knowledge, understanding and skills that underpin the education and training of healthcare professionals	C1	Knowledge and understanding
		C2	Skills including: information gathering, problem-solving, communication, numeracy, information technology
Benchmark Statement for Nursing			
A	The nurse as a registered healthcare practitioner; expectations held by the profession, employers and public	A1 A2 A3 A4	Headings as in health framework, but applied in the context of nursing
B	Principles and concepts: application to nursing practice	B1	Identification and assessment of health care need
		B2	Formulation of plans and strategies for meeting healthcare needs
		B3	Nursing practice
		B4	Evaluation
C	Knowledge, understanding and associated skills that underpin the education and training of nurses	C1	Knowledge and understanding: nursing; natural and life sciences; social, health and behavioural sciences; ethics, law and the humanities; management of self and others' reflective practice
		C2	Associated skills: communication and interpersonal skills; information gathering; care delivery; problem-solving and data collection and interpretation; information technology; numeracy
Diploma of Higher Education Level			*Honours Degree Level*
Statements in relation to the three headings above are presented to be commensurate with Dip HE, the threshold level for entry to the professional register			Statements in relation to the three headings above are presented to be commensurate with honours degree academic award and enhance the threshold standard for entry to the professional register

INTEGRATION INTO A CURRICULUM FRAMEWORK

The issues discussed earlier in this chapter all need consideration when beginning curriculum development and making decisions about development of a framework which will provide guidance for the detailed curriculum.

The identification of a curriculum framework is the necessary next step in developing the curriculum; it provides the skeleton on which the programme will be built and will also assist in clarifying the overall outcomes of the programme. The value of such a framework in providing a broad structure for the development of the curriculum is paramount. Some course teams identify a nursing or an educational model or an approach to curriculum delivery (e.g. problem-based learning) or more than one of these which is appropriate for the programme and congruent with the values and beliefs of the team.

An alternative approach is to use the agreed concepts, values and beliefs about nursing and the statutory body requirements and develop a simple framework which provides the overall structure for the programme. Figure 2.5 shows a possible framework for a pre-registration curriculum. The centre identifies the anticipated product from the course, that is, a

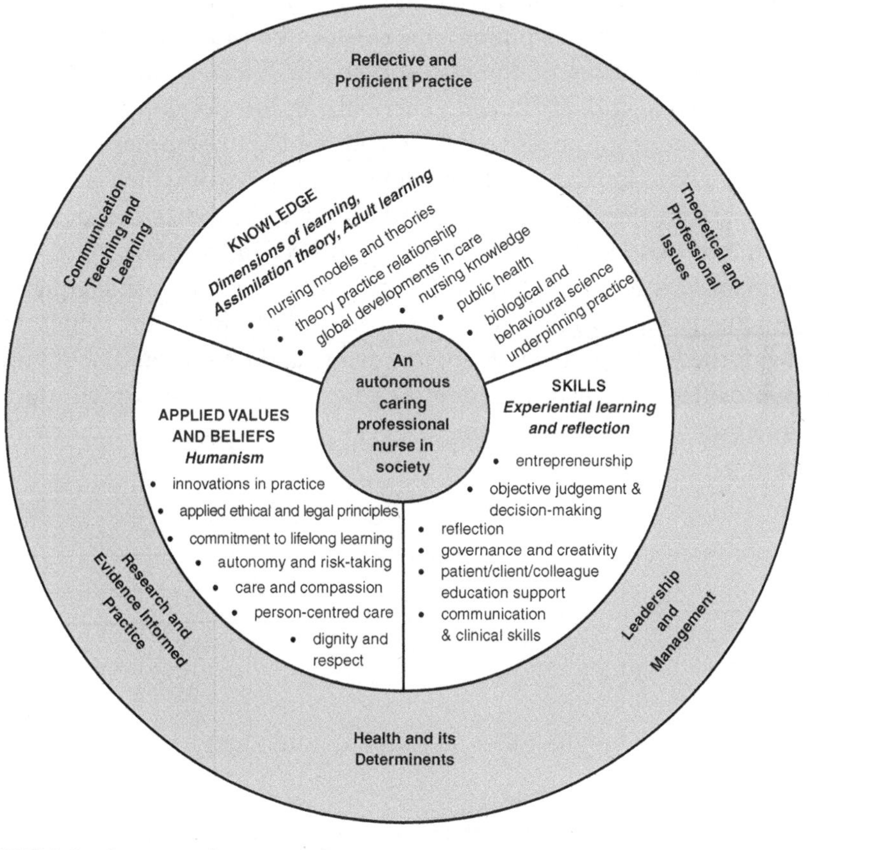

FIGURE 2.5 *Proposed Curriculum Framework Pre-Registration Nursing Education*

caring professional nurse in society, while the outer circle identifies six themes which run through the programme. Within each theme, knowledge ('knowing'), skills ('acting') and applied values and beliefs ('being') are indicated, which will be modified by the community requirements and statutory body standards for the particular programme. This structure facilitates the development of a spiral curriculum in which the themes are revisited at intervals through the programme at increasing levels of complexity. This structure also helps to minimise a major difficulty with a modular programme which is that students sometimes have difficulty in integrating content from the different **modules**. With any approach to curriculum delivery, the team needs to have a clear idea of the content which must be covered.

CHAPTER SUMMARY

A nursing curriculum is highly complex involving the integration of the nursing and educational philosophical issues considered in this chapter with the requirements of the statutory body. There is no single agreed theoretical framework for nursing curricula, and to develop a high quality curriculum the team needs to debate and resolve these issues early in the process. We have looked briefly at some of the ways in which nursing has been described through philosophy, theories and models and definitions and some of these will be considered again later in the book.

Humanism is recognised as a core value to underpin nursing education, and a schema for engaging with the curriculum is presented which marries with the values and beliefs about nursing and education. The statutory body provides a detailed description of the competencies which must be achieved and they are an essential check in the process of curriculum development.

3 PARTNERSHIP IN NURSING EDUCATION

INTRODUCTION

Nurses aim to provide care to patients, clients or communities, working with families, other nurses and professionals, and a range of statutory and voluntary bodies. Those undertaking a nursing education course will work with nursing and other healthcare practitioners in clinical areas overseen by nurse managers and will provide care for those now called 'service users'. The education programme provided will impact on all these groups and, thus, they all have a valuable perspective to share on the nature of the programme to be provided. Planning and delivering a curriculum needs to be carried out in partnership with a wide range of different stakeholders.

Planning a programme in partnership is not easy and needs careful thought and effort. While some individual aspects of partnership working have been written about, such as service users' involvement in nursing education, little has been written about the overall approach and principles of working in partnership in planning and delivering a curriculum in nursing education. In this chapter we will explore some of the principles we have been able to identify associated with partnership. We will discuss these in the context of the involvement of the different stakeholders in planning nursing curricula and providing the educational programme. In some countries, including the UK, partnership working in education is an absolute requirement of the validating body but even where this is not so there are many advantages to involving a number of people representing the different stakeholders from outside the educational institution. In particular they can contribute to the development of a curriculum which reflects local needs for the present and future of the community.

PRINCIPLES AND ISSUES IN PARTNERSHIP WORKING

Power and Engagement

The first issue to be considered is what is meant by partnership. In a true partnership all members are contributing equally, although differently, and the power is evenly distributed amongst the members of the partnership. However, in curriculum development and delivery, the power is distributed according to the contribution and degree of control of the different partners and will vary within the different aspects of the enterprise. The academic institutions and health service providers are the major partners in delivering a nursing curriculum. The nursing academic staff carry the primary responsibility for ensuring that the course is planned and delivered. The health service organisations are responsible for providing suitable practice learning placements and the necessary **mentor**ship for students. However, the appropriate standards will only be met if all partners contribute according to their expertise and resources. Thus, all partners hold equal power to make or break the quality of the programme

The key issue is to ensure that all partners recognise and accept the importance of their contribution and become fully engaged in the enterprise. The important beginning of this is in considering the philosophy, values and beliefs which underpin the whole programme. While this may initially be drafted by the nursing academics, it needs to be shared with all the different partners when new ideas may arise and the philosophy adjusted until it is acceptable to all concerned.

Sharing full information about the range of different developments during the planning of the curriculum with all those involved will help everyone to understand their contribution to the whole. There is increased likelihood that they will feel fully engaged in the process even though their contribution is in relation to just one part of the total exercise.

Costs and Benefits of Partnership

Writing about community health partnerships in which factors relating to the continued involvement of partners are explored, El Ansari and Phillips (2004) examined items under the headings of benefit, costs, satisfaction, commitment and sense of ownership. In the El Ansari Paradox they identified that, in order to get commitment to the project, the balance between benefits and costs had to be positive and a ratio of benefits to costs of 1.6 was perceived as favourable.

While the context of his study was quite different from that considered here, it is likely that at a general theoretical level the same principle about partnership applies in nursing education. Table 3.1 lists the costs and benefits for an organisation from outside the university becoming involved in a nursing curriculum planning team. While the idea of applying the 1.6 ratio may or may not be valuable, listing and openly discussing the costs and benefits in advance can be useful. If nothing else it articulates the expectations of organisations and helps the university to manage important relationships with other organisations and the individuals involved.

TABLE 3.1 *Costs and Benefits for External Organisations Participating in Curriculum Planning Team*

Benefits	**Costs**
Being part of a new initiative	Financial cost of travel to attend meetings
Developing collaborative relationships with other organisations	Time spent on partnership activities keeps individual from doing their own work
Getting to know other agencies and their staff and/ or meeting nursing staff with similar interest in area of care	The organisation does not get enough public recognition for work in the partnership
Gaining recognition and respect from others especially at national and/or international level	Too many similar organisations involved, no sense of being special or unique
Opportunity to influence content of the nursing curriculum and shape values of future employees	Individuals' skills and time are not well used in order to ensure full contribution
Potential to enhance the care of those with specific conditions requiring nursing intervention	
Opportunity to help students to understand the real life experiences of patients and carers	
The curriculum will ensure that students are suitably prepared for learning in clinical placement	
Ensures that curriculum takes account of placement availability in hospital and community	
Knowledge and skills will be adequate for working as a registered nurse on completion of the programme	
Suitable recognition and thanks to both individuals and organisations contributing to partnership and	
Professional development for clinicians and nurse managers involved in practice education	

In initiating discussions about partnership with the university it is a useful strategy to emphasise the benefits to the individual and their organisation, and to discuss how the costs will be minimised. Benefits may be tangible in the sense that the partnership will provide their organisation with nurses prepared well for their role in practice, but less tangible results may be that individuals feel valued and proud to be making a contribution to improve patient care in the future.

Managing Partnership in Curriculum Planning

Managing the involvement of this range of partners in curriculum development and delivery is complex. The aim is to enable all members of the partnership to make their contribution effectively and efficiently. We must ensure that there is an appropriate spread of representation and levels of expertise and consider how to enable busy people to feel included and valued while not taking up too much of their time. During curriculum development, some organisations need to be represented and fully involved at the strategic level. The input of other organisations and individuals is needed to assist in planning the individual theoretical and clinical modules and draws on participants' specific academic and clinical expertise and patient experience.

In setting up the partnership, it is necessary first to identify the different organisations whose inputs will be necessary and obtain their commitment to the enterprise, with an indication of the time commitment required. The individuals to participate in the different curriculum groups will be identified with their organisation. A guarantee that they will be able to attend meetings is essential and needs to include agreement that they will not be replaced with a substitute on occasions – a situation which has been found to be detrimental to the ongoing process of curriculum development.

In planning a large programme (such as a three-year pre-registration nursing course) a steering group will be needed to guide the work of different sub-groups. Within the UK a nursing education programme is 'owned' jointly by the Higher Education Institution (HEI) and the main service provider(s) (for example, National Health Service Trusts) and both must be fully involved at this strategic level. The other major groups also need to be represented. To enable this steering group to develop the overall programme structure and provide the necessary leadership to the various sub-groups, consistency in attendance is essential.

Depending on the curriculum framework being used by the team, a number of curriculum groups focusing on the themes running through the programme will be needed. Figure 3.1 shows an example of the groups involved within one curriculum planning process. These groups of nursing academics, subject specialists, clinicians with appropriate expertise and patient representatives as appropriate will be planning the course content and developing any teaching materials required. The chair or facilitator of each group should be a member of the steering group thus ensuring integration of the different themes into a coherent whole. In addition, groups focusing on key issues such as placement or assessment through the programme will be needed.

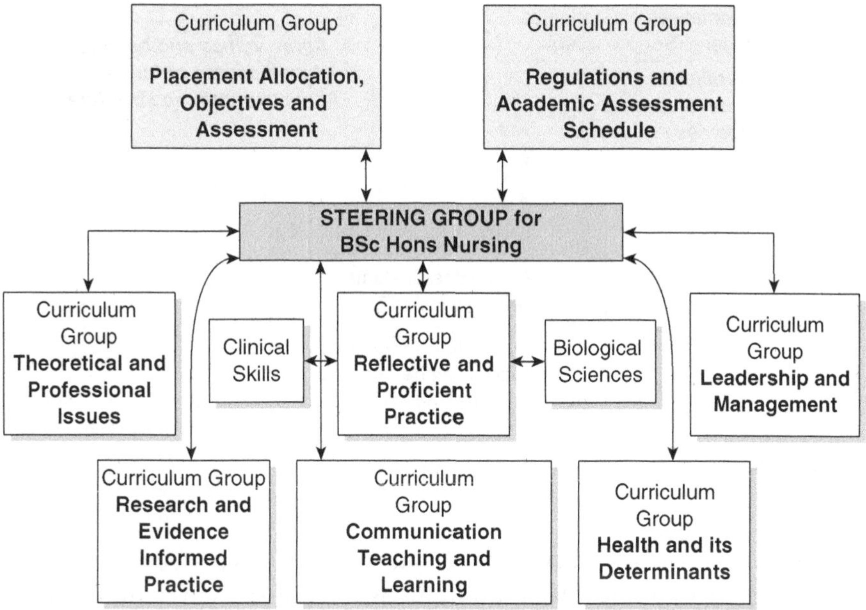

FIGURE 3.1 *Example of Curriculum Development Structures*

An individual experienced in curriculum development and with leadership qualities is necessary to lead this exercise, supported by other key academics with a particular interest in curriculum and service staff with specific roles in clinical education. However, it is also important to use approaches (Figure 3.2) which will enable all staff in the course team to feel involved and able to make a contribution, so that they will be committed to the new programme, even though in a large School it is unlikely that everyone will be intimately involved.

The use of whole day consensus conferences (see Box 3.1) including all stakeholders who can and wish to attend may be a valuable approach to develop the philosophy and curriculum framework, with the day ending with the setting up of curriculum groups. These groups will

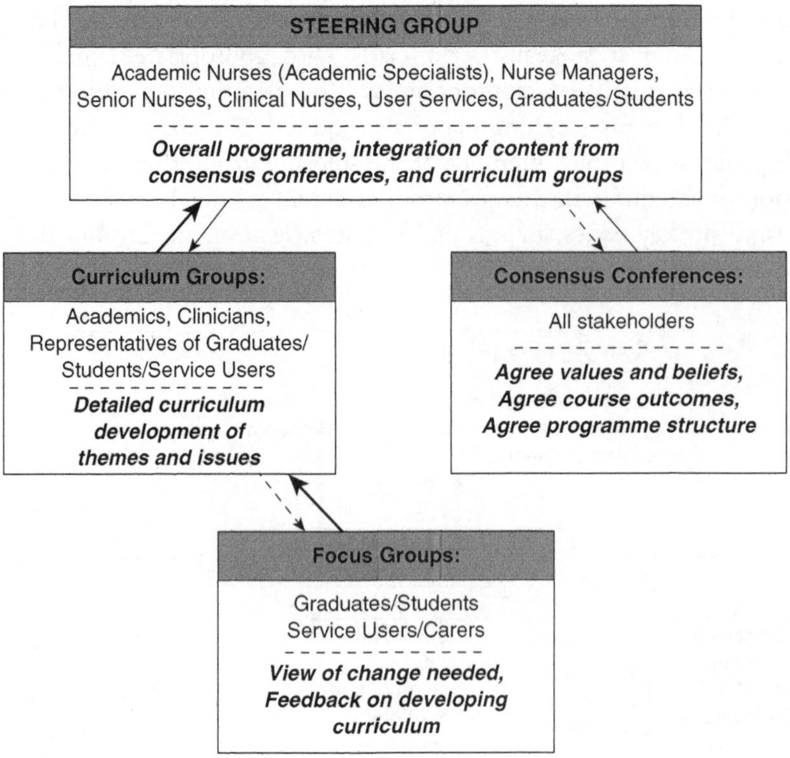

FIGURE 3.2 *Managing Partnership Working*

then meet at regular intervals (for example, every two weeks) and complete the development of the different aspects of the curriculum. A few additional whole day events can be held at key points in the curriculum planning to enable continued involvement of those unable to join one of the groups but who wish to present ideas for consideration. It may also be useful to have an agreed approach to enable all those interested to send proposals and ideas they would wish to see included in the programme to the steering group.

Box 3.1 Consensus Conference

Using a consensus conference approach in curriculum planning has not received much publicity but it can play a useful part in enabling different stakeholders to contribute to the final curriculum. To work effectively it needs to be planned and managed with care, working through the following stages:

- Set the objectives for the day with the steering group, framed to include input from all groups.
- Identify the participants to represent adequately the different stakeholder groups.
- Select a pleasant setting that is conducive to discussion and interaction.
- Identify individuals to fulfil roles of convening the meeting, introducing topic, chairing discussion groups, summarising the results.
- Prepare orientation and introduction to the work. This may include some short pre-reading materials.
- Set procedural guidelines e.g.:
    - all participants have the right to present their point of view;
    - statements can be questioned and rejected;
    - the communication between participants has to be a genuine dialogue;
    - any statement or comment has to be included in the deliberation;
    - any resolution, made in the CC, will be documented (Neilsen et al., 2006: 23).
- Participants in working groups discuss the issues, topics or questions allocated and reach a consensus.
- Feedback is shared through a short presentation from each group. Sometimes the three main points are reported but notes, sometimes on a paper tablecloth, left with the convenor are available for future use.
- Following the consensus conference, a report is prepared for the steering group which will influence further developments.

It is difficult for patients, carers, students and graduates to attend frequent numerous meetings but their input is important. Focus groups can be a useful method to obtain ideas and feedback to influence the development of the curriculum as a whole, or in relation to a particular aspect of the curriculum. Focus groups, mixed or each representing a particular stakeholder group such as students, graduates or service users, can feed information back through their representative on the steering group or to the appropriate curriculum group. These groups should review developments and comment at intervals.

Academics and clinicians are the two major partners in a nursing programme with the two groups working closely together. Academics primarily develop and provide the theoretical aspects of the programme; they also teach clinical skills in the university in preparation for practice learning and visit students in placement to ensure application of theory into practice. Clinicians are primarily responsible for the clinical part of the programme ensuring that students receive appropriate supervision and mentorship and achieve the necessary competencies. When possible clinicians should also contribute to the university based teaching. The importance of these two groups working together cannot be overemphasised in order to produce a programme in which theory and practice feed into each other.

A major issue to be discussed in relation to partnership in education is the involvement of the service users – patients/clients and carers. In relation to curriculum development a clear understanding of the patient experience and their requirements for care is invaluable in structuring the programme. In addition, using a range of approaches, they can make a valuable contribution to the teaching and other aspects of the programme provision.

Statutory, voluntary and private organisations may all be needed to provide the rounded curriculum through which we hope to prepare nurses able to provide holistic patient or client care in different settings. It is important to consider carefully the particular contributions that they can make and how this can be implemented effectively.

THE STAKEHOLDERS

There are a number of groups of individuals and organisations who have different contributions to make to curriculum development and educational provision.

The Academics

Academic staff in universities have three major roles, which are teaching, research and knowledge transfer, along with the necessary administration for these roles and, in addition, the NMC expects them to have 'clinical credibility'. However, Barrett argues that the '*expectation for nurse lecturers to carry out four distinct roles to a high standard – teaching, research, clinical, managerial – is unrealistic*' (2007: 372) and it is important to appoint staff with a range of different abilities so that individual lecturing staff in nursing may undertake specific roles depending on their strengths and interests. Some will be willing to carry the responsibility for managing programmes of study as Course Directors. Others will have major interests in clinical work, possibly holding joint appointments, and will be willing to undertake responsibility for the clinical skills teaching facilities and for teaching clinical skills. It is important in curriculum planning to ensure that all have the opportunity to contribute their expertise to planning new or updated programmes. Newly appointed lecturers are likely to be expert clinicians or researchers with an important contribution to make.

Leadership in curriculum development in nursing is provided by the experienced academics and clinical educators. The academic staff have the responsibility of accessing and sharing all the mandatory guidance from the statutory body and the HEI and guiding agreement of the values and beliefs underpinning the curriculum. They play an important role in the consensus conferences and in all the curriculum groups, while ensuring that input is procured from all relevant stakeholders. They will also ensure that the whole programme is coherent, progressive, interesting and future orientated. They have a key responsibility in helping all involved in curriculum development to understand the different approaches to curriculum delivery so that informed decisions can be reached. Academic staff also must undertake professional development activities to be able to participate in any new developments.

University academics in nursing play a major role in ensuring that the aspects of the programme required by the Statutory Body are included, but will also have to meet the standards of the HEI. An example of HEI standards is the expected inclusion of entrepreneurship within the undergraduate curricula in all science subjects (including nursing) within certain universities. Sometimes the HEI norms and Statutory Body standards are not entirely compatible and ingenuity is needed to achieve an acceptable structure: at the end of the day it is the Statutory Body requirements that must be met.

In addition to meeting the requirements above, the course may include some 'added-value' content within the curriculum. Particular expertise of staff within the School, which lies outside the usual content of pre-registration education, may be included and can add to the experience and later employability of the students. An example from the University of Ulster is disaster preparation and management and the inclusion of theoretical content and practical exercises in collaboration with the British Red Cross. The learning associated with this practical exercise relates to the objectives of the management placement during which it occurs. Other examples include an introduction to complementary therapies and teaching students massage to promote relaxation, and the opportunity to undertake an international elective.

Some of the sciences underpinning nursing may be taught by nursing academics or by academics who are subject specialists, depending on the resources available. In some universities the sciences underpinning nursing (such as the biological sciences) are taught by staff from those Schools to groups including students undertaking other degree programmes. It is important that the nursing academics ensure the appropriateness of the scientific content for the nursing programme, with a suitable balance between the pure and applied science. Nursing academics and clinicians play an important role in helping students to apply the knowledge of the sciences to nursing practice.

Teaching should draw on the research expertise and findings of the staff, as well as the published evidence. However, the expectations for research output, exemplified through the demands of the Research Excellence Framework (REF) (replacing the previous Research Assessment Exercise) in the UK, results in many very able nurse academics focusing on research to the detriment of teaching. This was exemplified in a description of **Professor**'s Responsibilities (Callanan, 2009) which totally omitted undergraduate teaching and curriculum development. Students usually receive an evidence-based education but one that may be lacking in the excitement of hearing about current research from those actually engaged in it and which does not open their minds to developing ideas in nursing. In some academic disciplines, professors draw on their breadth of knowledge and understanding of their subject area to teach first year students, and then teach final year students based on their research areas. It would be interesting to see a similar approach in nursing.

It is essential that nurse researchers contribute to pre-registration, as well as post-registration, education, but in a way that relates to their particular expertise and still enables them to have time to generate new knowledge through research to enhance patient care. Some approaches that have been used include:

- asking key researchers in the School to present their research to students through Celebrity Lectures at relevant points in the course;
- specifically requesting their involvement at stages in course planning that relate to their research area, and ensuring that this is time limited;
- involvement in development of elearning or other educational materials directly related to their area of expertise and presenting the most up-to-date ideas;
- some involvement in teaching research methods using examples from their own work.

All students are allocated to an academic as **Personal Tutor** or Adviser of Studies whose responsibility in this role is to facilitate the student in successful completion of their programme. The nursing academics will also play the major role in managing and providing the teaching based in the University, with the involvement of other partners as relevant.

Students and Graduates

Current students and recent graduates play an important role in developing a revised or new programme as they provide valuable information and ideas, with feedback on the developing curriculum being fed back into the curriculum planning groups and steering groups. Current students are able to reflect on issues in relation to curriculum, placement, teaching and assessment methods within the programme and may propose changes which could improve the student experience, without 'dumbing down' the curriculum. One important area in which they can help is the suitability of the preparation provided before practice learning groups and the support received during placement.

Recent graduates can also comment on similar aspects of the programme but it is particularly valuable to get feedback on their readiness for the role of a qualified nurse. Identification of any areas of skill or knowledge in which they felt deficient in their first clinical post and which could have been incorporated within the curriculum is important. It is also useful to ask them about the relevance of those aspects of the curriculum which provide added value, and can thus be modified without detracting from the required content.

Recent graduates who are (hopefully) in full-time jobs and current students undertaking a full-time programme will both have considerable difficulty in attending a lot of curriculum planning meetings. Consensus conferences and focus groups will meet fairly infrequently but student and graduate involvement in these will ensure that their views are considered. Inclusion in these activities will enhance their understanding of nursing education and act as a professional development opportunity. Helping them to recognise that their contribution is valued and will influence the education of future students and their contribution to patient care, as well as ensuring that participants are kept informed about the way in which their contributions are being used, are important in encouraging continued involvement and increasing the likelihood of continuing commitment. The HEI will need to negotiate with employers, all with a responsibility towards nursing education, to permit release from the workplace to contribute to this activity.

The involvement of students as peer mentors for new or more junior students in clinical practice settings is a valuable development (Aston and Molassiotis, 2003) from which both senior and junior students benefit. The junior students receive support and guidance from someone they see as less formidable than their mentor, while senior students begin to develop mentoring skills. This approach has been used with students of various healthcare disciplines but the preparation of students for their roles (as mentor and mentee) is important and approaches to dealing with conflict must be planned (Secomb, 2008). Clarity about the roles and responsibilities of students and clinical supervisor (mentor) is essential. The roles are demonstrated in Figure 3.3, but the mentor carries the overall responsibility for the success of this approach. Moving on from this, Burns et al. (2011) have reported the involvement of peer educators in portfolio development. A range of different approaches are now being used in peer-supported study.

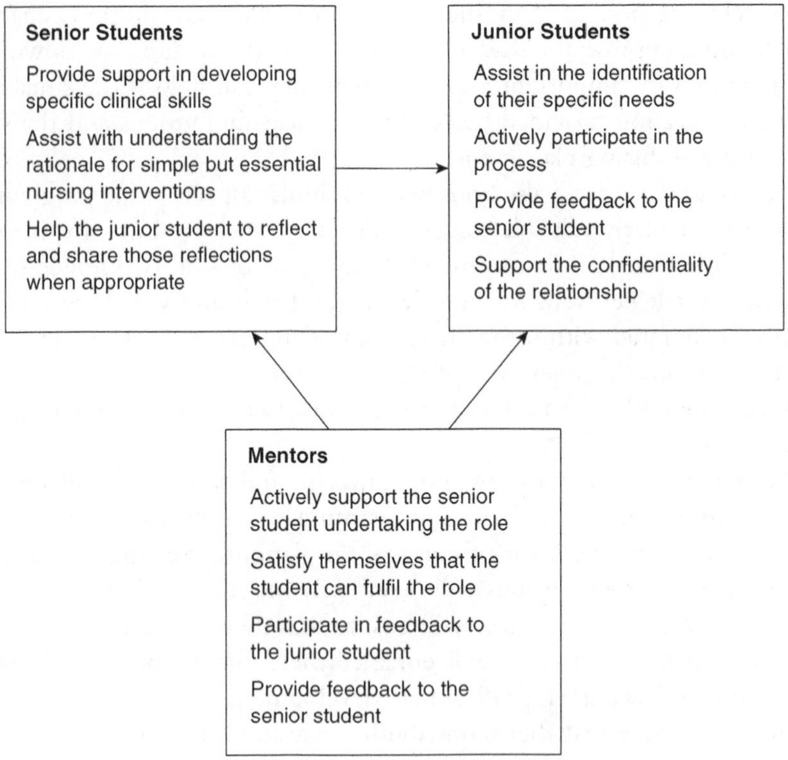

FIGURE 3.3 *Role Characteristics Between Students and Mentors in the Peer Support Scheme*

The NMC (2008b) encourages the involvement of students in the selection of future students. Although it is unlikely that students would be involved in formal interviews, they can play a valuable role in meeting with potential candidates and providing information about the course, the university, the clinical areas, the town as place to live, and answering any questions they may have.

Senior Nurses (Nurse Managers and Educational Facilitators)

Within health service organisations, nurse managers at different levels and those in roles such as Education Facilitators play a crucial role in planning for a smooth integration of the practical experience into the programme as a whole and in delivering the planned schedule. They need to ensure that the programme devised is manageable within the clinical facilities available and, most importantly, that at the end of their programme the graduates will meet the needs of service.

In particular senior colleagues from service are responsible for identifying and, in consultation with the academics, determining the optimum use of clinical areas to provide students with the necessary range of clinical experience. They will be responsible during the running of the programme for liaising with the university staff responsible for practice learning when any changes of use of clinical areas are planned, temporarily or permanently. This will permit necessary changes of student allocation. In addition, these nurse managers may be employing the graduates of the programme and know what they want to see in the students on completion of their programme and, thus, can identify issues which they consider essential for inclusion in the university parts of the course.

Educational Facilitators are employed in service to be responsible for ensuring that students are allocated to adequately prepared mentors who receive regular updating so that students will receive high quality teaching and supervision in developing their skills. They will also make certain that appropriate assessment of competence in practice is carried out. Their involvement in planning the curriculum is vital in determining that students go on placement with the necessary preparation to enable them to make the most of their clinical learning opportunities. Those who are involved in the training and support of mentors can provide an essential contribution. One Practice Education Facilitator described her experiences:

> It was really good that I was involved from the beginning. I was familiar with all the course content; this really helped me in the design and delivery of mentor training. Also I felt that I was able to influence the content so that future service needs could be addressed. At a personal level I felt my opinion was valued and this strengthened our working relationship with the University.

The benefits for senior nurses of partnership with the university in curriculum planning and in provision of clinical experience for students are mainly concerned with preparing high quality nurses able to fulfil the role of a Registered Nurse on graduation. Through their influence on the curriculum and on the course provision they can ensure that the quality of patient care in the future will, at a minimum, meet the required standards. They are making a valuable contribution to the future of the profession and the health service, but do need to attend regularly at course planning meetings and assure continuity of individual attendance. As managers of the nursing resource and clinical environment, they are also able to ensure that clinical areas are used appropriately and that the curriculum takes full account of placement availability in hospital and community.

Clinicians

Two specific groups of nurse clinicians play a particularly important role in nursing education: mentors and nurse specialists. In addition, a number of other health and social care professionals contribute to the preparation of students to work within the multiprofessional team.

Every student nurse on placement has a mentor who (in the UK) is responsible for ensuring student supervision, directly or indirectly, for at least 40% of the student's time in giving direct care. These specially prepared nurses have a valuable part to play in planning placement experience that will enable students to achieve the required competencies. However, their major contribution is when students are undertaking the practice learning components of their programme (50% of the course in the UK). Mentors ensure that students are exposed to experiences that enable them to meet the objectives of the particular placement, they supervise them in the clinical area, and they assess their competence in practice.

Nurse specialists can help to ensure that the theoretical and clinical content of the programme is based on the most up-to-date practice. Accompanying nurse specialists on their days' work is a stimulating experience for students who are able to see the high quality care and range of activities of the nurse specialist, recognise the influence of the specialist on the quality of life for patients and their families, and begin to see potential career pathways. Over the period of the students' programme, mentors also arrange for students to spend some time with other health professionals, thus developing their understanding of the contributions of the members of the multiprofessional health and social care team. Gaining an insight into the roles of the occupational therapist, the physiotherapist, speech and language therapist, the social worker and others will enable students to learn when and how to collaborate with the multiprofessional team members in providing 24-hour care and rehabilitation.

These groups of clinical nursing staff will have considerable demands on their time and are unlikely to be replaced while they contribute to course planning. Their involvement needs to be negotiated with nurse managers at an early stage to ensure that those selected can attend curriculum development meetings regularly. Their contribution is particularly important within the placement planning group where their intimate knowledge of the placement settings and the available educational opportunities is essential. In a programme using problem-based learning, clinicians can make a most valuable contribution to the development of scenarios as they can ensure that situations presented are true to life and will facilitate understanding of the complexity of the clinical context.

The benefits for these clinicians exist mainly in the influence they can have on the preparation of students before they begin particular clinical experiences, ensuring that they have the knowledge to care for patients with specific problems and conditions. They are able to ensure that graduates will have the necessary knowledge and skills to work as registered nurses on completion of the programme. The clinicians will also have the satisfaction of knowing that they are contributing to ensuring the future quality of care provided by the profession. For some of these clinicians the involvement in the education process acts as professional development and perhaps influences their future careers as they feel considerable satisfaction in their contribution. It is essential that they feel that the time they are contributing is valued; they need to perceive that the benefits exceed the costs of their contribution.

Patients, Clients and Carers (Service Users)

Those who use the health services as patients/clients, carers and families can contribute both to curriculum planning and to the teaching of students, while in some schools they are also involved in student selection (as recommended in the NMC (2008b) circular) and assessment.

The most important way in which service users can contribute in curriculum planning is in identifying those attributes of the nurse and aspects of care which they consider important in providing high quality care. Thus their involvement in developing the statement of values and beliefs is particularly important. They can also make valuable contributions to preparing the programme in relation to development of empathy and communication, as well as helping to develop the curriculum so that it gives students greater understanding of the patient experience in relation to various medical conditions.

However, they have a particularly important contribution during the delivery of the programme. Students learn from every patient they nurse but theoretical teaching is enlivened and enriched by the involvement of service users. While academic staff considered that the involvement of service users was essential and wanted to see this increase, they identified three barriers to achieving this:

- leadership and direction; … to drive creative solutions and sharing of good practice, evaluation and continuing development;
- links and networks; … identifying appropriate people, gaining access to local networks, … seeking to involve vulnerable people;

- organisational and cultural; ... managing appropriate payment, induction, support, liaison, training and informed consent. (Gutteridge and Dobbins, 2010: 510)

Detailed planning and preparation are essential and a whole system approach has been identified to promote service user and carer involvement, illustrated in Figure 3.4 (SCIE, 2007). While this has been developed for social care, it appears equally applicable to nursing. Key to introducing such a system is effective training for staff at every level '*from senior management to front line staff if they want to achieve meaningful participation*' (Gutteridge and Dobbins, 2010: 512). 'Meaningful participation' is identified by seeing that student learning is improved.

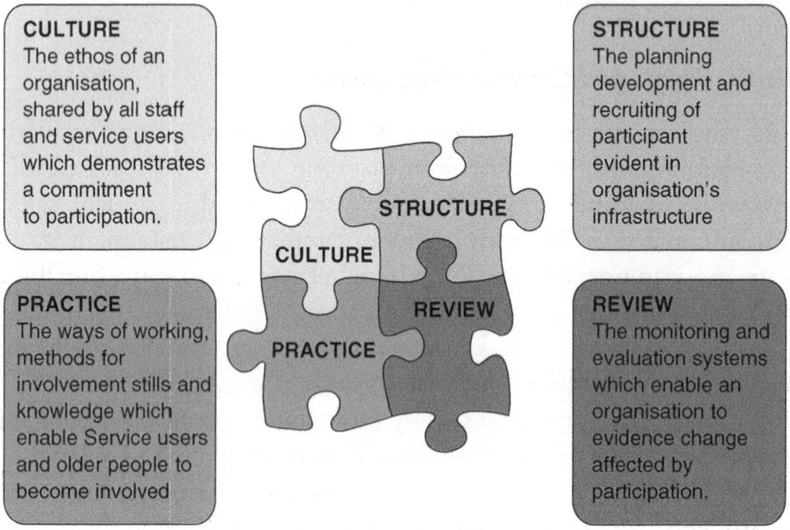

FIGURE 3.4 *A Whole Systems Approach to Service User and Carer Involvement* (SCIE, 2007:7)

In general, service users will contribute most effectively with small groups in which discussion can readily occur. However, it is important to work with the patients or carers to develop clear guidance on the content and management of the groups. This involvement can help students to gain an understanding of the patient experience, empathise with them and their carers and recognise how, as nurses, they can provide help and support. Ongoing involvement with the teaching team will enhance the contribution that service users are able to make. Experience indicates that service users who are accustomed to working with other organisations or advocacy groups find their role easier.

Other approaches involving service users can also be used to introduce the patient experience. For example the following were included in the pre-registration programme at the University of Ulster and could be used as stimuli to initiate problem-based learning:

- A number of patients agreed to be video recorded while they were interviewed about their illness. Video clips about the patient's experiences during illness and treatment were used in the development of elearning materials about pathophysiology. In this way students had immediate access to real lived experience which helped to root the biological sciences firmly within the holistic approach to care.
- The Lilliput Theatre Company, a professional theatre company consisting of adults with learning difficulties, present a series of educational sketches highlighting the discrimination that many adults with learning disabilities face today. These are used as a focus for discussion about inclusion and equality issues with students studying different fields of practice. As those with learning disabilities may also develop other conditions at any age, this is relevant to students preparing for working in any field of nursing.
- Students may be allocated to follow a patient with the family over a period of time (possibly one year), including following them between hospital and community. This enables them to begin to understand the complexity of the patient's and carer's experiences and the contribution required from professional healthcare workers.

Patients can also provide valuable feedback on student performance while working in the clinical area. Thames Valley University in the UK has involved patients in giving feedback on student performance on placement (Buckwell, 2010), after gaining consent from the patient. In particular, patients are well placed to provide feedback on students' interpersonal skills and have also been used in other healthcare professional education programmes (Davies and Lunn, 2009). However, service users may feel constrained in giving negative feedback on students providing their care, either because they feel their care may be compromised or because they do not want to upset the student. Students may also have reservations perhaps because they do not feel that patients are able to provide relevant judgements on their professional performance or may be biased. Clarification of what aspects of the student's performance the patient is judging and the criteria to be used should minimise the reservations of both parties.

Since 2008 the Nursing and Midwifery Council have encouraged direct or indirect involvement of lay people and students in helping to select entrants to nursing or midwifery programmes. One approach is to involve service users in assessing candidates, performance on interpersonal skills and knowledge of nursing demonstrated in group activities and discussions. Service users, academics and nursing candidates all considered that the service users brought a valuable perspective from the reality of receiving health care to the selection of future nurses (Rhodes and Nyawata, 2011). The importance of maintaining confidentiality, care with the information shared with lay interviewers, and the necessity for preparation were emphasised.

Patient and Client Councils (as exist in Northern Ireland, or the equivalent in other parts of the world) are often going to be the easiest way of finding appropriate representation from service users for a contribution to curriculum planning. The Patient and Client Council (2012) is an independent voice for patients, clients, carers and communities on health and social care issues. They will often welcome the opportunity to influence the content of the nursing curriculum with the potential to enhance the care of those with various conditions requiring nursing intervention. Developing a collaborative relationship with such Councils can often facilitate links with individual patients willing to speak to students or, in some other way to help students to understand the real life experiences of patients and carers. It is important to ensure that service users contributing to student learning are made well aware of the value of their contribution and that financial costs are covered.

Private and Voluntary Organisations

Student nurses gain clinical experience within private health organisations such as private hospitals and nursing homes and voluntary organisations. These must therefore be involved in curriculum development in the same way as discussed above for the senior nurses and clinicians: the NMC standards related to placement must still be met, including the requirement for preparation of mentors. The Registered Nursing Home Association (2011) may be a useful contact to identify suitable representation on curriculum planning groups.

In the UK, unlike most places in the world, nurses prepare to work in one of four fields of practice: adult, child, learning disability or mental health nursing. Key organisations related to some of these fields of practice are particularly valuable in planning programmes and contributing to nurse education:

- Organisations related to specific disorders, such as the Multiple Sclerosis Society or Diabetes UK, may be able to identify patients and carers willing to become involved in interacting with students to enhance their understanding of the adult patient experience and carers' needs.
- Mencap (2010) is the voice of learning disability and aims to promote valuing and supporting people with a learning disability, their families and carers. They may be able to identify clients, carers and professionals to contribute in different ways to nursing education.
- Similarly MIND (2010) endeavours to promote a society that protects good mental health for all – 'a society where people with experience of mental distress are treated fairly, positively and with respect' and may be able to identify individuals able to contribute to the education of both adult and mental health nurses.
- Barnardo's and other children-focused charities have valuable expertise to contribute in development of the child field of practice.

Some voluntary organisations may be able to offer placement experience in day centres or in relation to other activities.

When setting up a curriculum planning team involving voluntary organisations, if the project is to progress effectively it is necessary to be clear about the specific expertise of each organisation and the contribution they can make. An example of this is in planning the MSc course in Disaster Relief at the University of Ulster in which it is essential that students learn about the expertise of the different NGOs (Non-Governmental Organisations) and other organisations in disaster response and preparedness. A number of these were involved and were prepared to support the placement component of the course. Table 3.2 illustrates the specific expertise of different organisations involved in disaster relief.

TABLE 3.2 *Organisations in Disaster Response*

OXFAM	Rapid response and aid delivery in disasters; water purification
Concern Worldwide	Environmental health and nutrition
Merlin	Rapid medical response and rebuilding of in-country health services
International Federation of the Red Cross and Red Crescent	Health and community care in disasters
Medecins Sans Frontieres	Aid relief in complex emergencies
Red R	Aid relief worker recruitment and training
Islamic Aid	Health care and clean water
CARE	Poverty mitigation
World Vision	Capacity building in communities at risk of disaster
United Nations	International law and security in disaster situations
WHO	Global health issues and pandemic response

As with the other groups involved in curriculum planning and contributing to delivery of the programme, it is important to identify the benefits for each organisation and identify approaches to minimise the costs. The major benefits usually revolve around being able to influence the education of nurses in order to enhance the care they will be able to provide for the individuals with which each organisation is involved. In addition, they get to know other agencies and their staff and meet nursing staff with similar interest in their area of care resulting in collaborative relationships with other organisations.

Some groups may suggest having their logos on course documentation. In general this is not recommended, as the number of organisations involved could result in considerable complexities. However, it is important to ensure that they are given appropriate recognition for their assistance: a list of all members of the curriculum planning team, including users, should be included at the beginning of the programme document. This affirms ownership of the curriculum.

Statutory Organisations

Health is influenced by many aspects of living which come under the aegis of the local authorities and these may well have an interest in the education of healthcare workers, including nurses. While in Northern Ireland health and social care are integrated, in the remainder of the UK they are separately organised with social work, including child protection, under the control of the local council. But all nurses have a responsibility for protection of children and vulnerable adults and need to understand the roles and responsibilities of different professional groups for this aspect of care.

All nurses also have a health promotion aspect to their work. Much health promotion comes under the aegis of the local authority many of which are working towards recognition as a Healthy City within the Health Cities Project. This global project aims to engage local governments '*in health development through a process of political commitment, institutional change, capacity-building, partnership-based planning and innovative projects*' (WHO, 2011). Healthy Cities networks currently have more than 1,400 cities and towns across the WHO European Region as members and their commitment to the way forward has been confirmed through the Zagreb Declaration for Healthy Cities (WHO, 2009). The principles and values shown in Box 3.2 demonstrate a strong link with nursing and the importance of the input from local government is clear. It is important for nursing students to develop an awareness of local structures and how they impact on health care and educational preparation. The benefits for the local authorities lie in having a nursing workforce within their area with an understanding and equal commitment to the promotion of healthy living.

Box 3.2 Healthy Cities Principles and Values

- **Equity:** Addressing inequality in health, and paying attention to the needs of those who are vulnerable and socially disadvantaged; inequity is inequality in health that is unfair and unjust and avoidable causes of ill health. The right to health applies to all regardless of sex, race, religious belief, sexual orientation, age, disability or socioeconomic circumstance.
- **Participation and empowerment:** Ensuring the individual and collective right of people to participate in decision-making that affects their health, health care and wellbeing. Providing access to opportunities and skills development together with positive thinking to empower citizens to become self-sufficient.
- **Working in partnership:** Building effective multisectoral strategic partnerships to implement integrated approaches and achieve sustainable improvement in health.
- **Solidarity and friendship:** Working in the spirit of peace, friendship and solidarity through networking and respect and appreciation of the social and cultural diversity of the cities of the Healthy Cities movement.
- **Sustainable development:** The necessity of working to ensure that economic development – and all its supportive infrastructural needs, including transport systems – is environmentally and socially sustainable: meeting the needs of the present in ways that do not compromise the ability of future generations to meet their own needs.

Source: Zagreb *Declaration for Healthy Cities: Health and Health Equity in All Local Parties*. Copenhagen: WHO Regional Office for Europe, 2009: 2. www.euro.who.int/_data/assets/pdf_file/0015/101076/E92343.pdf

CHAPTER SUMMARY

This chapter has identified the major role of the partnership between academic and healthcare organisations in providing nursing education programmes, and the importance of the many groups which contribute as partners within nursing education. The importance of identifying the costs and benefits to the participants in aiming to achieve successful partnerships has been highlighted. The mode and importance of the contributions which can be made by the different groups have been considered. At the beginning of the curriculum process the questions in Box 3.3 in relation to partnership need consideration.

Box 3.3 Topics for Consideration

Within your own curriculum development situation:

- Who are the different partners you want involved and what do you want them to contribute?
- What are the benefits and costs to them of their involvement?
- What will be the best way of involving them in curriculum development?

In relation to the course that is to be offered:

- How do you envisage the different partners contributing to teaching?
- How will you support them in their involvement with students?
- How will you help them to prepare for their sessions with students?

4 EDUCATIONAL STRUCTURES

INTRODUCTION

Having developed the curriculum framework, determined the broad overall outcomes of the programme and engaged with the range of stakeholders, a number of strategic and structural issues need to be considered and decisions made before delving into the detailed development of the programme. The focus of this chapter is on setting the educational process in the national and international context. This will facilitate travel of students during their programme and achieve international recognition of professional qualifications on completion. To achieve the second of these, it is necessary that the equivalence of professional qualifications from different countries can be demonstrated and it is considered that teachers should have some understanding of the structures and processes involved. The Bologna Process, with the associated Tuning Project (2004), involves the countries of the European Higher Education Area (EHEA) and is having a major impact on higher education throughout Europe. It influences the structure of university courses and facilitates achievement of international recognition of professional qualifications. In writing this chapter, it has been interesting to note how the educational structures in Europe and in the UK have changed and continue to alter in pursuit of the goal of enhancing the educational experience for students. Every teacher needs to recognise the influence of these international agreements on education in their own country.

This chapter will focus mainly on nursing education in the UK as a case study of the application of the issues considered. In the UK the Quality Assurance Agency (QAA) is responsible for developing standards to help meet the Bologna Process outcomes. However, universities in the UK are independent institutions with freedom to determine the form of their own programmes of study, although with the QAA having a monitoring and advisory role. In addition many programmes also have to meet the requirement for professional accreditation.

Many of these issues overlap and need to be considered concurrently although they are examined separately in this chapter. HEIs often prescribe structural details such as semesters, modules, credit points etc. to fit the QAA standards which are compatible with the Bologna recommendations. In addition, the **Nursing Statutory Body** will specify requirements in relation to length, content and balance between theory and practice within a programme of nursing education and provides standards which have to be interpreted and implemented.

The Statutory Body and academic institution requirements both have to be managed, but sometimes are not easily compatible: those that cannot be modified are the professional parameters set by the Statutory Body. Nursing is a practice-based profession and, thus, practice is central to any nursing educational programme and plays a major role in determining the overall structure. Integrating the academic and professional sets of parameters to produce a programme which fulfils the professional and educational philosophies of the academic staff may take some creativity but is necessary. However, sometimes the HEI will have to accept situations outside the norm for the institution. As a result, nursing has often led the way in introducing change and flexibility in programme delivery to the universities.

Having said that this chapter is based primarily on nursing education in the UK, in reality much of the content is based on the education system in just three of the countries of the UK: England, Wales and Northern Ireland. Scotland has a somewhat different education system and the documentation for Scotland is differentiated from that of the rest of the UK.

In different ways, both systems are working towards implementing the Bologna Process standards as described by QAA. Other countries will have different education systems but much of the content of this chapter will be relevant.

IMPLEMENTATION OF THE BOLOGNA PROCESS (EURYDICE, 2010)

The Bologna Process started in 1998 with a joint declaration on Harmonisation of the Architecture of the European Higher Education System between four of the countries of the European Union (France, Germany, Italy and the UK). It was followed up by the Bologna Agreement in 1999 (with 29 countries involved) and five more ministerial conferences since then until the Leuven/Louvain-la-Neuve Communiqué in 2009. In the Bergen Communiqué the ministers responsible for higher education agreed that:

> We adopt the overarching framework for qualifications in the EHEA, comprising three cycles (including, within national contexts, the possibility of intermediate qualifications), generic descriptors for each cycle based on learning outcomes and competences, and credit ranges in the first and second cycles. We commit ourselves to elaborating national frameworks for qualifications compatible with the overarching framework for qualifications in the EHEA by 2010, and to having started work on this by 2007. (Bologna Process, 2005a: 2)

There are now 46 countries involved in the Bologna Process as members of the European Higher Education Area (EHEA). They are from the European Union, candidate members of the EU, the former USSR, and the European Free Trade Association (EFTA) and are all working towards the priorities set at Leuven until 2020 that:

- Each country should set measurable targets for widening overall participation and increasing the participation of under-represented social groups in higher education by the end of the next decade;
- By 2020 at least 20% of those graduating in the EHEA should have had a study or training period abroad;
- Lifelong learning and employability are important missions of higher education;
- Student-centred learning should be the goal of ongoing curriculum reform. (EURYDICE, 2010: 13)

The political objectives of the Bologna Process have been linked to higher education in large part through the Tuning Process (2004) which aims to enhance the quality of programmes through focusing on educational structures at subject level. The aim is not to achieve uniformity across European HEIs but to identify reference points and achieve common understanding. This process has resulted in considerable progress towards compatibility and comparability in educational processes through structures and tools which are being introduced and monitored throughout the EHEA. Other major areas of focus (EURYDICE, 2010) are in relation to:

- Quality Assurance (24);
- The Social Dimension of Higher Education (27);
- Lifelong Learning in Higher Education (34);
- Student Mobility (38).

Many of the developments through the Bologna Process are now incorporated into, or at least are compatible with, the guidance and standards produced by the Quality Assurance Agency for Higher Education (QAA) in the UK in relation to:

- quality assurance mechanisms;
- national qualifications framework;
- the three-cycle degree system;
- credit points and credit accumulation and transfer (CATS);
- diploma supplement.

Quality Assurance

Within the Bologna Process the importance of quality assurance is emphasised and most member countries of EHEA now have an agency independent of government which is responsible for ensuring quality. Within the UK, at present this is the QAA which is funded by the HEIs and has contracts with higher education funding bodies (QAA, 2009).

UK universities are independent, self-governing organisations which plan and provide educational programmes, and undertake activities in relation to research, scholarship, consultancy and knowledge transfer. Each university is self-regulating in terms of the quality of programmes offered but aims to work within the standards recommended by QAA. The quality of their educational activities is promoted by QAA which carries out two major groups of activities:

- external quality assurance through regular audits of HEIs' procedures to review their effectiveness in fulfilling their quality assurance responsibilities;
- guidance on maintenance and improvement of quality assurance processes and numerous aspects of course delivery.

Relevant publications include The Code of Practice (QAA, 2004–2010) published in 10 sections which provide guidance for Universities in assuring academic quality and standards (see Box 4.1). This is in the process of being replaced by the UK Quality Code for Higher Education.

As independent institutions, each university will have its own committee structure, roles in course management, quality assurance mechanisms, standard module sizes and examination regulations.

Box 4.1 The Code Of Practice

- Section 1: Postgraduate research programmes (2004)
- Section 2: Collaborative provision and flexible and distributed learning (including e-learning) (2004)
- Section 3: Disabled students (2010)
- Section 4: External examining (2004)
- Section 5: Academic appeals and student complaints on academic matters (2007)
- Section 6: Assessment of students (2006)
- Section 7: Programme design, approval, monitoring and review (2006)
- Section 8: Career education, information, advice and guidance (2010)
- Section 9: Work-based and placement learning (2007)
- Section 10: Admissions to higher education (2006)

National Qualifications Framework and Three-Cycle Degree System

The Framework for Higher Education Qualifications in England, Wales and Northern Ireland (FHEQ) (equivalent to the National Qualifications Framework of the Bologna Process) (QAA, 2008a) incorporates the three-cycle degree system of the Bologna Process (2005b) and credit points. The three cycles are the Bachelor's (or Baccalaureate) degree, the Master's degree, and the Doctorate degree, with short cycle programmes possible within the first and second cycles. In relation to examples of nursing qualifications in the UK, Table 4.1 shows the detailed credit point requirements for first, second and third cycle qualifications as well as the minimum number of credit points which must be achieved at the highest level within each award.

Academic Levels

The academic levels included in higher education range from 4 (first year undergraduate) to 8 (Doctoral level), with levels 1 to 3 being applicable to qualifications normally studied in Further (rather than Higher) Education Institutions. Level 3 is the usual standard for admission to higher education. Academic levels are one part of the description of the different components of a programme.

The nature and characteristics of the academic achievement expected at each level is specified by credit level descriptors (QAA, 2008a) presented in two parts:

- statement of the outcomes which the students will demonstrate they have achieved;
- statement of the wider abilities that students will be expected to have developed.

TABLE 4.1 *Higher Education Qualifications in Nursing in the UK (minimum credit points at specified level shown in brackets) (adapted from QAA, 2008b)*

Major HE qualifications	Examples of HE qualifications for Nurses	FHEQ level	Minimum UK Credit Points (minimum at highest level)	FQ-EHEA cycle
Doctorates	PhD/DPhil	8	Not usually credit rated	Third cycle (**end of cycle**) qualifications
	Professional Doctorates: DNSc, EdD		540 (360 at level 8)	
Master's degrees	MPhil	7	Not usually credit rated	Second cycle (**end of cycle**) qualifications
	MRes, MSc		180 (150 at level 7)	
	Integrated master's degree (e.g, MNurs: 4-year degree leading to initial nursing qualification(s) and meeting level 6 and 7 outcomes)		480 (120 at level 7, 120 at level 6)	
Postgraduate qualifications not meeting quantity of study for a Master's degree	Postgraduate diplomas (e.g. in Specialist Nursing)		120 (90 at level 7)	
	Postgraduate Certificate in Education for Nurses, Midwives and Health Visitors		60 (40 at level 7)	
	Postgraduate certificates (e.g. in Independent and Supplementary Prescribing)		60 (40 at level 7)	
Bachelor's degrees	Bachelor's degrees with honours (e.g, BA/BSc Hons in Nursing / Professional Development in Nursing	6	360+ (90 at level 6)	First cycle (**end of cycle**) qualifications
	Bachelor's degrees (BA/ BSc in Nursing) *(minimum level of qualification for RN in UK in courses introduced from 2011)*		300+ (60 at level 6)	
	Professional Graduate Certificate in Education		60 (40 at level 6)	
	Graduate diplomas/Graduate certificates		80 / 40 (all at level 6)	
	2nd year of Honours degree	5	*At least 120*	
	Foundation Degrees (eg, FdA, FdSc) *(minimum level of qualification for RN in UK, introduced 1989)*		240 (90 at level 5)	Short cycle (**within or linked to the first cycle**) qualifications
	Diplomas of Higher Education (DipHE)		240 (90 at level 5)	
	1st year of Honours degree	4	*At least 120*	
	Certificates of Higher Education (CertHE)		120 (90 at level 4)	

The credit level descriptors provide guidance for developing the outcomes for each level of a curriculum and are summarised in Box 4.2 (QAA, 2008b). These are compatible with the Dublin Descriptors of the FQ-EHEA (see QAA, 2008a, Annex B) which are generic statements of the achievements and abilities normally expected at the end of each of the three Bologna cycles. They are presented in five groups which are comparable to the graduate qualities which many institutions expect their undergraduates to achieve through their programme:

- knowledge and understanding;
- applying knowledge and understanding;
- making judgements;
- communication skills;
- learning skills.

Box 4.2 Summary of the England, Wales and Northern Ireland (EWNI) Generic Credit Level Descriptors

Learning accredited at this level will reflect the ability to:

Level 8

make a significant and original contribution to a specialised field of inquiry, demonstrating a command of methodological issues and engaging in critical dialogue with peers and accepting full accountability for outcomes

Level 7

display mastery of a complex and specialised area of knowledge and skills, employing advanced skills to conduct research, or advanced technical or professional activity, accepting accountability for related decision making, including use of supervision

Level 6

critically review, consolidate and extend a systematic and coherent body of knowledge, utilising specialised skills across an area of study; critically evaluate concepts and evidence from a range of sources; transfer and apply diagnostic and creative skills and exercise significant judgement in a range of situations; and accept accountability for determining and achieving personal and/or group outcomes

Level 5

generate ideas through the analysis of concepts at an abstract level with a command of specialised skills and the formulation of responses to well-defined and

(Continued)

(Continued)

abstract problems; analyse and evaluate information; exercise significant judgement across a broad range of functions; and accept responsibility for determining and achieving personal and/or group outcomes

Level 4

develop a rigorous approach to the acquisition of a broad knowledge base; employ a range of specialised skills; evaluate information, using it to plan and develop investigative strategies and to determine solutions to a variety of unpredictable problems; and operate in a range of varied and specific contexts, taking responsibility for the nature and quality of outputs

Level 3

qualification level for entry to HE

Honours Degree

Unlike most of the world, in the majority of UK universities the usual undergraduate award at the end of a three-year programme is an honours degree, although Scotland has a different education system with a four–year degree leading to honours. Box 4.3 shows the expectations of someone completing an honours degree.

An honours degree is classified into First, Upper Second, Lower Second, Third Class, (and some universities award Pass) degrees depending on marks achieved and, again in some universities, the proportion of marks within the classification boundaries. Universities vary in the latitude they permit around the boundaries for the classes of degree, as indicated in Table 4.2.

The usefulness of the degree classification in providing guidance to employers is being questioned and, at present, its future is under discussion with the possibility of moving towards a more detailed description of a student's achievement (see Diploma Supplement below) to replace the current system. It is considered that this would provide greater clarity about the outcome of higher education.

TABLE 4.2 *Honours Degree Classification*

Class of Degree	First	Upper Second	Lower Second	Third	Pass	Fail
Usual Mark Bands	70% >	60–69%	50–59%	40–49% OR 45–49%	Not Awarded OR 40–44%	< 39%

Box 4.3 The Honours Degree (Universities UK, 2007: 56)

Qualification descriptors usefully summarise that 'Honours degrees are awarded to students who have demonstrated:

- a systematic understanding of key aspects of their field of study, including acquisition of coherent and detailed knowledge, at least some of which is at or informed by the forefront of defined aspects of a discipline;
- an ability to deploy accurately established techniques of analysis and enquiry within a discipline;
- conceptual understanding that enables the student:
  - to devise and sustain arguments, and/or to solve problems, using ideas and techniques, some of which are at the forefront of a discipline; and
  - to describe and comment upon particular aspects of current research, or equivalent advanced scholarship, in the discipline;
- an appreciation of the uncertainty, ambiguity and limits of knowledge; and
- the ability to manage their own learning, and to make use of scholarly reviews and primary sources (e.g refereed research articles and/or original materials appropriate to the discipline)'.

A typical holder of an honours degree 'will be able to:

- apply the methods and techniques that they have learned to review, consolidate, extend and apply their knowledge and understanding, and to initiate and carry out projects;
- critically evaluate arguments, assumptions, abstract concepts and data (that may be incomplete), to make judgements, and to frame appropriate questions to achieve a solution - or identify a range of solutions - to a problem;
- communicate information, ideas, problems, and solutions to both specialist and nonspecialist audiences; and will have:
- qualities and transferable skills necessary for employment requiring:
  - the exercise of initiative and personal responsibility;
  - decision-making in complex and unpredictable contexts; and
  - the learning ability needed to undertake appropriate further training of a professional or equivalent nature.'

Thus, honours degree graduates will have acquired understanding of a complex body of knowledge, a wide range of high level skills and a broad level of experience.

A non-honours degree is awarded at a Pass level, or sometimes it is awarded with Commendation for those achieving a specified overall level, usually at 60%, while some universities also award Distinction for those with 70% or over. This degree only has to include at least 60 credit points at level 6 towards the end of the programme, compared to the minimum of 90 (and usually 120) level 6 credits in the honours degree.

Credit Points and CATS

Credit points are the second major part of the description of the modules comprising a programme and these reflect the amount of work involved. Most institutions now use modules as the unit of study and these are described in terms of academic level and credit points, or in the USA credit hours, as an indication of the amount of work required (QAA, 2008b) (see Box 4.4). While UK credit points are different from the European credit points, there is easy conversion between the two which are both based on a notional value of the amount of work expected for each credit point.

In contrast, credit hours are based on the time spent in class each week over a semester or a quarter and are not used in the UK. While many American academics seem to have an innate understanding of the value of credit hours, there is some controversy about their use (Blumenstyk, 2010) with Watkins and Schlosser (2002) proposing a Capabilities-Based Educational Equivalency Units model which appears to relate closely to academic levels (i.e. quality rather than quantity of study). Conversion between credit points and credit hours is not easy and will usually involve some degree of creativity. For example, nursing courses in Saudi Arabia which are validated by a UK university use an equivalence of four credit points to one credit hour in describing the programmes. Those arranging periods of study in the USA are able to estimate the amount of work undertaken.

The European Credit Transfer and Accumulation System (ECTS) is emphasised within the Bologna Process as a means to enhancing mobility of students within the EHEA and CATS is a recognised feature within the higher education sector in the UK (QAA, 2008b). It enables students to accumulate credits for the work completed and carry that to another institution and even a different area of study. The credits presented for recognition for another course/institution are considered for transfer in relation to:

- the proportion of credit which may be transferred;
- the currency or shelf-life of the credit;
- general credit, i.e. the overall amount of credit achieved;
- specific credit, i.e. the direct relevance of prior learning to the intended programme of study.

The accepting institution takes these factors into account when deciding how many credits student can carry into their new programme. Recognition of credits allows applicants to be considered for entry but the institution will accept or reject in relation to availability of places and suitability of the applicant for the programme.

Box 4.4 Credit Points and Credit Hours

UK Credit Points: Each credit point is equivalent to about 10 hours of study including formal hours of teaching, independent study and preparation of assessed work. Thus a 20 credit point academic module is equivalent to approximately 200 hours of study in total (sometimes referred to as 'effort hours'). However, if credit points are awarded to a clinical module, it is recognised that at least some of the time in practice is less easily identified as dedicated to learning. The credit points awarded will often be related to the amount of assessed work to be completed. For example a 6-week placement in which students will undertake a clinical assessment and submit an analysis of a clinical problem may be identified as a 20-credit point module.

EU Credit Points: Each EU credit point is notionally equated with 20 'effort hours', i.e. equivalent to 2 UK credit points. This enables equivalences to be readily calculated and facilitates student mobility across Europe.

Credit Hours: Used in North America and many countries throughout the world which have copied their system of education. A credit hour is a time measurement based on either a semester or a quarter: a semester is when the academic year is divided into two sessions, a quarter when divided into three (USA Education, 2010). A semester credit hour is based on 15 hours (1 hour per week for 15 weeks). Clinical time is often calculated as 3 to 1, ie. a 1 credit course would involve 45 hours. However, the Carnegie Unit is sometimes used and this includes 2 hours of homework with the one hour of lecture time per week (i.e. 3 hours per week) for a 16-week semester. It is possible to have more hours, but not fewer (ebookpedia, 2010).

Diploma Supplement

The members of the Bologna Process have also agreed that a Diploma Supplement will be provided to all students, and countries are at varying stages in its full implementation. In the UK the Burgess Report (Universities UK, 2007), in considering the continued viability of the honours degree, proposed that a Higher Education Achievement Report (HEAR) be introduced which would incorporate the requirements of the Diploma Supplement. It would run alongside the current Honours degree classification until or unless the honours degree became irrelevant and discarded. The intention is that the Diploma Supplement should be web-based and many institutions are intending to introduce the total package when new management systems are implemented. The Diploma Supplement should include the detail shown in Box 4.5.

Box 4.5 The Diploma Supplement (UK HE Europe Unit, 2006: 19–20)

1 Information identifying the holder of the qualification
  - 1.1 Family name(s):
  - 1.2 Given name(s):
  - 1.3 Date of birth (day/month/year):
  - 1.4 Student identification number or code (if available):

2 Information identifying the qualification
  - 2.1 Name of qualification and (if applicable) title conferred (in original language):
  - 2.2 Main field(s) of study for the qualification:
  - 2.3 Name and status of awarding institution (in original language):
  - 2.4 Name and status of institution (if different from 2.3) administering studies (in original language):
  - 2.5 Language(s) of instruction/examination:

3 Information on the level of the qualification
  - 3.1 Level of qualification:
  - 3.2 Official length of programme:
  - 3.3 Access requirement(s):

4 Information on the contents and results gained
  - 4.1 Mode of study:
  - 4.2 Programme requirements:
  - 4.3 Programme details: (e.g. modules or units studied), and the individual grades/marks/credits obtained: (if this information is available on an official transcript this should be used here)
  - 4.4 Grading scheme and, if available, grade distribution guidance:
  - 4.5 Overall classification of the qualification (in original language):

5 Information on the function of the qualification

5.1 Access to further study:
5.2 Professional status (if applicable):

6 Additional information

6.1 Additional information:
6.2 Further information sources:

7 Certification of the supplement

7.1 Date:
7.2 Signature:
7.3 Capacity:
7.4 Official stamp or seal:

8 Information on the national higher education system

At present some universities provide students with academic transcripts, along with a document providing the additional information to be included in the Diploma Supplement (UK HE Europe Unit, 2006). The academic transcript consists of information about modules studied, the credit point value and the marks or grades achieved for each module, and concludes with the overall class or level of award.

STRUCTURAL ISSUES IN NURSING PROGRAMMES

So far in this chapter we have been reviewing issues applicable to all disciplines. Here we are examining some of the same issues in the context of nursing education, in addition to other structural issues relevant to nursing.

There are three major patterns of nursing education:

- an apprenticeship system in which student nurses are a part of the workforce when undertaking clinical placements;
- a higher education system in which students are studying within a HEI which is responsible for ensuring their practice learning in collaboration with clinical services;
- a secondary education system in which students train as nurses as part of their secondary education.

Which of these patterns is in practice in any country is determined by government or the Statutory Body. In some countries one pattern will be more dominant than the others.

Most countries are moving towards a higher education system of nursing education as the profession becomes more aware of worldwide developments and the complexity of nursing activities increases.

International Professional Recognition

In most countries, the Statutory Body is responsible for reviewing international nursing qualifications and determining what, if any, additional preparation must be completed before recognition in their country. Within the European Union (EU, 2005) the directive on recognition of professional qualifications sets minimum standards for general nursing education programmes to permit recognition across Europe. The European standards specify that general nurse training programmes

> shall comprise at least three years of study or 4,600 hours of theoretical and clinical training, the duration of the theoretical training representing at least one-third and the duration of the clinical training at least one half of the minimum duration of the training. (Article 31, paragraph 3)

While formally the EU specifications only apply to general nurses (or adult nurses in the UK) the NMC also uses similar standards for education for mental health, children's, and learning disability fields of nursing.

The NMC sets standards for programmes leading to a qualification registered or recorded on the NMC Professional Register. Those related to the structure of the pre-registration nursing programmes are the most extensive and must be taken into account in planning such programmes. In the UK the NMC specifies an equal balance between theory and practice for pre-registration nursing programmes. However, there is considerable scope for variation in the way in which programmes can be planned within the overall EU standard. For example, in the Republic of Ireland pre-registration nursing education is currently a four-year programme, three of which are the usual academic years with a fourth extended year finishing with a 36 weeks period of internship (An Bord Altranais, 2005). The total programme fulfils the EU standards with a programme of approximately 44% theory (including self-directed study and examinations) and 56% practice.

Academic Award

A degree level qualification reflects the higher level of decision-making now required of newly qualified nurses in contrast to the many previous entrants to the profession who have developed this level of performance through experience and further study. The professional award is usually pre-determined by the Statutory Body or government, but the level of academic award often has some flexibility (as in the UK) and, within limits that the Statutory Body may set, is determined by the HEI.

Within the boundaries of the FHEQ one of the first issues to be resolved is to determine the academic level of the final award, and any appropriate and professionally acceptable lower awards. Since 1989, with the introduction of the Project 2000 programmes, a Diploma of Higher Education has been the minimum level qualification for entry to the nursing profession in the UK. The NMC has now specified that a (non-honours) degree will be the entry-level qualification to the nursing profession from programmes approved from 2011 onwards. However, it is up to the HEI to decide whether a higher level qualification will be offered, with or without a lower level award also being available.

UK universities differ slightly in their approach to the award of different levels of qualification. Some universities, particularly those who have offered honours degrees in nursing since the 1970s, will admit students to an honours degree but have the option to award a non-honours degree as a fall-back position for those who meet the professional requirements but struggle with the amount of level 6 work required for honours. Other universities will admit students to a non-honours degree with a possible option of transferring them to an honours degree programme if academic performance permits. It is also permissible to offer a four-year Master's degree which prepares students for an initial nursing qualification and which includes the requisite credits at academic levels 6 (Bachelor's level) and 7 (Master's level). This approach can be used to prepare nurses for two fields of practice, e.g. adult and mental health nursing.

The differentiation between a degree and an honours degree is specified by the number of credit points required at level 6: non-honours requiring at least 60 while honours students must achieve at least 90 and usually 120 credit points at this level. In many programmes this differentiation is reflected in a greater emphasis on research in the honours programme.

In reaching the decision about whether to offer honours or non-honours a number of factors must be taken into account:

- What this means in planning a programme, i.e. the level and quantity of academic achievement required.
- What are the potential implications for future career development?

There are potential implications in relation to the level of award. Specialist nursing qualifications are now offered at level 7 (Master's degree level) and the usual qualification required for entry to an MSc is an honours degree. However, most universities will accept students with a non-honours degree on to a Postgraduate Diploma (taught at level 7) completion of which usually meets the NMC requirements for the specialist nursing award. The PG Diploma is usually the first 120 credit points of the Master's degree and satisfactory performance in the PG Diploma will normally allow progression to complete the MSc through a 60-credit dissertation. Many students wish to complete the MSc, even without funding support. Thus no one completing a non-honours degree need be disadvantaged in career progression.

Number of Credit Points

An honours degree in most academic disciplines normally consists of 360 credit points: 120 at each of levels 4, 5 and 6 taught over two semesters in each of three academic years. However, full-time pre-registration nursing courses consist of considerably longer academic years of 45 weeks (often including some weeks of independent study time). So how many credit points should the programme be worth?

Different universities approach this in varying ways. Some conform to the system of allocating 120 credit points per academic year, with each credit point notionally worth significantly more than the standard 10 hours. Others use the notional value of one credit point equivalent to 10 effort hours for university-based work and a lower value for placement with the overall number of credits in the course exceeding 360 credits (for example 410 credits). This still fits within the Bologna Process (2005b) recommendation that a first cycle qualification should be represented by 180–240 ECTS credits which is equivalent to 360–480 UK credits.

The NMC now states that there must be equal weighting in the assessment of practice and theory in contributing to the final award. However, the interpretation of this is difficult: it does not necessarily mean an equal number of credit points for theory and practice in calculating the level of the final award. The essential requirement is to demonstrate that theory and practice are recognised as equally important. In addition, the NMC now states that practice learning will be assessed formatively in practice leading up to a summative assessment of performance at the progression point, or completion of the programme, at the end of each year (Figure 2.4).

Practice Learning (Clinical Placement)

Experience in clinical placements to enable practice learning plays a central role in nursing education and successful implementation of this important part of the curriculum is dependent on successful partnership between the academic staff of the HEI and managers and clinicians in practice settings. Students need experienced nurses to act as mentors in relation to placement experience in order to ensure that adequate learning takes place in practice (in the UK preceptors support newly qualified nurses). A major consideration for many Schools of Nursing is finding enough suitable clinical settings, with prepared mentors, for the number of students undertaking the programme.

For some institutions the restricted clinical facilities available may be the major factor influencing the overall practice/theory pattern. For example, in a three-year programme it may not be possible to have all three years of students undertaking practice learning at the same time and, within each student group, students will have to rotate through a number of different clinical areas in order that no clinical area is overloaded with students.

The selection and organisation of clinical settings needs to take account of demographic changes and the resulting societal needs. The population is growing older and medical technology continues to develop, resulting in:

- a growing incidence of chronic diseases;
- an expanding number of people needing care in the community;
- an increasing level of acute interventions occurring on a day-case basis and in the community;
- an increasing proportion of those patients who are in hospitals requiring critical care or high dependency nursing.

Nurse educators and practitioners have to plan programmes which will prepare nurses with the knowledge and skills, decision-making ability and confidence to provide and be accountable for the care required.

The clinical placement schedule needs to be planned so that each student gains a good balance of the key areas of practice. Community based experience is becoming increasingly important and it is essential to enable students to gain an understanding of the different types of practice in the community: care of those with long-term conditions, acute care, palliative care, public health, practice nursing, and protection of children and vulnerable people. Acute care skills which previously have only been applied in hospital are now also being used in community care and practice learning needs to be arranged to ensure that students are able to develop competence in these skills by selective use of community and hospital settings.

It is also necessary to prepare nurses able to provide care for the acutely ill including those needing critical care and high dependency nursing. A question which Schools of Nursing may wish to consider is whether some level of specialisation should begin within pre-registration education. Clearly all pre-registration students must learn about the principles of care in the range of settings and will need both community and hospital experience. However, is it reasonable that some could have a greater focus on community care and others an enhanced emphasis on acute care?

The length of each clinical experience needs to be sufficient for students to get used to the environment and to be able to take full advantage of the learning opportunities to which they are exposed. A key element in planning is ensuring that students receive appropriate preparation before each practice learning placement and debriefing afterwards to help them to reflect upon their learning.

Modular Structure

In most universities, a programme consists of a number of modules (sometimes called units of study or courses) each of which focuses on a major concept or a few related concepts. Modules may be theoretical, clinically based or a combination of the two. In pre-registration nursing programmes, modules are mainly or all prescribed, although some institutions are able to offer a few optional modules. If the proposal to permit students to focus mainly on caring for those with chronic illness in the community or on those requiring acute care is accepted, then there will be a necessary degree of optionality within the programme in relation to both theory and practice.

As already indicated, a module is defined by two parameters – academic level and number of credit points – each of which must be taken into account in developing content and materials for a module. The level should be clearly demonstrated in the learning outcomes written for each module, and should also incorporate the generic graduate qualities.

Module size may be specified by the institution and modules often carry 10, 15, 20 or 30 credit points, or equivalent European credit points (5, 7.5, 10 or 15). With each UK credit point nominally equivalent to 10 effort hours (and ECTS credits 20 effort hours), the modules above need to be planned with an estimated workload in mind – 100, 150, 200 or 300 hours for the examples above. Within a programme, academic modules of comparable credit value should be equitable in workload. Placement modules are also allocated credit points but the hours of placement do not usually relate to credit points in the same way. Instead these are allocated according to a judgement about the amount of learning and assessment taking place during the experience. For example, a 12-week clinical placement during which the student completes a portfolio demonstrating the learning which has taken place may be allocated 30 credit points although, in terms of hours for a 35-hour week, it would be worth 42 credit points.

In a programme such as pre-registration nursing, many of the themes identified run through the programme and are revisited at intervals in a spiral curriculum. Modules may be too large to facilitate this arrangement so some other structure has to be devised. Within a theme the planning team may identify several portions or units of study, the later ones building on the earlier. These can be used effectively to prepare a spiral curriculum and units from different themes which all relate to a particular focus, e.g. chronic illness, can be grouped to form a module (discussed in Chapter 6).

Within a normal academic semester, 60 (or 30 European) credit points is the usual modular load studied which may be made up in a number of ways thus permitting a considerable degree of flexibility (see Box 4.6).

Box 4.6 Usual Modular Load for One Academic Semester

The usual load for one academic semester is 60 credit points (or 30 European credits) which can be made up in numerous ways. Most UK Universities will not permit 5 credit modules.

UK Credits		European Credits	
20 credit modules x 3	= 60	10 credit modules x 3	= 30
20 credit modules x 2 10 credit modules x 2	= 60	10 credit modules x 2 5 credit modules x 2	= 30
15 credit modules x 4	= 60	7.5 credit modules x 4	= 30
15 credit modules x 2 30 credit modules x 1	= 60	7.5 credit modules x 2 15 credit modules x 1	= 30
30 credit modules x 1 20 credit modules x 1 10 credit modules x 1	= 60	15 credit modules x 1 10 credit modules x 1 5 credit modules x 1	= 30
10 credit modules x 6	= 60	5 credit modules x 6	= 30

Progression and Integration

In any programme key issues are progression through the different academic levels and integration of the different aspects of the programme into a coherent whole.

In a degree programme, students progress through academic levels 4, 5 and 6, roughly in line with years 1, 2 and 3 of the course, normally achieving at least 120 credits at each level for an honours degree. In relation to the learning outcomes of clinical experience, the outcomes specified as students progress through the course also need to demonstrate progression through the three levels. At later stages of the programme, the HEI will expect students to demonstrate enhanced sophistication in clinical assessment in relation to the level of application of knowledge, use of evidence, decision-making and leadership skills in clinical practice.

The NMC (2010a) now specifies that, in the programmes being introduced from 2011, two progression points must be included dividing the three-year course into three stages, normally of one year each. Each stage of the programme must include at least 40% and not more than 60% practice learning with a period of at least four weeks clinical experience taking place towards the end of stages one and two, and 12 weeks towards the end of the three-year programme.

Students must achieve minimum requirements detailed by the NMC and be assessed in clinical practice (although some may be through simulation) by the end of stages one and two, and at the end of the programme for entry onto the Professional Register. These will be integrated with the HEI's requirements for academic progression.

It is sometimes argued that the modular structure predisposes to students having difficulty in integrating curriculum content from different modules. However, integration of the curriculum can be facilitated by:

- ensuring that students understand the themes of the curriculum framework and can see how these relate to the whole of the course;
- making clear links between concurrent modules;
- clarifying the relationship between current and previous and succeeding modules;
- ensuring that placement modules are preceded by appropriate theoretical content to enable students to learn from experience;
- link lecturers helping students on placement to relate previously gained knowledge to clinical practice;
- holding debriefing sessions following placement to relate clinical experience to previous learning and to introduce material to be considered next.

CHAPTER SUMMARY

Although the Bologna Process appears bureaucratic and perhaps of limited relevance to nursing educators it has played an important role in enabling national and international recognition of professional qualifications and in promoting recognition of nursing as a worldwide profession. This chapter has considered a number of structural issues arising from the Bologna Process, their implementation within the UK and application within nursing education. An explanation of the different levels of learning and credit weighting provides an understanding of the basic structure of programmes. In addition the requirements of the NMC and the centrality of clinical placement linked with academic content within nursing education programmes have been emphasised.

5 CURRICULUM APPROACHES

INTRODUCTION

In this chapter and the next the selection and organisation of curriculum content will be discussed. Much of the content will be determined by the outcomes to be achieved as specified by the Statutory Body. However, the HEI has the responsibility for determining the content required to meet the Statutory Body outcomes, and other content identified as desirable by the programme team, for grouping the material appropriately, and preparing a curriculum for validation and delivery. Some concepts will be included in all nursing programmes while others will be determined by the specific nature of the programme.

Based on the philosophical beliefs of the staff group about education and nursing, decisions need to be made about the overall approach to the curriculum, which will then determine the work to be undertaken in its development. A number of different approaches to curriculum design will be discussed in this chapter and we will also look at the way in which these relate to the hoped for outcomes of the programme and the abilities which students will develop during their period of study to support them through lifelong learning. Constructive alignment is critical to this process.

Within the approach taken, the framework developed earlier (see Chapter 2) becomes invaluable as the themes from that framework, which incorporate the domains identified by the NMC (2010a) (Table 5.1), provide a structure for identifying the content. The NMC domains could be used as the framework but within a university context, the analytical approach used by academics identifies the distinctiveness of the six themes, and the importance of the theme of research and evidence-informed

TABLE 5.1 *NMC Domains and Framework Themes*

NMC Domains	**Framework Themes**		
Professional values	Research and evidence-informed practice	Theoretical and professional issues	Health and its determinants
Communication and interpersonal skills		Communication, teaching and learning	
Nursing practice and decision-making		Reflective and proficient practice	
Leadership, management and team working		Leadership and management	

practice in the preparation of graduates is paramount. It is important to recognise that each of the themes relate to all the others and the student must be able to integrate the content from them all.

In most HEIs, programmes are prepared as a series of modules which, between them, will meet the course aims and objectives/outcomes. However, there are various ways in which module content can be arranged to achieve the goals of the programme. A number of decisions must be made in relation to the direction of the curriculum and a number of issues are discussed here which will influence content and delivery.

Future Planning

The curriculum planned must at least be up-to-date, but preferably should be innovative and forward looking: it is certain that the context and knowledge underpinning health care will change during a graduate's career in nursing. Thus selection of content needs to take account not just of the requirements for practice at registration, but should also provide the basis for the registrants' future development and potential changes in practice during their professional career. The following list shows some examples that can be identified now:

- Increasing numbers of qualified nurses are undertaking roles as independent or supplementary prescribers. Pre-registration education needs to provide a good understanding of pharmacology as the basis for this post-registration specialisation.
- Some knowledge of genetics will be necessary to understand the personalised drug regimes which are being developed and are likely to appear in clinical practice in the near future.
- The growing number of older people and those with chronic illness will shape nursing practice to increase the focus on community care within the professional lifetime of those now being prepared.

- Enhanced technological development in medical treatment will result in increasing demands for critical and high dependency care, to which nurses need to be able to respond.
- Growing incidence of mental health issues, including suicide, among young people will increase the need for nurses with skills in working with this client group.

It is essential that students thoroughly understand the material being taught so that in their future careers they can develop their knowledge from a firm base and apply it in novel situations. In addition, it is imperative that the skills for lifelong learning are achieved and that students develop the motivation to continue to learn.

Worldwide Nature of Nursing

Nursing is a worldwide profession and there is value in reflecting the vision of national and international bodies for nursing in the future. Students need to develop an awareness of cultural and global issues affecting the profession as well as to be able to apply this understanding in practice within multicultural communities. Staff involvement in relevant local, national and international working parties and committees can contribute to achieving global awareness and cultural sensitivity in the curriculum and preparing graduate nurses able to participate in the range of professional activities.

Academic Depth and Progression

This is an important issue to come to grips with throughout the whole curriculum. In the previous chapter the issue of the level of academic award to be achieved was discussed. However, it is also necessary to specify the academic level of each component of the programme and to develop each module with learning outcomes and content of the appropriate intellectual demand. Achievement in clinical practice must also reflect the academic level expected, demonstrated through evidence-based practice and level of decision-making. As students progress through the programme the academic demands increase until, by the end of the programme, students are performing in both theory and practice at the level of the academic award.

Creativity of Staff and Students

It is important to encourage creativity among the teaching staff so that, while the curriculum is covered, there is enough flexibility available to enable innovation in teaching. In addition, students are being prepared for working in a healthcare context in which patient needs are changing and approaches to care must adjust. Entrepreneurship is now recognised as an important area of competence needed in nursing and is firmly based on creativity and innovation. Approaches to selection of content and teaching methods that encourage creativity are to be welcomed and some of the curriculum approaches discussed below facilitate this.

Added Value

In addition to the outcomes specified by the Statutory Body, each course planning team must consider what 'added value' they can provide through the contributions of staff with specialist expertise. Some examples might be:

- a research group on person-centred care can contribute to development of the curriculum framework and prepare materials to facilitate learning about this approach to care;
- staff with expertise in learning disability nursing could develop the curriculum and learning materials to enable students to develop skills in working with this client group in general, mental health or children's nursing;
- a team with expertise in disaster relief may include an introduction to the relevant theory and apply management principles in a disaster field exercise with students;
- several staff with expertise in alternative therapies could offer an introduction to their inclusion in nursing and teaching basic massage skills.

COURSE AIMS AND OUTCOMES

The first step in writing the curriculum is to develop the overall aims and objectives or outcomes of the programme. These are stated in broad terms, providing an outline picture of what the course will examine, and must incorporate all the Statutory Body requirements. The detail of the programme is developed later within the different themes and modules influenced by the approach to the curriculum which is selected.

The aim (or aims) of a programme provides a broad statement of the overall goal of the course. It will usually indicate what completing students will be able to undertake on completion and what can be expected of them. An example of a statement of the aims of a pre-registration nursing honours degree programme is shown in Box. 5.1.

Box 5.1 Example of Aims for Pre-Registration Nursing Programme

The overall aim of this pre-registration programme is to prepare graduate nurses who:

- will provide high quality, person-centred, evidence-based care;
- are able to reflect systematically upon their practice;
- can contribute to the development of nursing knowledge and practice within their field of practice.

It is anticipated that many of the graduates of this programme will develop into leaders within the profession.

The programme outcomes specify the major components of what will be achieved by the end of the programme. How these are written may be determined by the institution but must be compatible with the level descriptors for the endpoint of the programme, as discussed in Chapter 3. One approach is to write an outcome (or outcomes) in relation to each theme within the curriculum framework. Some HEIs now require outcomes to be presented within groupings which relate to the qualities expected of graduates as specified by the institution in relation to: knowledge and understanding, intellectual qualities, professional/practical skills

TABLE 5.2 *Course Outcomes within the Theme of Leadership and Management Showing Graduate Qualities*

Knowledge and understanding	Demonstrate understanding of the principles of leadership and management and the ability to apply these competently, within the context of the multidisciplinary team, in managing the provision of high quality safe care for a group of patients.
	Understand the role of the entrepreneur and the potential for the application of entrepreneurial skills in health and social care.
Intellectual qualities	Enhance the professional development and safe practice of others through peer support, leadership, supervision, and teaching.
	Assess and analyse the needs of a patient/client group, and identify the skills and resources (including financial) required to meet those needs.
Professional/ practical skills	Contribute to the protection of individual patients/clients and the public through the exercise of sound clinical judgement across a range of contexts, and through risk assessment and quality assurance.
	Plan, implement and evaluate changes in clinical care or a new patient/client care initiative.
Transferable skills	Operate within different roles, including that of leader, within the uni-professional and multidisciplinary teams and critically analyse the dynamics of team life.
	Demonstrate a willingness to be creative and innovative in practice.

and transferable skills. Table 5.2 shows an example in relation to one theme of an appropriate outcome for each of the four sets of graduate qualities. However, other institutions are satisfied with course outcomes which integrate these different types of quality. Table 5.3 shows an example of course outcomes of this kind for a pre-registration nursing programme.

TABLE 5.3 *Example of Course Outcomes for Pre-Registration Nursing Programme*

Theme	Outcome
Reflective and proficient practice	Use critical analytical thinking, understanding of the sciences underpinning nursing, and decision-making skills in assessing, planning and evaluating care for individuals and groups of patients and demonstrate a high level of clinical skills in providing care within a specified field of practice. Use reflection in and about practice to continue to improve professional performance.
Theoretical and professional issues	Understand the regulation and development of the profession and professionals as practitioners, policy-makers, researchers, leaders, innovators. Discuss how models and theories of nursing in combination with personal insights and tacit knowledge inform their own practice. Participate in ethical decision-making. Work collaboratively in problem-solving and demonstrate the skills and motivation for lifelong learning and continuing professional development.
Health and its determinants	Identify factors which influence health status and uptake of health services and apply principles and skills of public health and health promotion to enhance the health of individuals, groups and communities, while demonstrating respect for the values and cultures of others.
Communication, teaching and learning	Use understanding of communication and teaching/learning theories in using oral, written and IT skills to develop therapeutic relationships, provide appropriate teaching with patient/clients and carers, and empower individuals, families and groups to participate in health-related decisions, and to work collaboratively with others.
Leadership and management	Demonstrate principles of leadership and management through peer support, leadership, supervision and teaching to enhance professional practice of others within the context of the multidisciplinary team, and through sound clinical judgement, risk assessment and quality assurance ensure provision of high quality safe care for a group of patients. Be creative in practice and use the knowledge and skills of entrepreneurship to identify need and introduce changes in clinical care or a new patient/client care initiative.
Research and evidence-informed practice	Use understanding of research methods to enhance professional practice by identifying and implementing appropriate evidence, and by asking research questions and proposing research methods to investigate clinical issues.

CURRICULUM APPROACHES

As the extent of knowledge continues to grow and healthcare provision becomes ever more complex, it is clear that it is not possible to teach within a three-(or even four-) year programme everything that nurses will need to know at qualification, let alone throughout their careers. One of the key elements of pre-registration education is to provide students with a firm foundation for their future career and this includes learning to learn, and enjoying that learning.

In developing a curriculum that will enable student learning, it is necessary to understand the principles underpinning the different approaches and advantages and disadvantages of each. When considering the curriculum, it is necessary not only to decide what students should know and the clinical skills they will be able to use, but also the transferable skills they will develop for current and future use.

Uys and Gwele (2005) identify three broad approaches to curriculum design and delivery: content-based, process-based and outcomes-based. Whichever approach or combination of approaches is used, the outcomes required by the Statutory Body incorporated within the course aims and outcomes must be achieved. In addition, the changing healthcare environment results in the necessity to consider a community-focused programme.

CONTENT-BASED APPROACH

This is still the commonest and most traditional curriculum approach used in nursing education in which the teaching staff decide upon and deliver the content. The major teaching method is lectures with some discussion or seminar sessions, with nursing skills teaching and practice learning in the clinical environment. Students are expected to assimilate the knowledge presented in the formal teaching sessions. The assumption is that they will be able to repeat it in examinations and to apply this knowledge in practice even though the lectures may not show any direct relevance to practice.

The major advantages of this approach are that a lot of material can be covered in a relatively short time, it is easy to organise and it is sparing of staff time. The focus on research within HEIs, particularly in the context of the Research Excellence Framework (REF) in the UK, makes this a particularly attractive approach to those institutions which aim for excellence in research. However, several disadvantages can be identified:

- Over-teaching may occur, with students being presented with more material than they can reasonably be expected to remember and understand.
- Students may find it difficult to apply in the practice context the material they have been taught.

- The independent learning skills needed for lifelong development may not be acquired.
- Some of the teaching may be seen as irrelevant.

PROCESS-BASED CURRICULA

These approaches are based on theories of adult education (andragogy) as discussed by Knowles et al. who describe this as '*a set of core adult learning principles that apply to all adult learning situations*' (2011: 2) which are student-centred in nature. In the development of the andragogical model they draw on a number of different educationalists and identify several key assumptions. In most countries nursing students are adults and, thus, these are important to enhance student learning:

- *The need to know:* Adults need to know why they need to learn something before they will undertake to do so. Thus, a key role of the teacher/facilitator is that of helping students to recognise why they need to learn.
- *The learners' self-concept:* Adults are responsible for their own lives and resent being treated as incapable. Thus, the formal educational setting of a lecture theatre in which they are taught may invoke the dependency experienced in their previous schooling. It is important to develop learning opportunities in which the learners are self-directing.
- *The role of the learners' experience:* A group of adult learners will have a wide range of different experiences which can be drawn upon for the learning of the whole group. However, they may have acquired habits and attitudes which need to be examined and, perhaps, challenged.
- *Readiness to learn:* Adults are ready to learn what they need to know to be able to cope with their situation. In the context of nursing education, if the next placement is to be in intensive care they will be ready to learn about the care of patients on assisted ventilation and about the importance of working through families to minimise stress in patients.
- *Orientation to learning:* Adults tend to be orientated to learning material that will help them to carry out real-life tasks or deal with problems that they encounter. In nursing education the programmes that will have the best results are those that are focused on examples of real-life clinical situations, including the use of simulations and case studies.
- *Motivation:* External rewards may be important but, for adults, internal factors associated with job satisfaction, self-esteem or quality of life are likely to be of greater value.

In this section, Problem-Based Learning (PBL) is discussed in some detail, with Enquiry-Based Learning (EBL), Case-Based Learning (CBL) and

Task-Based Learning (TBL) considered more briefly. These last three methods have some similarities with PBL but are used rather differently. The key element in PBL is that students are given the problem or situation to be explored at the beginning of the process. In these other approaches, there is some variability in the process.

Problem-Based Learning

PBL was introduced in medical education at McMaster University in Canada in the 1960s. Since then it has been used as the key curriculum approach in many healthcare and other professional programmes. It has been described by Barrows as a closed loop process of

> encountering the problem first, problem-solving with clinical reasoning skill and identifying learning needs, self-study, applying newly gained knowledge to the problem and summarizing what has been learned (cited by Glen and Wilkie, 2000: 11).

PBL is founded on adult learning principles in which self-directed learning is central – students learning what they are interested in learning and what they can see as relevant. Self-directed learning has been defined as:

> A process in which individuals take the initiative, with or without the help of others, in diagnosing their learning needs, formulating learning goals, identifying human and material resources for learning, choosing and implementing appropriate learning strategies, and evaluating learning outcomes. (Knowles, 1975, cited by Kocaman et al., 2009: 286)

This is clearly congruent with the principles of PBL.

In this approach to curriculum design and delivery the major factor is that the programme is student- rather than teacher-focused and learning is self-directed. The key elements are shown in Box 5.2.

A series of problems are prepared that will present students with scenarios that should lead to identification, understanding of the concepts, and development of the knowledge and skills that will achieve the specified outcomes for the relevant component of the programme and contribute to achieving the goals of the whole programme.

Box 5.2 Key Elements of Problem-Based Learning (Boud and Feletti, 1997)

- Scenarios are planned to focus students' discussion on an important problem, question or issue;
- Scenarios are presented as a simulation of professional practice or a 'real life' situation;
- Students work cooperatively in the PBL group, sharing exploration of issues in and between group meetings, and have access to a tutor who can facilitate group learning;
- Limited resources require students to decide on effective use of available resources;
- Students learn from defining and attempting to resolve the given problem, identifying their own learning needs and how to achieve them;
- This new knowledge is applied to the original problem and its wider application considered;
- Evaluation of their learning processes can stimulate critical thinking.

Benefits of PBL

One of the major benefits of this approach to the curriculum is considered to be the active engagement and self-direction of students in their own learning. This enables them to develop the skills necessary for lifelong learning which will carry them through different roles and areas of practice throughout their careers (Wilkie and Burns, 2003). In support of this hypothesis, Shin et al. (1993, cited in Glen and Wilkie, 2000) found that PBL-educated doctors held up-to-date knowledge in the years after graduation, compared with a negative correlation between knowledge and time since graduation in non-PBL educated doctors.

Six months following qualification, nursing students from both PBL and non-PBL programmes considered that they had achieved the 'entry-to-practice competencies' but graduates from PBL programmes identified critical thinking, self-directed learning and teamwork learned through PBL as helping them to achieve this level of practice (Applin et al., 2011). In addition, an ethnographic study with graduates from a UK PBL programme found that they considered that they had a responsibility, even a duty, to challenge some of the abiding assumptions and practices in nursing (Biley and Smith, 1998).

In life, let alone in nursing, some degree of conflict is common and can lead to creativity and be generally beneficial but can also lead to stress, be dysfunctional and be generally unhelpful. Group working will result in some disagreement and conflict and the group has to develop the skills to evolve into an effective team. Those educated through PBL were found to have more effective conflict resolution skills than other nursing students (Seren and Ustun, 2008).

Using a quantitative approach Ozturk et al. (2008) demonstrated enhanced critical thinking in PBL students using the California critical thinking disposition inventory, with the subdimensions 'open-mindedness' and 'truth-seeking' also being higher than their conventionally educated peers. However, a systematic review (Yuan et al., 2008) does not confirm enhanced critical thinking resulting from a PBL programme.

Jones and Johnston (2006) examined the influence of a PBL curriculum on student wellbeing and performance. Their study did not demonstrate any enhancement in academic performance but did show improved student wellbeing and adaptation to higher education. Students have also described PBL as '*fun, exciting, interesting, and motivating*' (Cooke and Moyle, 2002). However, it has not been shown to have any influence on anxiety related to clinical practice (Melo et al., 2010).

Difficulties with PBL

There are a number of potential difficulties with using PBL as the sole method of learning in a professional programme. Glen (in Boud and Feletti, 1997) cited a number of studies which identified less than adequate knowledge in students on PBL courses. There are likely to be difficulties in undertaking PBL when students have no initial knowledge on which to build, such as at the beginning of a programme or when they do not have the necessary skills and motivation. Many entrants to nursing come to university straight from school, where the encouragement of self-directed learning is uncommon and students have not developed the necessary competencies to participate effectively in PBL. Some of these students identify a desire for teacher-centred, rather than student-centred, learning particularly at the beginning of their programme (Levett-Jones, 2005). Teaching students the skills for self-directed learning in PBL may be as important as ensuring that they learn the necessary content. However, Kocaman et al. (2009), in a longitudinal study, found that students developed the necessary competencies over the four years of the programme with the highest scores in the Self-Directed Learning Readiness Scale at the end of the programme.

Another issue to be considered is the workload associated with working with small groups or teams of students, with 7 to 12 students per PBL team performing '*optimally in the group tasks of problem-solving, cohesion and individual productivity*' (Curzon, 1985, cited by Glen and Wilkie, 2000: 23).

However, when necessary, one staff member can work with more than one group (Barrett and Moore, 2011). Other resources needed are enough small rooms to accommodate the PBL teams, access to laboratories when clinical skills development is part of their identified learning, internet and library facilities, and experts who can be consulted as appropriate.

The remaining major potential difficulty is related to the readiness of the staff to change their role from their usual mode of functioning to that of facilitator of learning. Most lecturers in nursing are experts in their subject area and good at teaching about it to pre- and post-registration students of nursing. PBL requires them to develop skills in facilitating learning in all areas being covered and support from the staff development department will be necessary. Some will be enthusiastic about their new roles and skills development; others may be reluctant to participate. Facilitators who fall back into the traditional mode of teaching with the teacher in control will cause difficulties for students in getting to grips with their new roles (Lekalakala-Mokgele, 2010).

How PBL can be Implemented

PBL can be used in different ways within the curriculum. Savin-Baden (2003, cited in Barrett and Moore, 2011) has described seven approaches to using PBL:

1 a single module in the final year of the programme;
2 PBL on a shoestring, when some lecturers use it in a few modules at minimal cost;
3 the funnel approach, when it is used for the full final year;
4 the foundation approach, when students are introduced to concepts and principles in year one, followed by limited exposure to PBL followed by full PBL, in the final year;
5 the two-strand approach, in which it is combined with a variety of learning methods;
6 patchwork PBL, when PBL is used in all modules but without a fully integrated framework;
7 in an integrated programme the whole programme uses a PBL framework which is applied through all modules.

Different approaches can be used as an introduction of PBL into a programme, allowing evaluation by staff and students, before extending its use to the final stage where it is fully integrated into the whole programme.

In planning a programme and its delivery all these dimensions need to be considered. The decision whether to develop a fully PBL curriculum, a hybrid form or not to use it at all will be determined by:

- the philosophy of education espoused by the staff of the school. PBL is based on the principles of adult learning in which the real-life relevance of the problems presented is central in promoting willingness to learn;
- an understanding of the nature of PBL, including the problems, PBL tutorials, and PBL assessment (discussed in later chapters);
- the enthusiasm of individual staff members;
- resources available.

Figure 5.1 illustrates the total curriculum approach to PBL and identifies the key stages in developing and delivering the curriculum. While presented in stages it is important to consider the totality of the programme at all the different stages.

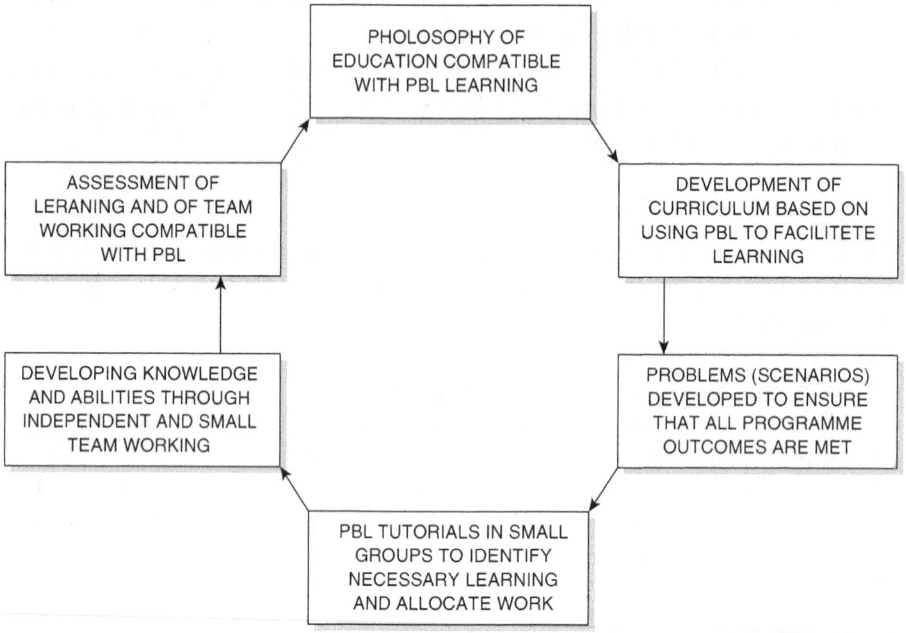

FIGURE 5.1 *The Dimensions of PBL*

Hybrid approaches are planned in different ways to meet the resources, expertise and wishes of the nursing staff group and some examples are shown in Box 5.3

Staff groups considering using PBL in a new curriculum are recommended to consult some of the books written about PBL such as: Barrett and Moore (2011), Boud and Feletti (eds) (1997), Glen and Wilkie (2000), Price (2003), Wilkie and Burns (2003).

Box 5.3 Examples of Hybrid Approaches in PBL in Nursing

- PBL can be used as a module alongside others in the semester or year to encourage integration of materials taught using traditional methods in previous and concurrent modules.
- Using a PBL module or modules in the final year can encourage integration of all material studied in the programme.
- PBL can be used as the mode of learning in a strand through the programme, e. g. ethics, biological sciences.
- PBL can be supported by lectures focused on the particular problem, elearning materials, clinical skills sessions etc.
- PBL can be used during practice learning periods to help students integrate their university-based teaching into clinical practice

Enquiry-Based Learning (EBL)

This term is used in different ways. For example it can be used to cover PBL as discussed above, plus field work, case studies, workshops, projects (individual and group) and research activity (Kahn and O'Rourke, 2005, cited by Barrett and Moore, 2011). The term is sometimes used synonymously with PBL but Price (2003) distinguishes between PBL and EBL while recognising the similarities in approach. PBL mainly uses clinical problems about which facts can be identified and solutions found. EBL, on the other hand, aims to enhance understanding of the nature of professional practice and to recognise the principles which may be applied in different situations. The topics and the conclusions drawn are much broader and less specific than in PBL as indicated in a number of questions identified by Price (2003) which might be investigated through EBL (see Box 5.4).

Box 5.4 Examples of Questions for EBL (Price, 2003)

- Why do we practise in this way?
- Under what conditions or circumstances, do our approaches change?
- Are there situations when we should rethink our approaches?
- Where we operate differently as practitioners, should we consider consolidating nursing approaches? If so, to what purpose?
- How do others see our nursing approaches - are there advantages/disadvantages, challenges or opportunities here?

Case-Based Learning (CBL) (Uys and Gwele, 2005)

Cases can be used in different ways to enhance teaching and learning:

- Cases can be presented either before or after a lecture to illustrate the content of a teaching session.
- Students can be presented with a case to promote learning through reflection.
- In clinical contexts, students are often asked to prepare a case study for discussion with their mentor or link lecturer.
- An integrated case-based curriculum can be presented.

An integrated CBL curriculum has some similarities with a fully PBL curriculum with a series of cases prepared to ensure that all the necessary content is integrated into them. Often student learning is guided through requiring them to answer a number of questions related to the case presented. Students use analytical and decision-making skills while actively participating in considering realistic situations. Case studies can also be used to enable students to develop skills in applying theoretical models of nursing in realistic situations (DeSanto-Madeya, 2007), one of the areas which students often find difficult. However, the major difference from PBL is that in CBL students are applying theoretical knowledge already learnt. CBL can be differentiated from PBL by the way in which the cases are presented and used in teaching (see Table 5.4).

TABLE 5.4 *Comparison Between a Problem-Based and a Case-Based Curriculum (Uys and Gwele, 2005)*

	Problem-based curriculum	**Case-based curriculum**
Focus	The focus is strongly on the process of learning. PBL through module is planned to cover required content	Often part of a module and content, process and outcomes are all important
Information given	Students given limited information initially. Additional information is released as students explore problem	Before the group session complete information about the case is provided
Confronting the case	In group working, students analyse the scenario together and decide who will study and collect data on individual aspects	Students individually study the information provided then discuss it in class in a large group or in sub-groups
Group size	Usually 8-12 students to one facilitator (who may be facilitating more than one group)	May be used with large classes split into smaller groups for initial discussion in which groups then feed back conclusions to whole group

This is a method with benefits for both staff and students. In general students respond well to the use of cases which enables them to see the direct applicability of their new knowledge and increases motivation to learn. In relation to staff, this approach provides more flexibility than PBL and can be used in a range of different situations.

Task-Based Learning (TBL)

TBL has been used in medical education (Glen and Wilkie, 2000) and could be equally applicable in nursing education. Instead of a case or a problem, a clinical task is the focus for student activity. As in PBL, students work in small groups to identify the relevant issues, carry out the individual tasks and share their new learning. Learning how to do the 'task' is carried out in practice learning in role play and in the clinical setting. The TBL activity requires the students to learn about the why and when they would carry out this task, what they might learn about their patient in the process, and how this may be used in providing high quality nursing care.

OUTCOMES-BASED CURRICULA

Outcomes-Based Education

Using outcomes based education (OBE) is discussed by Mtshali (in Uys and Gwele, 2005) and three approaches in their development are described. She clarifies that the outcomes specify what the student is expected to be able to do on completing the programme. As mentioned earlier, some universities expect course outcomes to be written in terms of: knowledge and understanding, intellectual qualities, professional/practical skills/transferable skills but in some universities module objectives are also expected to be written under the same headings (University of Ulster, 2010a).

Traditional OBE

This is similar to content-based curricula described earlier. The focus is still on subject-focused knowledge but the clear statement of outcomes helps students to focus their learning. The major disadvantages are that students learn content, but linking content from different subjects is not facilitated.

Transitional OBE

These programmes still focus on the academic subjects, but there is greater emphasis on integrating material from different areas of study and students are encouraged to develop the necessary skills for professional practice. It contains elements of both traditional and transformational OBE.

Transformational OBE

These programmes are based on critical outcomes through achievement of which graduates will be able to perform their roles in professional practice and will continue to learn through their careers. The curriculum is modified in response to external changes and lecturers function as facilitators. Characteristics of transformational OBE are shown in Box 5.5, but the key characteristic is that the learner knows from the beginning exactly what they have to learn, and this is followed through in the curriculum structure.

Box 5.5 Transformational Outcomes-Based Education (adapted from Uys and Gwele, 2005: 196–7)

- The expectations for current practice within the workplace and for continuing professional development are factors in determining curriculum content
- From the beginning of the programme students are given clear instructions about the required learning
- The academic staff member's role is primarily that of a facilitator to enable active, enthusiastic students to achieve the specified outcomes
- Students are expected to achieve the ability to use and apply the knowledge, skills and attitudes they have acquired
- Continuous assessment using authentic learning experiences (discussed in Chapter 12) helps students to remain motivated to learn through experience
- A range of different learning and assessment strategies meets all students' needs
- The aim is for students to acquire 'applied competence'; that is the ability to demonstrate understanding and adaptability in undertaking tasks in differing situations. This includes:
  - Practical competence: i.e. ability to do the task
  - Foundational competence: i.e. understanding of the underpinning knowledge and the rationale for the particular behaviour
  - Reflexive competence: i.e. ability to use reflection to evaluate quality and appropriateness of the action (Chapter 8), and identify learning needed

Behavioural Objectives Models

This approach developed by Tyler (1949, cited by Quinn and Hughes, 2007) is used widely. It is often used in conjunction with the content-based approach discussed earlier with the outcomes expected of each student expressed in behavioural terms. Behaviour in this context includes thinking and feeling as well as doing, although Tyler's focus on behaviour of students has tended to result in limiting behavioural objectives to *'observable, measurable changes in behaviour, leaving no room for such things as "understanding" or "appreciation"'* (Quinn and Hughes, 2007: 111).

Behavioural objectives specify what the student is expected to be able to do as a result of their learning and thus must contain a word which identifies the measurable or observable action. It is suggested that a behavioural objective should have three parts:

- a verb indicating what the student will be able to do (e.g. write, demonstrate, describe);
- specification of the conditions under which the action will be performed;
- the standard of performance.

The Behavioural Objectives Model often uses the levels of behaviour described in Bloom's taxonomy. Within this taxonomy three types of learning are identified: cognitive, affective and psychomotor. The cognitive domain has six main classes, the affective and psychomotor five classes. The cognitive (Bloom, 1956) and affective (Krathwohl et al., 1964) domains have been developed in detail with each class subdivided into a number of subclasses. The most utilised of these taxonomies is the cognitive domain which has been updated by Anderson and Krathwohl (2001) with nouns converted to verbs, and modification of the levels. As the original cognitive classification is still in use, both versions are included in Figure 5.2.

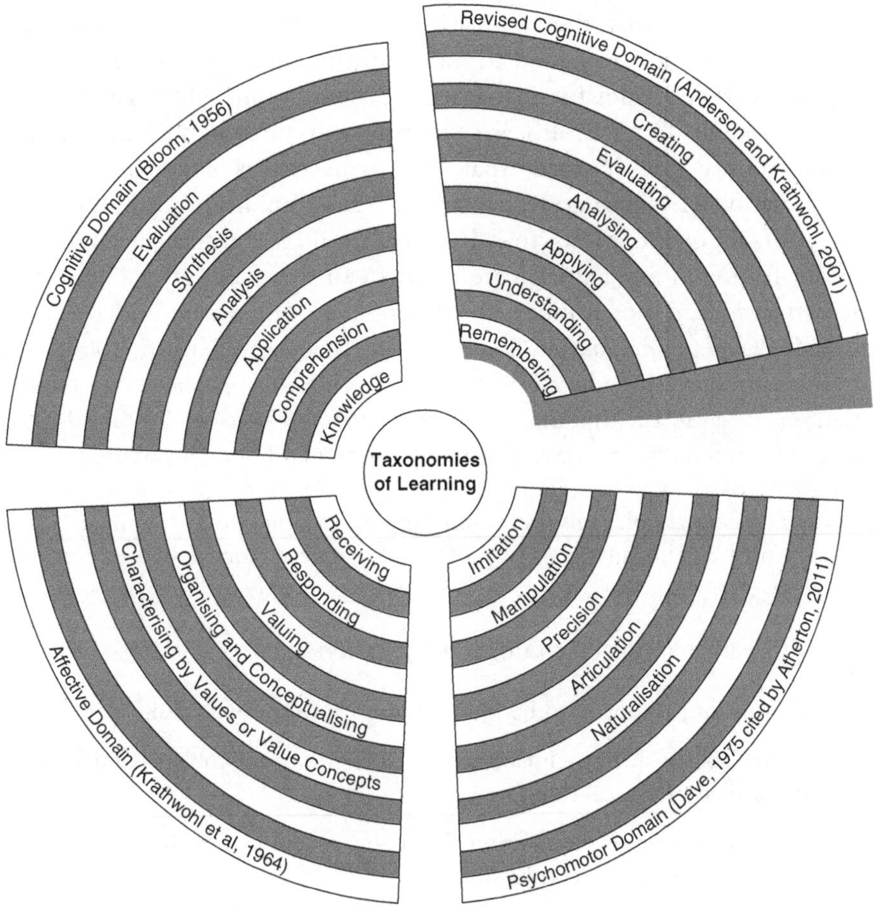

FIGURE 5.2 *Taxonomies of Learning (based on and cited by Atherton, 2011)*

Many institutions require behavioural objectives to be prepared for each module using the graduate qualities of knowledge and understanding, intellectual qualities, professional/practical skills and transferable skills (e.g. University of Ulster, 2010a). These objectives must then be assessed.

Caring Curriculum (Bevis and Watson, 2000)

Bevis and Watson (2000) have argued that the behavioural approach to nursing curricula that Tyler promoted has served nursing well in endeavouring to achieve high quality education. However, they also suggest that while it can prepare competent and even skilled clinical nurses, it falls short in developing the *'educated, caring scholar-clinicians capable of meeting the complex needs of today's society'* (2000: 29).

They propose that the standard form of education is '*maintenance-adaptation'* in nature, designed to maintain the status quo through learning methods and rules for managing usual situations. However, it is no longer suitable for a healthcare environment in which change is the only certainty. They propose that what is needed is '*anticipatory-innovative'* learning in which creativity and imagination are promoted to prepare nurses for situations that may occur in the future, even in the distant future, in a changing care context. In this form of teaching participation is key (not unlike in Process-Based Curricula) and needs to include *'cooperation, dialogue, and empathy'* (Bevis and Watson, 2000: 41).

This approach to education has been promoted in the USA by the National League of Nursing (cited by Bevis and Watson, 2000: 39) in a series of conferences reviewing nursing curricula. They emphasised

> 'nursing's essential role, mission, commitment and function of human caring and a return to the human aspect of nursing and a moral-based educational perspective' .

This alternative approach to nursing education aims to:

- enable nursing graduates to be more responsive to societal needs;
- be better able to bring scholarly approaches to client problems and issues – more capable of critical thinking;
- be more successful in humanising the highly technological milieus of health care – more caring and compassionate;
- be more insightful about ethical and moral issues and better able to advocate ethical positions on behalf of clients. (Bevis and Watson, 2000: 348)

Constructive Alignment

In essence this sounds similar to the previous outcomes-based approaches used but is presented by Biggs and Tang (2007) as a '*marriage between a constructivist understanding of the nature of learning and an aligned design for teaching that is designed to lock students into deep learning*' (2007: 54). Deep learning occurs when students build on previous learning and combine it with new learning to achieve understanding of the concepts and principles and their interrelationship within the subject. They are constructing their own cognitive map of the subject area through their own activities for learning. Figure 5.3 indicates how Intended Learning Outcomes (ILOs) are prepared which shape the Teaching/Learning Activities (TLAs) and Assessment Tasks (ATs). This approach can be combined with some of the earlier approaches through the development of the ILOs to be achieved.

Biggs and Tang identify the four stages in designing a course using constructive alignment:

- Describe the learning outcomes in the form of a verb (learning activity), its object (the content) and specify the context and a standard the students are to attain;
- Create a learning environment using teaching/learning activities that address that verb and therefore are likely to bring about the intended outcome;
- Use assessment tasks that also contain that verb, thus enabling you to judge with the help of rubrics if and how well students' performances meet the criteria;
- Transform these judgements into standard grading criteria (Biggs and Tang, 2007: 54–55).

Intended Learning Outcomes (ILOs)

ILOs need to be expressed in a way which identifies the level of work required as described in Box 4.2 in relation to the generic credit level descriptors (QAA, 2008b). Several taxonomies are available which can be used to select appropriate descriptions for the different levels of academic activity.

The SOLO (**S**tructure of the **O**bserved **L**earning **O**utcome) Taxonomy may be useful (Biggs and Collis, cited in Biggs and Tang, 2007). This

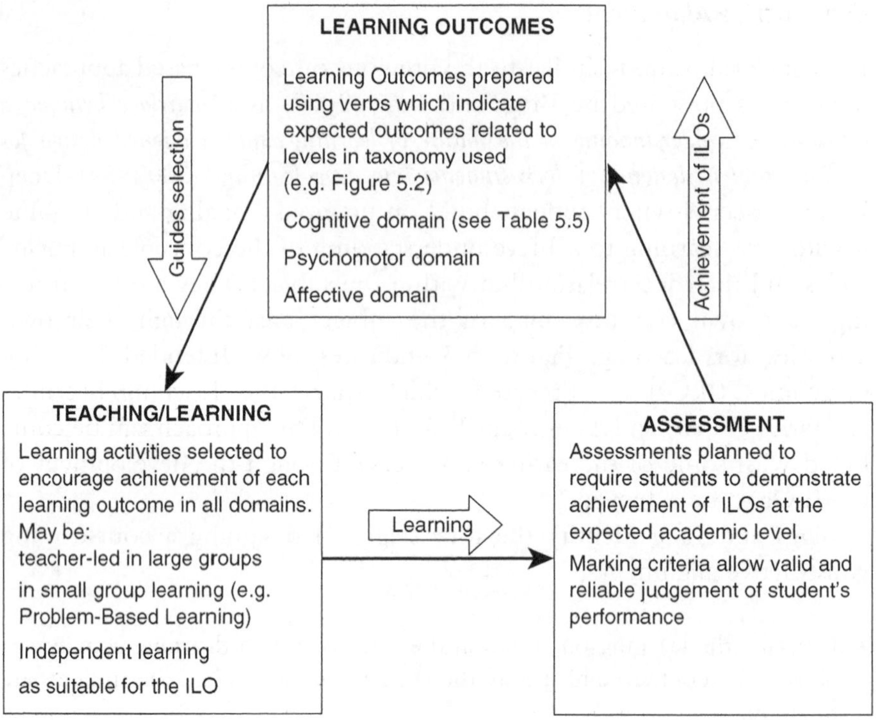

FIGURE 5.3 *Constructive Alignment: Learning Outcomes, Teaching and Assessment*
Source: Biggs and Tang, (2007). *Teaching for Quality Learning at University*.

identifies a hierarchy of approaches to learning and which move through stages of:

- quantitative learning where the amount of knowledge acquired increases through to
- qualitative changes where knowledge acquired is restructured as the different items of learning are integrated and moves to another dimension with creative thinking at the highest level.

Figure 5.4 shows this hierarchy of learning.

One of the commonest taxonomies used is Bloom's Taxonomy, as shown in Figure 5.2, for which appropriate words can be selected which relate to the different levels of activity for the three domains: cognitive (or revised cognitive), psychomotor and affective. Table 5.5 identifies numerous verbs which are applicable to levels in relation to the cognitive domain in Bloom's revised Taxonomy. Selecting the topics to be included is considered in the following chapter. Succeeding chapters examine teaching and learning (chapters 7–11) and assessment (Chapters 12 and 13) in both the academic setting and in clinical practice.

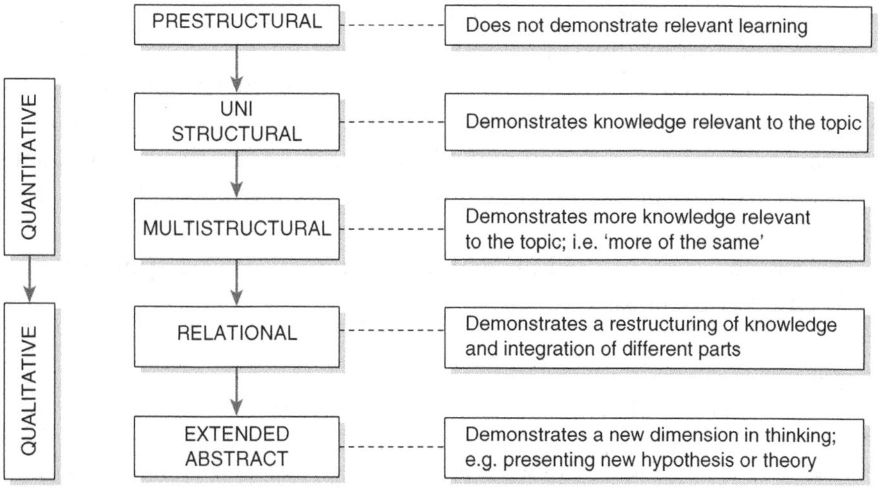

FIGURE 5.4 *The Solo Taxonomy – A Hierarchy of Learning*

Source: Biggs and Tang (2007) *Teaching for Quality Learning at University*. © Reproduced with the kind Permission of Open University Press. All rights reserved.

TABLE 5.5 *Selected ILO Verbs Applicable to Bloom's Taxonomy: Revised Cognitive Domain*

Remembering	Define, describe, recognise and identify, draw and label, list and order, match, name, quote, recall, recite, tell, narrate, write, imitate
Understanding	Classify, compare and contrast, draw conclusions, demonstrate, discuss, explain, identify, illustrate by example, interpret, paraphrase, predict, report, select and sequence, outline, summarise (précis)
Applying	Apply, change, select and use, compute, dramatise, implement, interview, prepare, produce, role play, show, transfer, integrate, predict, make a plan, debate, construct
Analysing	Analyse, characterise, classify, compare, contrast, debate, deconstruct, deduce, differentiate, discriminate, distinguish, examine, organise, outline, relate, research, separate, structure, conclude, review, argue, transfer, differentiate, review and rewrite, translate, paraphrase, solve a problem
Evaluating	Appraise, argue, assess, choose, conclude, critique, decide, evaluate, judge, justify, predict, prioritise, prove, rank, rate, select, monitor, make a case, reflect
Creating	Construct, design, develop, generate, hypothesise, invent, plan, produce, compose, create, make, perform, theorise, generalise, originate, prove from first principle, make an original case

Succeeding chapters examine teaching and learning (Chapters 7–11) and assessment (Chapters 12 and 13) in both the academic setting and in clinical practice.

COMMUNITY-FOCUSED CURRICULUM

With the increased prevalence of chronic illness and demographic changes resulting in an increase in the number of elderly people in the population, community-based care is growing in importance. This is an area in which there is considerable variation across countries in the quality of services available in terms of provision of nursing care and in relation to promotion of public health. In general, pre-registration nursing programmes prepare graduates to work within the hospital context but the value of community- focused programmes is now being considered in the UK and elsewhere.

The issues to be focused on within a community-focused programme will vary according to:

- the health status of the population;
- the current provision and structure of community nursing and public health;
- the resources available;
- the field of nursing (i.e., adult, child, mental health or learning disability in the UK);
- the availability of post-registration specialist education for community nursing.

Mtshali (in Uys and Gwele, 2005) discusses the development of a community-based nursing education programme. In countries where major health problems exist, these can be minimised by public health measures; a major focus for students will be working with the local community leaders and the population to promote healthy living, for example, the use of insecticide-impregnated mosquito nets, ensuring clean water and safe sewage disposal, maternal and child health. While nursing the sick will be a part of the programme, public health will be a major focus.

In countries such as the UK with relatively well-developed community nursing and public health services, the focus will be on health promotion to minimise chronic disease and on the promotion of self-management through empowerment of individuals, their families and communities. In addition, students will learn to contribute to the acute care provided in the community. In any nurse education programme students will also be prepared to work within institutional settings.

In planning a community-focused programme, students would gain practice learning experience in a variety of community settings through the period of the programme. Table 5.6 shows some suggested practice learning experiences for a student of adult nursing undertaking a community-focused programme.

As more acute care moves into the community, it is essential that students have opportunities to become competent in clinical skills. Within a district nursing placement, exposure to any one skill is likely to be limited, thus it is essential to build into the programme specific opportunities to

TABLE 5.6 *Possible Practice Learning Experiences in a Pre-Registration Community Nursing Programme*

	Community experience	Institutional experience
Year 1	Home visits to well elderly people Family visits with children Day centres for people with learning disabilities	Care of elderly people Maternal and child health
Year 2	General practice setting including primary care team Health promotion settings and health visiting Mental health team District nursing experience	General adult nursing experience Attachment to specialist nurse in chronic illness (e.g. diabetic nurse, stroke nurse, respiratory nurse)
Year 3	Acute care team Management of community nursing	Minor injuries units Day procedure units

develop psychomotor skills. For example, specific outcomes can be written for time with a practice nurse during which students will become competent in venepuncture.

THEORY AND PRACTICE LEARNING

The curriculum approach selected will have a major influence on the organisation of the knowledge component of the course and the development of intellectual and transferable skills. Linked to this, the arrangement of

TABLE 5.7 *Sequencing of Learning*

Sequence	Example
Health to illness	Examining health and factors enhancing health before moving on to consider illness
Simple to complex	At the beginning of the programme focusing on care of one patient or client, moving through managing care for a few patients and then takings responsibility for leading a team providing the care for a group of patients
Chronological	Focusing initially on child care and moving on to adult care and care of older people
Use of taxonomies	Using Bloom's taxonomies (cognitive, affective, psychomotor) to structure achievement through levels
Whole to parts	Gaining overall picture of community resources, then experience in different aspects of community care and learning about influences on health and policy determining healthcare services
Parts to whole	In relation to understanding of the human body, starting with the cell, moving on to organs, systems and total organism

practice learning opportunities must be considered and organised to integrate with the academic aspects of the programme. Table 5.7 shows a number of possible sequencing frameworks.

Some of these may be used for the programme as a whole while others are more appropriate for individual modules within the programme. The selection of the order of concepts to be considered needs to take into account the focus of the programme, the clinical experience available for practice learning, and attractiveness to students. A sequence of health to illness for the programme may be intellectually attractive to staff but many students of nursing enter the course because they wish to care for sick people. They find it easier to appreciate the importance of understanding health and developing competence in health promotion when they have cared for sick people and recognise the importance of preventing illness. A combination of types of sequencing may be used for different aspects of the programme.

Pre-registration nursing programmes have to take into account clinical experience and different HEIs will manage this in varying ways. The geographical location of the HEI and the availability of clinical facilities will influence how theory and practice are managed within the programme. If students will have to travel considerable distances to their clinical placement, then it is not feasible to include both HEI-based and practice learning within the same week. In this situation, it is likely that some modules will focus on theoretical learning with others entirely focused on practice learning; students will spend blocks of time based in clinical environments. In other situations, it may be possible to combine theory and practice learning within the same modules.

CHAPTER SUMMARY

This chapter has considered a number of approaches to planning the curriculum which have different philosophical underpinnings and varying implications for the teaching/learning and assessment methods used. The decision about which approach to use for a new programme is important and careful consideration is needed. If a single approach is to be used throughout the whole programme it must be accepted by the whole course team. However, in many situations such agreement may not be reached and in many programmes a combination of approaches may be used. In this situation it is essential that:

- there is clarity about what approach is being used within each module;
- the selection of approach is appropriate for each of the different areas of study;

- the use of different approaches is planned through the curriculum to develop the knowledge and skills expected in graduates;
- the outcomes achieved for the course are aligned with those required by the Statutory Body, the graduate qualities and the module outcomes;
- teaching and learning methods and assessment activities fit the outcomes to be achieved thereby adhering to the principles of constructive alignment.

6 CURRICULUM CONTENT

INTRODUCTION

In this chapter the selection and organisation of curriculum content will be discussed. While much of the content is specified by the Statutory Body and influenced by the approach to the curriculum discussed in the previous chapter, it still has to be organised to make a coherent, developmental and interesting programme. At this point the framework developed earlier becomes invaluable as the themes from that framework can be used as the major organising structure for the curriculum content within the curriculum approach. (The relationship between the six themes of that framework and the four domains of the NMC (2010a) are shown in Table 5.1 in the previous chapter.) The content then has to be aggregated into modules of study and, with practice learning opportunities, organised into a programme incorporating the necessary knowledge, skills and values which equate with the knowing, acting and being discussed in Chapter 2 (Barnett and Coate, 2005). It will fit within the period of time specified by the Statutory Body for the curriculum, or longer if the HEI chooses.

In this chapter some of the issues determining the content, its organisation and its presentation will be considered. While much of the content is fairly standard, there are some topics which merit discussion. One of the key issues that all lecturers must deal with is ensuring that the content included is based on appropriate evidence.

STATUTORY REQUIREMENTS

The pre-registration nursing programme must at least cover the topics specified by the Statutory Body and must meet the outcomes specified.

How these requirements are met is decided by the HEI. Table 6.1 shows the content to be covered by the end of the programme which underpins practice, and the content in relation to meeting the needs of patients as specified within the UK standards (NMC, 2010a).

TABLE 6.1 *Expected Requirements for Pre-Registration Nursing Education in the UK (linked to themes in Figure 2.5). Most of this content is taken from Standards for Pre-Registration Nursing Education,* NMC, 2010a)

Content to underpin practice (NMC, 2010a: 73–4)	Content in relation to essential and immediate needs of all people and complex needs of people in their chosen field (NMC, 2010a: 74–5)	Themes of study
life sciences (including anatomy and physiology) pharmacology and medicines management causes of common health conditions and the interaction between physical and mental health and illness best practice essential first aid and incident management	identity, appearance and self-worth autonomy, independence and self-care maintaining a safe environment eating, drinking, nutrition and hydration comfort and sleep moving and positioning continence promotion and bowel and bladder care skin health and wound management infection prevention and control clinical observation, assessment, critical thinking and decision-making symptom management, such as anxiety, anger, thirst, pain and breathlessness	Reflective and Proficient Practice
theories of nursing and theories of nursing practice professional codes, ethics, law and humanities	equality, diversity, inclusiveness and rights	Theoretical and Professional Issues
communication and healthcare informatics	communication, compassion and dignity emotional support	Communication Teaching and Learning
principles of national and international health policy, including public health social, health and behavioural sciences	public health and promoting health and well-being	Health and its Determinants
principles of supervision, leadership and management principles of organisational structures, systems and processes	risk management medicines management supervising, leading, managing and promoting best practice	Leadership and Management
research methods and use of evidence healthcare technology	information management	Research and Evidence-Based Practice

In addition, the NMC specifies the outcomes to be achieved at the end of each stage in relation to their four domains and in relation to the essential skills clusters (see Figure 2.4). The NMC (2010a) has specified detailed criteria (98–101) which must be achieved by the first progression point (usually at the end of year 1). These criteria are related to the public's expectations around competence in fundamental skills, communication with vulnerable people, and ensuring dignity. These cover:

- safety, safeguarding and protection of people of all ages, their carers and their families
- professional values, expected attitudes and the behaviours that must be shown towards people, their carers, their families, and others. (NMC, 2010a: 97)

By the second progression point (usually at the end of year 2) students must be able to show that they are able to work with less direct supervision as they progress towards being *'confident and fit for practice'* by the point at which they enter the register. The minimum criteria specified for continuation into the third stage of the programme are much broader than at the earlier progression point and do not indicate necessary content, rather they emphasise the student's development in confidence and competence. These criteria are:

- works more independently, with less direct supervision, in a safe and increasingly confident manner;
- demonstrates potential to work autonomously, making the most of opportunities to extend knowledge, skills and practice (NMC, 2010a: 102).

THEMATIC CONTENT

The six themes introduced in Chapter 2 provide a useful structure for identifying the relevant content for a pre-registration nursing curriculum. The content of each theme can be developed as a number of 'units' of study. It is helpful if each unit is worth a specified number of credit points, usually 5, 10 or 15, determined by the work required. Within topic areas, each unit builds on earlier ones and is combined with units from other themes to produce congruent modules of study. The different themes are all important in the education programme and students need to recognise how they all link together. In addition to these themes, students moving into higher education need to develop appropriate study and other skills to be a successful nursing student.

Reflective and Proficient Practice

This is the theme which provides the core of the programme and is much the largest. Its focus is the clinical activity of providing knowledgeable, safe and skilled patient care. It can be subdivided into several sub-themes of:

- biological sciences;
- patient safety and personal care;
- care of those with differing needs and in different contexts; and
- clinical skills.

Table 6.2 shows an outline of the content of this theme for those studying to become an adult (or a general) nurse.

TABLE 6.2 *Outline of Topics within Theme on Reflective and Proficient Practice*

Biological sciences	Anatomy, physiology, biochemistry, nutrition, pathophysiology, pharmacology, genetics
Patient safety and personal care	Infection control Risk assessment - falls, DVT, pressure sores Medicines administration Hygiene and skin care, eating and drinking, breathing, elimination, mobility Complementary and Alternative Medicine (CAM)
Care of those with differing needs and in different contexts	Care of those with chronic illness Care of those receiving surgical intervention Care of the acutely and critically ill Care of the mentally ill Care of those with learning difficulties Rehabilitation Maternal and child care Care in the community Care in intensive and high dependency care settings
Clinical skills	Patient assessment Wound care Nutritional and fluid balance Management of enteral and parenteral fluids Aided elimination (catheterisation, stoma care) Injections Venepuncture Management of life support equipment (e.g. ventilators, dialysis) and other skills appropriate to clinical setting

Biological Sciences

The biological sciences are an area of study which many nursing students find difficult but which are essential underpinnings for safe practice. Considerable thought needs to go into helping students to understand how the human body works, and one of the important issues is who will teach this area of work. Sometimes nursing students are taught within a multidisciplinary class of health professionals but this can be difficult as needs of the various professional groups differ. For example, physiotherapists need detailed knowledge of the musculoskeletal and neurological systems, while nurses require less detailed knowledge of these systems but do need a good overall understanding of how the body works, including the digestive and endocrine systems. In addition, most healthcare professions require 'A' level biology as an entrance requirement, while many nursing programmes do not, and thus many students lack the background to cope unaided with the science aspects of the programme. In universities, a subject specialist from the relevant academic department may be asked to teach human biology but it is important that nurse academics ensure that the material is appropriate for nursing students, and that students are able to apply it in the context of patient care.

The selection of a recommended textbook(s) for pre-registration nursing students is an issue for consideration. Some publications are too detailed for many nursing students but *Ross and Wilson Anatomy and Physiology in Health and Illness* (Waugh and Grant, 2010) provides a good foundation for further study of pathophysiology.

Pharmacology and genetics are both subjects growing in importance in relationship to nursing. Growing numbers of qualified nurses are becoming independent or supplementary prescribers and a solid understanding of how drugs work is essential (see McGavock, 2005). Students can supplement this with using the British National Formulary (BNF, 2012) or other drug manual to learn about the drugs in use. A growing understanding of pharmacogenetics is leading towards the probable introduction of personalised medication in the near future. Understanding of genetics will be important for participating in this aspect of care, and is necessary now to recognise the genetic contribution to disease, and thus, the importance of health promotion in those at risk. Recommended genetics competencies at the point of registration are shown in Box 6.1 and an appropriate syllabus for pre-registration nursing students has been developed (Kirk et al., 2011). The other area of particular importance in the biological sciences is nutrition, which has been an area of care in which deficiencies have been identified.

Box 6.1 Genetics Nursing Competencies (Kirk et al., 2011)

1 Identify clients who might benefit from genetic services and/or information through a comprehensive nursing assessment:

- that recognises the importance of family history in assessing predisposition to disease, and recognises the key indicators of a potential genetic condition;
- taking appropriate action to seek assistance from and refer to genetics specialists and peer support resources;
- based on an understanding of the patient pathways that incorporate genetics services and information.

2 Demonstrate the importance of sensitivity in tailoring genetic information and services to clients' culture, knowledge, language ability and developmental stage:

- recognising that ethnicity, culture, religion, ethical perspectives and developmental stage may influence the clients' ability to utilise these.

3 Advocate for the rights of all clients to informed decision-making and voluntary action:

- based on an awareness of the potential for misuse of human genetic genomic/information and
- understanding the importance of delivering genetic/genomic education and counselling fairly, accurately and without coercion or personal bias;
- recognising that personal values and beliefs of self and client may influence the care and support provided during decision-making.

4 Demonstrate a knowledge and understanding of the role of genetic/genomic and other factors in maintaining health and in the manifestation, modification and prevention of disease expression, to underpin effective practice.

5 Apply knowledge and understanding of the utility and limitations of genetic/genomic testing and information to underpin care and support for individuals and families prior to, during and following decision-making, that incorporates:

- awareness of the ethical, legal and social issues related to testing and recording of genetic/genomic information;
- awareness of the potential physical, psychological and social consequences of genetic/genomic information for individuals, family members and communities.

6 Examine one's own competency of practice on a regular basis in order to:

- recognise areas where professional development related to genetics/genomics would be beneficial;

(Continued)

(Continued)

- maintain awareness of clinical developments in genetics/genomics that are likely to be of most relevance to the client group, and
- based on an understanding of the boundaries of one's professional role in the referral, provision or follow-up to genetics services.

7 Obtain and communicate credible, current information about genetics/genomics, for self, clients and colleagues:

- using information technologies and other information sources effectively to do so, and
- applying critical appraisal skills to assess the quality of information accessed.

8 Provide ongoing nursing care and support to patients, carers and families with genomic healthcare needs:

- being responsive to changing needs through the life-stages;
- demonstrating awareness about how an inherited condition, and its implications for family members, might impact on family dynamics;
- working in partnership with patients, carers, family members and other agencies in the management of conditions;
- recognising the expertise of patients and carers with enduring genomic healthcare needs that develops over time and with experience.

Published with the permission of the NHS National Genetics Education and Development Centre.

The other areas of this theme are equally important but rather more straightforward in selecting the material to be considered. One exception that is worth considering is that of CAM (Complementary and Alternative Medicine) in conjunction with nursing care. A number of HEIs incorporate some teaching about these therapies and teaching massage techniques in which all students experience giving and receiving massage has been reported (Cook and Robinson, 2006). Results of evaluating this innovation were very positive with 95.5% of respondents feeling that massage skills would benefit their practice as a nurse and would have positive patient outcomes. The experiential learning of this skill was received positively.

Theoretical and Professional Issues

The focus of this theme is the theoretical and professional context in which nursing practice occurs and Table 6.3 identifies the main topics within this theme. Graduates of a pre-registration programme are joining a profession and it is hoped that they will contribute to its development based on understanding the characteristics of a profession and how nursing has developed into its current structure. One of the important elements is *'cultural competence'* in working with both colleagues and patients from different cultures (Leininger and McFarland, 2002). The Consortium of Higher Education Institutes in Health and Rehabilitation in Europe (COHEHRE), consisting of institutions from five different cultures, is designing a programme to enable European nurses to provide culturally competent care (Richardson, 2011).

TABLE 6.3 *Topics within Theme on Theoretical and Professional Issues*

Nursing as a profession	Outline history of nursing, key influences on development, changes in educational provision, role development
	Professional attributes, statutory and professional organisations, professional regulation and legislation (UK and Europe), nursing worldwide
	Role of individual professionals in ensuring high quality care, cultural competence in care
	Legal issues: organisational and professional issues in a legal context, legal status of the Registered Nurse
	Current issues in nursing: continuing professional development and lifelong learning, practice development; advanced practice; importance of research and development
Values	Personal and professional values, the value of caring
	Dignity, privacy, cultural sensitivity, religious needs
	Respect for patients, their families, nursing and multidisciplinary colleagues
	Valuing diversity, non-discrimination and good practice in the NHS
Ethics	Key concepts of ethical reasoning and discernment; Professional Codes, Ethical Nursing practice: individuals' rights and risks; ethical issues arising in practice, concept of informed moral decision-making, valid consent to care
	Ethical frameworks and theories
	Human Rights: legislation, rights and resources, quality of life issues, Advance Directives; patient empowerment; anti-oppressive practice
	Ethical dilemmas: including refusal of informed consent and compulsory treatment; allocation of scarce resources; highlighting poor performance
Theories and models of nursing	What are theories and models? The Nursing Metaparadigm
	Contribution of theories and models in understanding and guiding nursing
	Possible study of different models and theories in relation to different areas of practice

Graduates will also have a clear perception of professional ethics including the importance of respect for individuals, patients in particular but also their families and nursing and multidisciplinary colleagues. Ethical principles are important in providing care but also in relation to management of care, and in research. Nurses are expected to behave in all situations within the code of professional conduct (NMC, 2008c) and the guidance for students (NMC, 2010b).

In the UK, theories and models of nursing have been considered to a greater extent since nursing education first moved into higher education. Now referred to as 'grand theories' (Fawcett, 1989; Meleis, 2011; McEwen and Wills, 2011) rather than 'models', such frameworks have an important part to play in conceptualising nursing. Most fields of nursing are moving towards more multidisciplinary frameworks of assessment and more '*eclectic*' approaches that draw on a range of frameworks and theoretical perspectives (Dyer, 2003). The philosophical ideas of person-centredness (McCormack and McCance, 2006), holism, human autonomy and human dignity (Jacobs, 2001), all of which are inherent in most of the early grand theories of nursing, have recently been given a new vitality in nursing curricula. Inclusion of such ideas in a modern curriculum and across all fields of nursing is important if teachers wish to stay current. How grand theories should be used in pre-registration education is still under debate with HEIs taking different approaches. In the early years of nursing education in HEIs one grand theory may have been enough to convey key concepts of nursing to other disciplines (see Meleis, 2011 and McEwen and Wills, 2011 for early history of nursing models in universities within the United States). Using one conceptual framework to articulate the discipline of Nursing is no longer feasible. A more pluralistic approach that exposes students to a range of grand theories and conceptual frameworks across the curriculum is more appropriate and Table 6.4 identifies clinical areas to which particular theories and frameworks relate.

TABLE 6.4 *Possible Nursing Grand Theories within the Curriculum*

Area of Practice	Appropriate Theory or Model
Fundamentals of care	Activities of daily living (Henderson, 1966; Roper et al., 2002)
Care of those with chronic medical illness	Orem's self-care model of nursing (Orem et al., 2003)
Care of those having surgical interventions	Roy adaptation model (Roy, 2008)
Critical care nursing	Neuman healthcare systems model (Neuman and Fawcett, 2010), Mead model (McClune and Franklin, 1987)
Mental health nursing	Peplau's theory of psychodynamic nursing (Peplau, 1993) Barker's tidal model of mental health recovery (in Alligood and Tomey, 2010)
Learning disability nursing	Activities of daily living (Henderson, 1966; Roper et al., 2002) Orem's self-care model of nursing (Orem et al., 2003)
Children's nursing	Casey's model of children's nursing (Casey, 1995; Gibson et al., 2003)
Maternal and child health	Models of midwifery care (Bryar and Sinclair, 2010)
Leadership and management of care	Transformational leadership models (Bowles and Bowles, 2000)

Communication Teaching and Learning

Nursing as a practice profession is dependent on communication and developing caring, empowering relationships with individuals, families, groups and communities. Working within the complexity of the healthcare system, communication skills are also essential to ensure care by all members of the multidisciplinary team is coordinated and high quality care provided. Table 6.5 identifies a range of areas to be considered within this theme.

TABLE 6.5 *Topics within Theme on Communication, Teaching and Learning*

Year 1	Psychology for healthcare to understand patient behaviour in health and illness
	Communication as skilled performance, basic communication skills for taking nursing history in assessment, communication within multidisciplinary team
	Therapeutic relationships for working with all patients based on genuineness, acceptance and empathy
Year 2	Information giving for perioperative care
	Patient and family teaching of knowledge and skills for self-management
	Coaching to support behaviour change in patients with chronic illness
	Writing patient reports
	Communicating with severely ill patients, providing support following bad news
	Communicating with families, helping them to communicate with unconscious or ventilated patients
Year 3	Communication for leading a small team and directing care
	Teaching more junior staff and providing support and correction as necessary
	Giving report and handing over to next shift
	Coordinating care with multidisciplinary team
	Transferring patients to other care contexts
	Dealing with complaints
	Preparing applications for posts and developing skills for interviews
	Participating in clinical supervision

One of the major methods through which nurses aim to improve quality of life and health status is through promoting behaviour change through communication. Teaching individuals and their families or carers the knowledge and skills they need to become real partners in their personal decision-making and care is an important aspect of nursing: every nurse is a teacher.

However, perhaps more important is helping people to change their behaviour to enhance or maintain their health in, for example, chronic diseases such as diabetes mellitus, but the evidence for the long-term effectiveness of the usual education programmes is slight. An exploratory trial study at stage 2 of the evaluation of complex interventions (MRC, 2000, cited by McGloin, 2012) indicates that wellness coaching over a three-month period can help patients to change their behaviour. At follow-up at six and twelve months the effects on empowerment and diabetes distress were maintained although by twelve months exercise levels had dropped in most of the participants (McGloin, 2012). It is possible that some level of continued support is necessary to maintain the changed behaviour. The approaches used in coaching build on those of therapeutic relationships and aim to empower the individuals concerned. They are relevant to working with patients with chronic diseases or with unhealthy lifestyles.

Health and its Determinants

In the latest standards for pre-registration nursing education the NMC emphasise the importance of promoting health and preventing illness in two statements about expectations of a new nurse:

- act on their understanding of how people's lifestyles, environments and the location of care delivery influence their health and wellbeing
- seek out every opportunity to promote health and prevent illness. (NMC, 2010a: 5)

Table 6.6 shows an outline of topics which are relevant in relation to this area of the curriculum. This is an aspect of nursing which is often not seen as relevant by students initially and they need to be motivated to incorporate this into their practice. It is important that students recognise how health promotion is an integral part of their role within hospital or community settings, with those who have acute or chronic illness, with the individual patients/clients and their families. As an example, consider a middle-aged man who has had a heart attack: the nurse looking after him should also be helping his wife to understand the importance of encouraging a healthy diet and exercise for children.

Leadership and Management

Within this theme, most of the content will be covered towards the later part of the programme. However, it is important that students begin to think about some of the concepts that will be applied relatively early within their first practice learning experiences, including such topics as:

- team working;
- creativity and imagination in individual patient care;

TABLE 6.6 *Outline of Topics within Theme on Health and its Determinants (from Carr et al., 2007)*

Understanding health	Defining health, illness and disability, health and wellness across the lifespan
	Factors influencing health, biological, social, vulnerable groups
	Inequalities in health and disease
	Relevant elements from sociology, social policy
	Introduction to epidemiology and public health
Health services	Political, social, cultural and economic influences on healthcare
	Health enhancement and healthcare delivery services, statutory and non-statutory organisations, non-health organisations
	Health service funding, alternative funding systems, pressures and constraints
	Community care, Primary Health Care teams and nurses in local commissioning
	Uptake of health services, equity of access to healthcare
	WHO and provision of health for all
Health promotion	Theoretical principles of health promotion
	Health promotion services and public health
	Principles of screening
	Principles of health education, health beliefs, assessment of need
	Selecting appropriate, effective, economic, evidence-based and ethically sound approaches to meeting identified need, empowerment
	User/community participation, community development
	Protection of vulnerable groups including child protection
Nurse as health promoter	The nurse as a role model for healthy living
	Promoting wellness within illness or disability
	Stress management: complementary therapies

- organising their own work to ensure all patients are cared for;
- maintaining patient safety.

This theme is about leadership (aiming to do the right thing) and management (doing things right) and the roles can be differentiated as follows:

- A manager:
  - has an *assigned position within the formal organisation;*
  - has *power due to delegated authority;*
  - carries out *specific functions, duties and responsibilities;*
  - has an emphasis on *control, decision-making … and results;*
  - manipulates *people, the environment, money, time, and other resources;*
  - has greater *formal responsibility and accountability … than leaders;*
  - directs *willing and unwilling subordinates.*

(Marquis and Huston, 2012: 31)

- A leader:
  - *often do(es) not have delegated authority, works through other means e.g. Influence;*
  - has a *wider variety of roles than managers;*
  - may or may not be part of the formal organisation;
  - focuses *on group processes*, information gathering, feedback and empowering others;
  - emphasis on *interpersonal relationships;*
  - directs *willing followers;*
  - May *have goals that do not necessarily reflect those of the organisation.*

(Marquis and Huston, 2012: 32)

TABLE 6.7 *Outline of Topics within Theme on Leadership and Management*

Making informed decisions	Definition, theories and characteristics of decision-making Decision-making principles and techniques Ethical factors in decision-making Problem-solving approaches and skills in the decision-making process Collaboration in decision-making
Teams	Roles and professional boundaries in the multidisciplinary team Interprofessional education Multi-agency working Cross-boundary working practices; primary, secondary and tertiary care Oral and written communication networks
Entrepreneurship and implementing change	Social enterprise, creativity, innovation, opportunities; changing health care environment, entrepreneurship in promoting best practice Identification and analysis of need for change Planning change: theories of change, risk analysis, project planning, change agents and entrepreneurial team, resources for change Implementing and evaluating change
Leadership	Differentiating between leadership and management; theories, models and dimensions of leadership and management Leadership styles and strategies; motivation; individual, group and organisational goals
Management	Management styles *Managing care*, setting priorities, skill mix, patient dependency, record keeping, legal issues, organising care, discharge planning *Managing teams*, team development and support, group dynamics; power and influence; roles, responsibilities and accountability *Managing people*: authority, responsibility and accountability, delegation and supervision, clinical supervision; managing conflict *Managing quality*: patient-focused, total quality management; quality improvement; standards, guidelines and frameworks; clinical risk management, clinical incident reporting; care pathways *Management issues*: risk assessment and management, managing emergencies, resource management, legal issues
Governance	Corporate governance; issues in clinical governance, political uses of quality, frameworks to support clinical governance

Perhaps more than the other themes within a pre-registration programme, this theme needs to provide a foundation on which graduates will build at later stages in their career. As newly registered nurses, graduates are primarily involved with managing care for individual and small groups of patients. With progression in their career, they may move into positions with responsibility for larger groups of patients and for institutional management. The overall goal of a manager at any level within the organisation is to achieve goals already set, working within the parameters of their specific role. However, at any level in an organisation, any nurse may be a leader who uses creativity and innovation to introduce change and enthuse others to follow. Table 6.7 indicates topics for inclusion within a pre-registration nursing programme. Those moving into more senior management positions in health care will need to develop further their knowledge and skills about different aspects of management.

Interprofessional education (IPE) is an important issue for inclusion within the curriculum. The Universities of Sheffield and Sheffield Hallam prepared a set of learning outcomes (which they described as capabilities) to be achieved in pre-registration nursing education shown in Box 6.2. These will make a good starting point for developing the curriculum in collaboration with academic staff from other healthcare professions. Bennett et al. (2011) found considerable enthusiasm amongst a number of healthcare academics for implementing IPE using e-technology to overcome some of the difficulties. A number of topic areas have been identified as suitable for IPE including: community health, ethics, communication, critical appraisal, epidemiology, evidence-based practice, informatics, project management and mental health.

Box 6.2 Capabilities for Interprofessional Practice (CUILU 2010, cited in Barr et al., 2011)

The practising professional should be able to:

- lead and participate in the interprofessional team and wider inter-agency work, to ensure a responsive and integrated approach to care/service management that is focused on the needs of the patient/client;
- implement an integrated assessment and plan of care/service in partnership with the patient/client, remaining responsive to the dynamics of care/service requirements;

(Continued)

(Continued)

- consistently communicate sensitively in a responsive and responsible manner, demonstrating effective interpersonal skills in the context of patient/client-focused care;
- share uniprofessional knowledge with the team in ways that contribute to and enhance service provision;
- Provide a co-mentoring role to peers of own and other professions, in order to enhance service provision and personal and professional development

Entrepreneurship is an activity which is now recognised as important for nursing although for many nurses the terminology used is not obviously relevant to professional practice. However, much of the knowledge and skills identified as being *'entrepreneurial'* are very similar to those applied in the identification of need, planning an innovation in care, and implementing and evaluating such change (Boore and Porter, 2011).

Research and Evidence-Based Practice

This is the theme which is likely to differ the most between an honours and a non-honours degree programme. Table 6.8 shows the topics suggested for this theme.

TABLE 6.8 *Topics within Theme on Research and Evidence-Based Practice*

Information technology	For learning, clinical care, management, searching for evidence, research
Evidence and research in nursing	Evidence to support professional practice; selecting and evaluating evidence, nature and types of evidence
	Research use; barriers/facilitators to implementation of evidence/research-informed practice
	Research governance, implications for role of clinical nurses
The research process	Stages and functions of research process:
	literature review, researchable questions, statement of hypotheses, theoretical framework;
	research design and methods, samples and sampling, ethical issues;
	analysis and presentation of data; discussion, conclusions
Research methods	Use of qualitative, quantitative methods and mixed methods
	Qualitative methods: types of approach; value, uses and limitations; trustworthiness; analysis of data; scope of conclusions
	Quantitative methods: range of design and methods; value, uses and limitations of different methods; reliability and validity: analysis of quantitative data using statistical package; tables and graphics in presenting results; drawing conclusions
Preparation for research	Research governance
	Developing research proposal including all stages of research process
	Preparation of dissertation, writing papers

The essential element in this theme, because of its influence on the quality of care provided, is the ability to find, evaluate and implement evidence to support practice, whether in the clinical context, management, education or policy development (Parahoo, 2006). All pre-registration students should be learning enough about research to be able to read and evaluate research papers, understanding whether the conclusions drawn are supported by the results presented, and the implications of the paper for practice. During the process of completing this unit all students should develop the skills to be able to search the literature related to a particular topic, critically analyse, synthesise and evaluate the literature, and make recommendations for practice.

In most HEIs honours degree students will develop a greater understanding of research design and methods and in many institutions will complete a research proposal or other research-based activity as their honours level dissertation.

ORGANISATION OF CONTENT

The content in a curriculum can be organised in different ways but, in most institutions in the UK, must be presented in the form of modules.

Traditional Organisation

In many academic disciplines each module deals with a specific topic. As the academic levels progress, content becomes more complex and intellectual skills expected are more demanding. However, the complexity of nursing and the importance of developing a qualified nurse with the necessary level of knowledge and skills in a range of areas makes this traditional organisation difficult to apply in a pre-registration programme. Many topics need to be introduced early in preparation for initial clinical experiences and developed further at later stages in the programme as students mature in their professional role.

Spiral Curriculum

A spiral curriculum is used in many healthcare curricula. It has a structure in which topics are revisited through the curriculum, on each occasion building on earlier work and achieving greater depth of understanding. The key elements, identified by Harden and Stamper (1999), are:

- topics are revisited on several occasions;
- there are increasing levels of difficulty;
- new learning is related to previous learning;
- the competence of students increases.

An example of a spiral curriculum in relation to the theme on communication is shown in Figure 6.1.

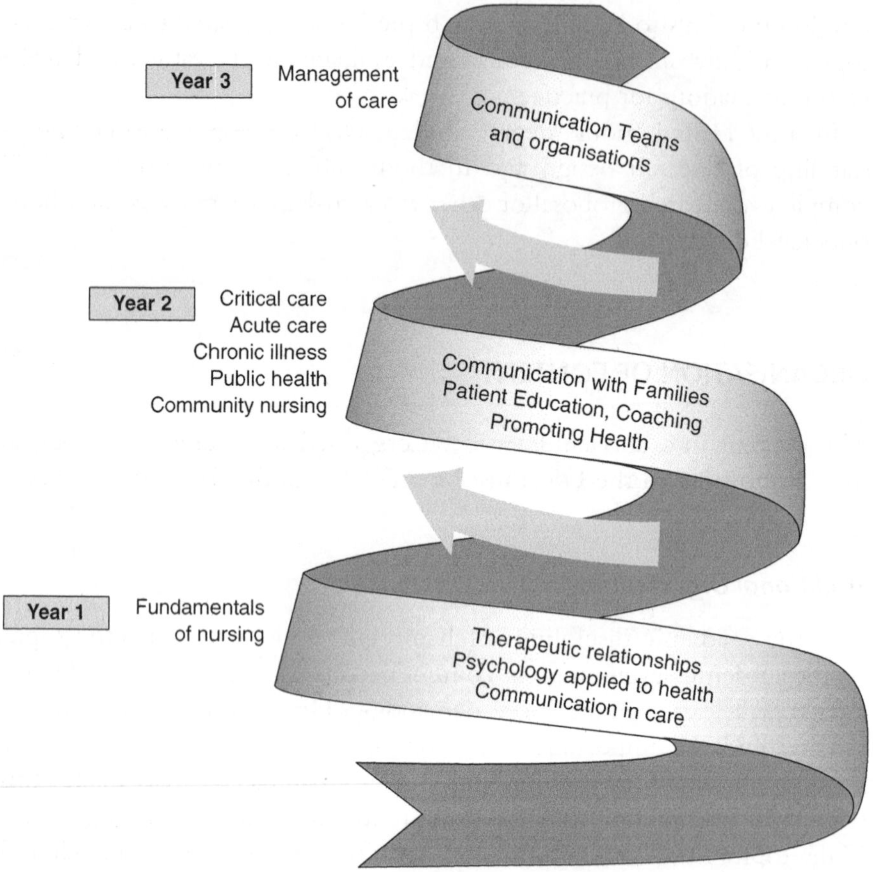

FIGURE 6.1 *Spiral Curriculum: Communication, Teaching and Learning*

Harden and Stamper (1999) also identified a number of valuable attributes of this curriculum structure:

- Reinforcement of learning occurs through repeated exposure to the topic.
- A move from simple to complex helps students to develop a good understanding of the topic at increasing levels of complexity.
- Integration of topic areas is easier with this structure as topics are not taught in large chunks.

- A logical sequence of topics is studied.
- Higher level objectives are achieved as students progress through the programme.
- Flexibility is greater than the more traditional structure and facilitates credit transfer.

Writing Modules

In the UK, most HEIs require a programme to consist of a number of modules of study and completion of the series of modules enables achievement of the course outcomes. Module outlines are included within the curriculum document for evaluation of a new programme or revalidation of a revised programme. Each HEI will have specific guidelines for preparation of the documentation (e.g. University of Ulster, 2010a) although this may be modified somewhat if a joint evaluation event is to be undertaken with the Statutory Body.

Each module is at a specified academic level (4, 5 or 6 in a Bachelor's degree programme) and carries an agreed number of credit points, and thus an expected amount of effort hours. The content of a module must match the academic level and the anticipated amount of work necessary to complete it. Modules of the same credit value should be similar in the amount of content. In most institutions, the assessment of each module must allow the student to demonstrate the achievement of every learning outcome for that module.

In most subjects, each module normally deals with a specific topic area. In nursing this may be problematic as topics often need to be revisited at a higher degree of sophistication at different stages of the curriculum. However, a module can be made up of small 'units' of learning on topics from more than one of the themes within the framework which together create a coherent whole. An example of an outline for a 20 credit module is shown in Table 6.9, with content from three different themes but all related to the same patient group.

The composition of a module will vary according to the curriculum approach used. For example, within PBL a module will consist of a

TABLE 6.9 *Module on Caring for those with Chronic Illness*

Themes	Units of study	Credit points
Reflective and proficient practice	Pathophysiology of chronic illness	10
Communication teaching and learning	Patient education and coaching to promote self-management of chronic illness	5
Health and its determinants	Epidemiology and chronic illness	5
	TOTAL	**20**

number of problem situations studied in turn over the period the module is running. These are written to lead the students to learn about, integrate and apply selected content from several themes of study. Table 6.10 shows an outline of a possible PBL module.

TABLE 6.10 *PBL Module on Caring for those with Chronic Illness*

Problem	Content	Themes	Credit points
Elderly woman after a stroke	Pathophysiology of these chronic illness	Reflective and proficient practice	6
Sixty-year-old man with chronic respiratory disease	Drug therapy and other therapeutic approaches	Communication teaching and learning	6
Middle-aged man with Type 2 diabetes	Patient education and coaching to promote self-management of chronic illness	Health and its determinants	
	Epidemiology and chronic illness	Leadership and management	8
	Specialist services for these patients		
		TOTAL	**20**

Those preparing the PBL modules must be conscious of the outcomes in terms of content and skills specified for the module and ensure that the foci of the problems presented will enable students to achieve those outcomes. Within an overall programme, students must achieve the competencies and cover the content specified by the Statutory Body.

Each module outline is expected to include some recommended reading or examples of resources which students will need to access. The specified reading associated with a module should take into account the anticipated effort hours required for the credit points allocated and what is reasonable to expect of students. A three-page list of reading material attached to a 10-credit module will not all be read and the size of the list may well discourage students from reading anything.

At the end of the process of writing the curriculum it is important to return to the individual modules in the context of the whole programme and check the following:

- Is each module coherent and meaningful?
- Does it conform to the principles of constructive alignment?
- Are the reading lists relevant and appropriate?
- Are modules carrying the same credit points comparable in relation to workload, credit rating and detail provided? It may be necessary to cut detail.
- Does the assessment for each module examine achievement of each learning outcome?

CHAPTER SUMMARY

This chapter has considered a number of issues in relation to the content to be included within a curriculum and its organisation and has considered briefly the six themes of the curriculum framework from Chapter 2. At the end of writing a course document for a new or revised programme it is essential to review the complete documentation to answer the following questions:

- Are links between modules clear?
- Is overlap with previous modules reduced to that essential to help students to make the links with earlier work?
- Is the programme as a whole coherent?
- Have all the course outcomes been achieved through the sum of the individual modules?
- Have all the Statutory Body requirements been met?

7 UNDERSTANDING LEARNING AND TEACHING

INTRODUCTION

Previous chapters have examined issues concerned with planning a programme and making decisions about content. This chapter moves on to examine ways of understanding teaching and learning. It returns to some of the educational theorists and philosophical and theoretical issues arising from education introduced in Chapter 2 which will enhance the lecturer's understanding of teaching and learning and guide approaches to working with adult learners. It prepares the groundwork for the following four chapters on different aspects of teaching and learning. Understanding some of these issues enables the course team to make appropriate decisions about approaches to teaching which will enhance learning within their particular student population.

CONTEXT OF EDUCATION

The world of higher education has changed radically in the past 20 years. The proportion of school leavers in the UK who move into higher education has dramatically increased and many students are less focused on study for the sake of enlightenment, but are working under pressure to gain employment. The teaching methods used have had to adapt in order to promote learning in student groups of mixed ability and motivation, with a much wider range of academic and social backgrounds than used to be common. The introduction of fees has resulted in a consumer mentality among students demanding results from lecturers, while not always being prepared to accept responsibility for learning. While most nursing students do not have to pay fees, many will consider (with justification) that they have a right to high quality teaching and a wide range of teaching methods.

Jarvis (2002) discusses how the role of lecturers has changed to become much broader than in the past, incorporating pastoral care and counselling within their educational and administrative responsibilities. The QAA, Statutory Body and HEI all impose standards that impact on the role of the lecturer and leave reduced time available for the development of knowledge through research, although this expectation is still held by HEIs.

TEACHING OR LEARNING

The role of the lecturer and the methods used in achieving the goals of the curriculum will vary with the curriculum approaches selected, the size of student groups and how the School conceptualises teaching and learning. To teach is a 'teacher-focused activity' and is defined as being to:

- impart knowledge to or instruct (someone) in how to do something, especially in a school or as part of a recognised programme;
- give instruction in (a subject or skill);
- cause to learn by example or experience. (OED, 2006)

On the other hand, to learn is 'student-focused' and defined as being to:

- acquire knowledge of or skill in (something) through study or experience or by being taught;
- commit to memory;
- become aware of by information or from observation. (OED, 2006)

While academic staff in HEIs will virtually always state that their aim is to enable students to learn, whether teaching or learning activities are the major focus within a programme will be determined by the educational philosophies and beliefs held by the staff group. The traditional approach to delivering an educational programme is by teaching, and hoping that students thereby learn, while the more innovative methods such as problem-based learning focus on enabling students to learn.

One of the key issues to consider in determining methods of teaching is that the amount of knowledge needed for professional practice has grown enormously, and continues to grow, so that a student cannot learn and remember everything that will be needed for a complete professional career. The most important aspect of a programme has to be facilitating students in learning to learn and developing a foundation for lifelong learning which is now a requirement for healthcare professionals. Within pre-registration education, it is essential that the necessary skills and attitudes for continuing professional development are acquired.

TYPES OF LEARNING

Gagné (cited in Knowles et al., 2011) identified a hierarchy of eight types of learning (see Table 7.1) of which the higher levels are most relevant to nursing education. In particular, the aim is to enable graduates to use their learning at lower levels in problem solving within the clinical context.

TABLE 7.1 *Gagne's Distinctive Types of Learning (adapted from Knowles et al., 2011)*

<table>
<tr><th></th><th>Learning type</th><th>Description</th><th colspan="2">Example in Nursing/Nursing Education</th></tr>
<tr><td>1</td><td>Signal learning</td><td>A general diffuse response to a signal</td><td>Raised temperature can be caused by several factors</td><td rowspan="4">Applied in achieving higher levels of learning including problem-solving in clinical practice</td></tr>
<tr><td>2</td><td>Stimulus-response learning</td><td>A precise response to a specific stimulus</td><td>Infected wound produces pus and feels hot to touch</td></tr>
<tr><td>3</td><td>Chaining</td><td>A chain of two or more stimulus-response connections</td><td>Raised temperature leads to increased pulse rate</td></tr>
<tr><td>4</td><td>Verbal association</td><td>Learning of chains that are verbal</td><td>Descriptions of pressure area grades</td></tr>
<tr><td>5</td><td>Multiple discrimination</td><td>Different particular responses to many different, more or less similar, stimuli</td><td colspan="2">Differentiating between grades of pressure sore and selecting the correct intervention</td></tr>
<tr><td>6</td><td>Concept learning</td><td>A common response to a class of stimuli which may vary in appearance</td><td colspan="2">Selecting an appropriate dressing for a particular wound taking into account the characteristics of the wound and the range of dressings available</td></tr>
<tr><td>7</td><td>Principle learning</td><td>A chain of two or more concepts which result in specific behaviour</td><td colspan="2">Recognising the link between pressure and/or friction and the development of a pressure sore and introducing a turning schedule</td></tr>
<tr><td>8</td><td>Problem solving</td><td>Combining previously learnt concepts and principles through thinking to produce appropriate decisions and actions</td><td colspan="2">Developing a learning resource for health care assistants to help them learn about causes and prevention of pressure sores</td></tr>
</table>

Deep and Surface Learning

In an outcomes-led programme, students are expected not just to acquire information but also to develop a conceptual understanding of their discipline. Effective learning enables students to achieve an overall understanding of the structure and concepts of their discipline, and thus changes how they perceive their profession and its practice.

Biggs and Tang (2007) discuss two main types of learning with different implications for level of understanding: surface learning and deep learning. Surface learning is when the student learns at a superficial level through, for example, memorising content and regurgitating it when required without necessarily understanding the meaning. Table 7.2 summarises factors of student and teacher which are likely to lead to surface learning.

TABLE 7.2 *Factors Encouraging Surface or Deep Learning*

Surface Learning	**Deep Learning**
	Student
Has cynical view of education and intends to obtain a minimum pass	Interested in subject and determined to do well by engaging with task meaningfully and appropriately
Non-academic priorities greater than academic	Appropriate background knowledge
Insufficient time: too high a workload	Preference and ability to work conceptually
Misunderstands requirements, thinks factual recall is adequate	Can focus at high conceptual level, working from first principles
Unable to understand specific content at deep level	
	Teacher
Does not clarify intrinsic structure of discipline	Explicitly brings out structure of topic or subject
Does not require active engagement of students	Elicits active response from students
Teaches piecemeal	Builds on what students already know
Inadequate focus on ensuring students' understanding	Confronting and eradicating students' misconceptions
Assesses independent facts, short answer and Multiple Choice Questions	Assessing for structure rather than independent facts
Teaches/assesses in way that encourages cynicism	Teaching and assessing in way to encourage positive working environment, students learn from mistakes
Provides insufficient time for task, emphasises coverage rather than depth	Emphasizing depth of learning, rather than breadth of coverage
Creates undue anxiety or low expectations of success	Using teaching and assessment methods that support explicit aims and outcomes of course

Source: Biggs and Tang (2007) *Teaching for Quality Learning at University*.

Deep learning, on the other hand, is when the student wants to fully understand the material being presented and to be able to see where it fits in the broad framework of the discipline. Here, students are aiming to build on previous learning and add new knowledge to the structure of their discipline that they have already developed through comprehending the main ideas, themes and principles of the subject. They are constructing their own understanding. Table 7.2 summarises approaches of student and lecturer to achieve such learning.

A third type of learning, known as strategic learning, has also been identified in which students make a strategic choice about using deep learning for some topics and surface learning for others, depending on their perceived importance for success (Race, 2005). It can be argued that those who focus their learning on cues picked up from lecturers and past examination papers are making sensible choices for success.

Threshold Concepts and Troublesome Knowledge

In considering types of learning, Meyer and Land (2006) discuss threshold concepts and the notion of troublesome knowledge, which are both useful for teachers in understanding how their students may be struggling with learning. A threshold concept is described as

> 'akin to a portal, opening up a new and previously inaccessible way of thinking about something. It represents a transformed way of understanding, or interpreting, or viewing something without which the learner cannot progress'. (Meyer and Land, 2006: 3)

These are usually described as core concepts and are important components of the curriculum. A threshold concept may have the following characteristics:

- *transformative* – in that it changes the way in which the learner views the subject area, often through modification in values or feelings;
- probably *irreversible* – in that it is unlikely to be forgotten;
- *integrative* – which demonstrates relationships between concepts;
- *bounded* – usually has boundaries with other areas of knowledge;
- potentially *troublesome* (Meyer and Land, 2006: 7).

What is described as troublesome knowledge is that which is *problematic or troublesome for learners* (Meyer and Land, 2006: 9) and several types are identified:

- *Ritual knowledge* is routine and tends to appear meaningless to students unless put into the wider context. In nursing an example could be how to calculate drug dosages, which only becomes meaningful in the clinical context.

- *Inert knowledge* is learnt but not used or remembered until something calls it forth. For example, students learn physiology but many will not see the use of it until they are caring for a patient with a physiological condition, when the care required is understood in the light of the disordered physiology.
- *Conceptually difficult knowledge* is, as it sounds, knowledge which students find difficult. For many students, research is an area of the curriculum which they find difficult and which can seem irrelevant to their practice. Emphasising the importance of evidence-based practice, with examples of changes in practice because of research, helps students become motivated to focus on this aspect of their learning.
- *Alien knowledge* is that which is foreign and appears irrelevant to their discipline. Research methodology, already identified as conceptually difficult, is also identified by some students as the subject which seems least relevant to their nursing degree.
- *Tacit knowledge* is knowledge which is not readily transmitted and tends to be acted upon without the individual recognising the knowledge behind the action.

Eraut (2000) discusses the implicit learning which takes place and results in tacit knowledge, which Polanyi defined as *'that which we know but cannot tell'* (cited by Eraut, 2000: 118), although others have discussed making it explicit. It is suggested that tacit knowledge can be identified when some stimulus brings it to the surface, such as in a situation when experiences and comments are being discussed. In the Dreyfus model of skills acquisition (see Table 7.3), one of the characteristics of the 'expert' is an *'intuitive grasp of situations based on deep tacit understanding'* (Eraut, 2000: 126). Benner (1984) applied the Dreyfus model in nursing in discussing the development of qualified nurses from novice in a new clinical setting to expert after several years experience and with a high level of clinical expertise. This model is also relevant to the development of the nurse lecturer. However, some HEIs use Benner's model as a framework for assessing nursing students' progress in clinical practice although only the first three levels, possibly four for very good students, are applicable to learners.

To help students cope with this troublesome knowledge, the teacher has to find ways of engaging students with the topic and identifying approaches to help them learn. Of the types of troublesome knowledge, tacit knowledge is the most difficult to teach, although the principles of tacit learning and its use can be imparted. Tacit knowledge has been identified in three forms – tacit understanding, tacit procedures and tacit rules:

- *Situational understanding:* This is developed through all five levels and is based largely on experience and remaining mainly tacit.
- *Standard, routinised procedures:* This is developed to competence level for coping with demands of work without suffering information overload. Some begin as

TABLE 7.3 *Summary of Dreyfus Model of Skill Acquisition (Eraut, 2000: 126)*

Level 1: Novice	Rigid adherence to taught rules or plans Little situational perception No discretionary judgment
Level 2: Advanced Beginner	Guidelines for action based on attributes or aspects (aspects are global characteristics of situations recognisable only after some prior experience) Situational perception still limited All attributes and aspects are treated separately and given equal importance
Level 3: Competent	Coping with crowdedness Now sees actions at least partially in terms of longer-term goals Conscious deliberate planning Standardised and routinised procedures
Level 4: Proficient	See situations holistically rather than in terms of aspects See what is most important in a situation Perceives deviations from the normal pattern Decision-making less laboured Uses maxims for guidance, whose meaning varies according to the situation
Level 5: Expert	No longer relies on rules, guidelines or maxims Intuitive grasp of situations based on deep tacit understanding Analytic approaches used only in novel situations, when problems occur or when justifying conclusions Vision of what is possible

explicit procedural knowledge then become automatic and increasingly tacit through repetition, with concomitant increases in speed and productivity.

- *Intuitive decision-making*: Pattern recognition and rapid responses to developing situations are based on tacit application of tacit rules. These rules may or may not be explicit or capable of reasoned justification, but they are tacit at the moment of use. (Eraut, 2000: 127)

HOW DO PEOPLE LEARN?

A number of authors have written about how people learn and this section introduces some of this work. The main aim here is to encourage academic staff to think about their own approaches to teaching.

Ausubel

In considering how the programme is to be presented, it is important to understand something about how people learn. The work of Ausubel et al. (1978) draws on cognitive psychology and is highly relevant to nursing education. He identifies two independent dimensions of learning:

Rote learning and ⟷ Meaningful learning
Reception learning ⟷ Discovery learning

The rote learning end of the continuum relates to surface learning, while meaningful learning is comparable to deep learning. Most areas of learning in nursing education involve both dimensions. Rote learning is much easier if it is first made meaningful, for example explaining how the skeleton functions makes it easier to learn the names of the major bones. Reception learning, as in lecturing to enable students to acquire knowledge and understanding, is the main method used within higher education. Complete discovery learning, where students find out for themselves, takes a considerable amount of time which is not readily available within a three-year course of theory and practice. Figure 7.1 illustrates how a number of different teaching/learning methods used in nursing fit within these dimensions.

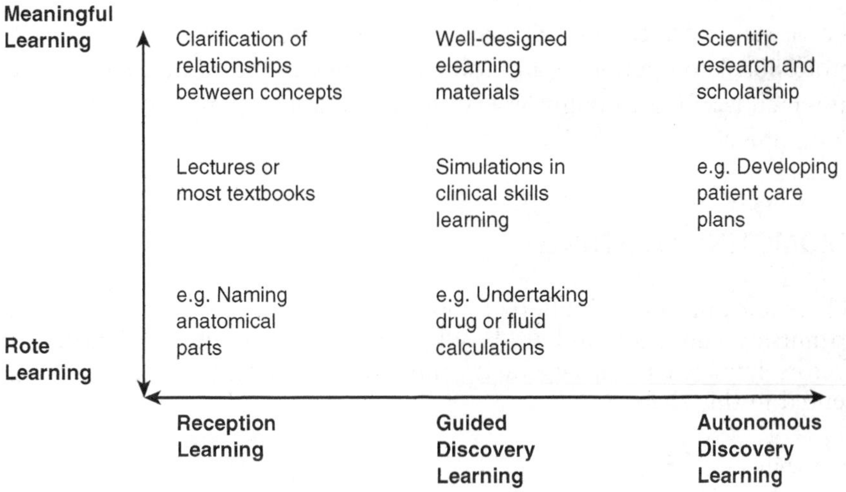

FIGURE 7.1 *Dimensions of Learning (adapted from Ausubel et al., 1978)*

Ausubel also presented assimilation theory in which previous knowledge (or cognitive structure) is built on through the assimilation of additional knowledge to achieve meaningful learning. An example of this would be learning about the requirements for individual cell function and linking on to this, knowledge about how the different body systems maintain the requirements for cell function.

Bandura

Bandura (1986) is associated with social learning theory (or social cognitive theory). He describes four processes through which learning occurs by observation in the social environment.

- *Attention* determines what is learnt by observation and is influenced by: properties of the activity to be modelled (clearly visible, uncommon, technically skilled); characteristics of the observer (previous knowledge providing a framework, intellectual ability, interest in the subject); functional value of the activity (relevance, importance); attention guided by mentor or preparation for the experience.
- *Retention* and rehearsal by using some mechanism (e.g. symbolic representation) to remember and relate this learning to previous learning. Reinforcing learning through rehearsal including cognitive (going over activity in one's mind) and active rehearsal.
- *Production* of the activity based on the representation of the activity previously achieved. Learning is enhanced by '*making the unobservable observable*' (1986: 66) through receiving feedback and explanation. The simpler components are learnt first.
- *Motivation* determines the effort put into learning. The incentives for doing an activity effectively may be internal (e.g. personal satisfaction from undertaking the skill smoothly without pain to the patient) or external motivation such as achievement of objectives for placement assessment.

These stages are highly relevant when planning for students to develop professional competencies and role proficiency in the clinical environment in which learning through observation, imitation and modelling is a major component.

PROMOTING LEARNING

There are a number of different approaches to learning which are relevant to nursing education and are briefly considered here. Race identifies five factors involved in successful learning which relate to other work presented in this chapter:

- wanting to learn;
- needing to learn;
- learning by doing;
- learning through feedback;
- making sense of things – or digesting (Race, 2005: 26).

In aiming to encourage learning, these factors help the lecturer to structure the educational context and activities for students to achieve the anticipated learning.

Behaviourism is the scientific study of behaviour and is based on an understanding that learning is shown through behaviour, and focuses on the forces which change behaviour. This has a useful, but limited, role in nursing education in which acquisition of skills is important. However, it does not recognise the critical thinking and decision-making which occur before the visible behaviour and are developed through the process of nursing education.

Discovery learning in its purest form is when the student is given complete freedom to decide what and how to learn. More common is guided discovery in which the teacher asks questions or identifies problems to which the students will find the answers. Bruner (1966, cited in Knowles et al., 2011) states that this is based on a will to learn and he identifies four benefits of this type of learning: it increases intellectual growth; students move from needing extrinsic rewards to intrinsic rewards; they learn how to discover things for themselves; the learnt material is remembered more effectively. Problem-based learning is a variant of discovery learning.

Experiential learning is a major issue in nursing education in which clinical experience plays a major part: in the UK the NMC requires that pre-registration nurse education is 50% practice. Kolb (1984, cited in Knowles et al., 2011) played a major part in clarifying the process of learning through experience by identifying a model of experiential learning (see Figure 7.2). The importance of reflection on and in practice (Schön, 1987) for effective learning is recognised now in all UK nursing programmes.

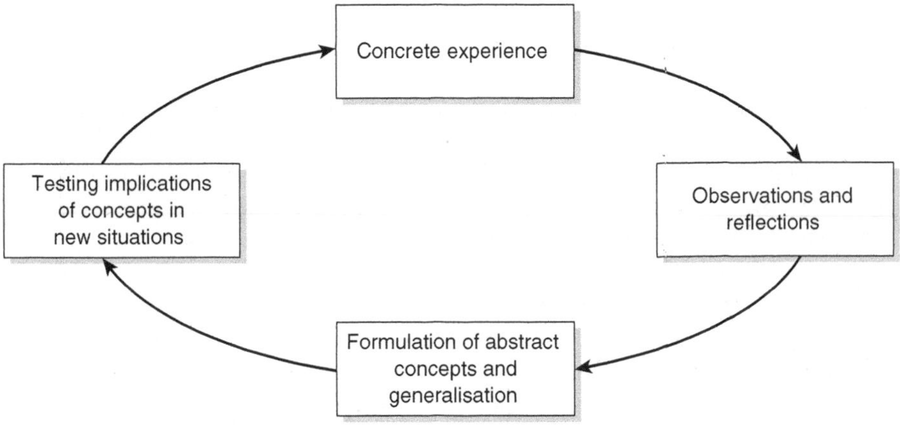

FIGURE 7.2 *Kolb's Experiential Learning Model (Knowles et al., 2011)*

The balance between experience and reflection is important, as shown in Figure 7.3, and the quality of the experience and of the reflection is equally important. It is clear that good experience without good reflection and vice versa, are likely to result in ineffective learning. Adaptation of the old adage can be stated as '*I am a nurse who has had 10 years' experience, not a nurse who has had one year's experience ten times*'.

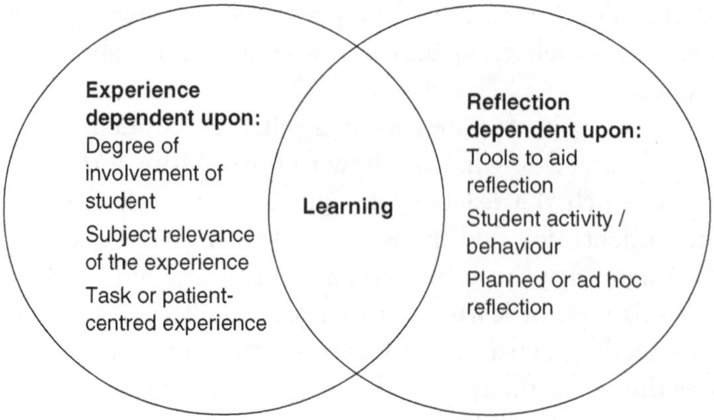

FIGURE 7.3 *The Balance Between Experience and Reflection*

Fowler (2008) discusses facilitating factors and barriers to experiential learning. Facilitating factors are identified as:

- a teacher who deliberately intervenes to provide an experience and prompt reflection;
- a student who deliberately sets out to reflect on experience;
- a random occurrence resulting in experience interacting with reflection.

The barriers specified are:

- other work priorities distracting the nurse from combining reflection with the experience;
- personal or social problems draining the energy needed for combining the two elements;
- active resistance on the part of the individual towards the situation.

Strategies to promote effective learning from experience can be selected for use within the four stages of Kolb's model. Concrete experience can be provided through demonstration of skills and simulation exercises leading up to experience within the clinical environment. Students can reflect on observations within small group discussions or with their mentor or link lecturer, and thus acquire the ability to reflect individually. Within group discussion students can develop generalisable understanding of their experience which they can then apply in different clinical situations. Reflection is discussed in greater detail in Chapter 8.

TEACHING

This section looks at how the lecturer may apply some of the knowledge from the learning theories above in order to promote learning. Students are being provided with the stimuli to build on what they already know and to help them construct their own knowledge.

Levels of Teaching

Biggs and Tang (2007) discuss levels of teaching which teachers tend to move through as their career progresses. These are:

- Level 1: Focus – what the student is. The teacher imparts information and what the students do with it is up to them. They may be good students who attend all classes, learn what they are meant to and give in good assignments, or bad students who don't do all these things. The outcomes depend on student ability and motivation. Essentially, this is a *blame the student theory* (Biggs and Tang, 2007: 17).
- Level 2: Focus – what the teacher does. At this level, the teacher uses a range of approaches to transmit concepts and ensure that students understand the material. The teacher is competent in planning classes and presents them clearly and coherently but the focus is on what he or she is planning and doing. If the outcomes are inadequate, it is the teacher's fault.
- Level 3: Focus – what the student does. The key point is how well the outcomes are achieved, indicating how well the student understands the material. The teacher identifies the learning activities which students undertake to achieve the outcomes. The emphasis is on what the student does, rather than what the teacher does.

These levels broadly illustrate the approaches to teaching which can be identified in many HEIs. However, a more sophisticated way of looking at approaches to teaching is reported by Trigwell et al. as:

- Approach A: A teacher-focused strategy with the intention of transmitting information to students;
- Approach B: A teacher-focused strategy with the intention that students acquire the concepts of the discipline;
- Approach C: A teacher/student interaction strategy with the intention that students acquire the concepts of the discipline;
- Approach D: A student-focused strategy aimed at students developing their conceptions;
- Approach E: A student-focused strategy aimed at students changing their conceptions (Trigwell et al., 1999: 58).

Approaches A and B both use a strategy which assumes that students learn by being told about things. While B and C have the same intended outcomes, approach C involves student engagement in the process of learning although it is still teacher directed. The last two approaches described involve students constructing their own conceptual view of the subject. Prosser and Trigwell (1999) identify the physical setting, the context (School and HEI) and the students as being the situation which influences how the teacher functions and the way the teacher functions influences what and how the students learn. A reciprocal relationship between perceptions of teacher and students develops and influences the methods with which the teacher is comfortable. These descriptions of approaches to teaching, in conjunction with the work on the learning environment below, provide a guide for new lecturers to develop their own abilities in helping students to learn.

The Learning Environment

Gagné (cited by Knowles et al., 2011) described functions of the educational environment which must be managed by the teacher to enhance student learning (see Table 7.4). The eight stages identified help the lecturer to identify what to focus on in preparation for teaching.

TABLE 7.4 *Functions of the Learning Environment (Knowles, 2011)*

1	The situation or stimulus is presented	Stimuli must identify the type of learning expected, e.g. a clinical situation to use in problem-based or enquiry-based learning, or a range of different dressing types when learning about wound care, or clear presentation of knowledge to be acquired
2	Methods are used to direct students' attention	Questions are asked or students complete activities to guide learning
3	A model is provided of final performance	Ensures that the learner knows what he or she is expected to achieve
4	External prompts for learning are used	Additional information assists students in making links between different aspects of the stimulus or differentiating between similar stimuli
5	Direction of thinking is guided	By giving hints or suggestions to help students avoid irrelevant hypotheses
6	Encourages application of knowledge in other contexts	Helping students to apply the learnt knowledge and competencies in a novel situation through discussion or other approach
7	Assesses learning	Students are asked questions to identify learning and its application
8	Provides feedback	Students find out whether they are right or wrong, adequate or inadequate in what they have learnt

CHAPTER SUMMARY

This is the first of five chapters which examine different aspects of teaching and learning. Theoretical issues which help to explain how people learn and how teachers facilitate learning have been the primary focus.

8 INTELLECTUAL SKILLS FOR LEARNING AND PRACTICE

INTRODUCTION

It is clear that students need to develop a number of ways of thinking which are important for skilled professional practice and lifelong learning and professional development. The aim in this chapter is to provide guidance for teachers on how to help students develop particular ways of thinking: reflection, critical thinking, creativity, problem-solving and decision-making. This includes enhancing clinical judgement for patient care.

Judgement has been defined as: '*the ability to compare or evaluate alternatives to life situations and arrive at an appropriate course of action*' (Daniels et al., 2010: 1731). Four types of judgement have been described by Lamond et al.

> A Causal judgements (diagnosis): ... expressing a state or condition based on the presence of attributes which are used to explain a problem;
>
> B Descriptive judgements: ... expressing a state or condition based on the presence of attributes which had been observed directly or obtained from another source;
>
> C Evaluative judgements: ... expressing a qualitative difference in a state or condition based on the presence of attributes which had been observed directly or obtained from another source;
>
> D Inference judgements: ... expressing the presence of a state or condition which is not based on any information gathered from or about the patient. (cited by Thompson and Dowding, 2002: 49)

In the context of clinical practice, a combination of the skills considered in this chapter is used in clinical judgement in determining the professional care to be implemented, thus they are essential skills for students to learn and apply in practice learning. These are skills they will require throughout their professional career.

REFLECTION

Underpinning much learning, but particularly that achieved in practice, is experiential learning based on Kolb's Experiential Learning Model (see Figure 8.1) in which observation and reflection, thinking about experiences, are central. Schön (1987) introduced the ideas of reflection in and on action and emphasised the importance of preparing a reflective practitioner. Reflection **in** action is thinking about what one is doing while doing it, relating it to previous experience and what has been learnt, and applying this to the current situation. Reflection **on** action occurs after the experience is over, when it is reviewed and areas for future learning are identified.

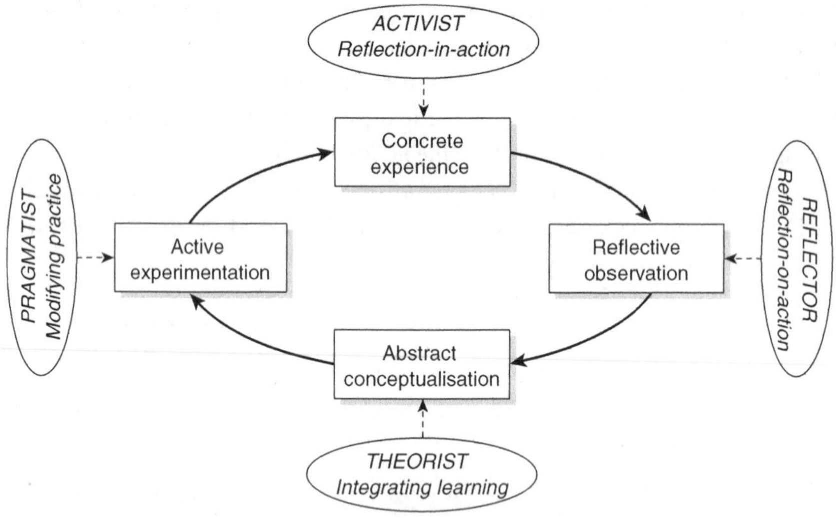

FIGURE 8.1 *Learning Styles and Reflection within Kolb's Experiential Learning Model*

Considering what happened in a particular situation and what could be improved is probably the most important activity available to enhance learning. Reflection is essentially structured thinking used to direct further learning, and is now recognised as an essential skill for student nurses and for lifelong learning in qualified professionals. Burnard (2002) discusses the place of reflection in experiential learning and the different ways in which reflective practice, that is the application of reflection, is used to enhance the quality of care. However, understanding the process of reflection is not easy; it has been described in numerous ways which together contribute to understanding its rationale and process. Based on the literature and research, Kember describes reflection as follows:

- The subject matter of reflection is an ill-defined problem – the type of issues and cases dealt with in professional practice.
- In professional practice the process of reflection may be triggered by an unusual case or deliberate attempts to revisit past experiences.
- Reflection can occur through stimuli other than problems or disturbances to the normal routine. The stimuli may be encouraged or arranged.
- Reflection operates through a careful re-examination and evaluation of experience, beliefs and knowledge.
- Reflection most commonly involves looking back or reviewing past actions, though competent professionals can develop the ability to reflect while carrying out their practice. (Kember, 2001: 174)

The process of reflective practice has been described by Gopee (2010: 53) in a way that provides helpful guidance for students learning to undertake reflection in and on their practice:

Describing the incident	→	Exploring associated feelings (or emotions)	→	Examining the incident in the context of existing publications, policies and experience	→	Generating new ways of dealing with such incidents	→	Generalising and applying the learning to new situations

Along the same lines, Sharples (2009) identifies the different learning styles of activist, reflector, theorist and pragmatist, and ways of thinking in relation to the four stages of Kolb's experiential learning cycle (see Figure 8.1). While students may start with different learning styles, this figure identifies that all these differing learning styles are needed for the various stages of experiential learning, and students need to become competent at all types of learning.

Table 8.1 clarifies the different styles of learning and thinking (Honey and Mumford, cited in Sharples, 2009) and identifies how these relate to the stages of Kolb's cycle. Through their programme, students need to develop their reflective skills and the content of this table can help to focus their learning.

TABLE 8.1 *Learning Styles and Reflection at Stages in the Experiential Cycle (Sharples, 2009)*

Concrete experience	*ACTIVISTS* – involve themselves fully and without bias in new experiences. Open-minded, not sceptical, enthusiastic about anything new. Act first, consider consequences afterwards. Thrive on challenge of new experiences, but bored with implementation and longer term consolidation. ***Reflection-in-action:*** reflection on experience while taking place: past experiences, values, opinions and expectations. Relate learning experience to outcomes.
Reflective observation	*REFLECTORS* – stand back and ponder. Collect data from self and others, think thoroughly before reaching conclusion. Are cautious, thoughtful people who consider all possible implications before acting. Listen to others before contributing to discussion. ***Reflection-on-action:*** reviewing the experience after it is over. Considering experience from many perspectives, to enable thinking and practice to move forward. Discussion with mentor to provide guidance.
Abstract conceptualisation	*THEORISTS* – adapt and integrate observations into logically sound theories. Think through problems in step-by-step logical way. Perfectionists. They analyse and synthesise. Like basic assumptions, principles, theories, models and systems thinking. They prize rationality and logic. Uncomfortable with subjective judgements, lateral thinking, ambiguity. ***Integrating learning:*** making sense of the experience following reflection. Linking to past experiences, integrating with what they already know, testing for validity and accepting learning. Recognise strengths and weaknesses, identify learning needs.
Active experimentation	*PRAGMATISTS* – keen on trying out new ideas. Enjoy experimenting with applications. Act quickly and confidently on ideas that attract them. Essentially practical, down-to-earth people who like making practical decisions and solving problems. Problems and opportunities are 'a challenge'. ***Modifying practice:*** applying knowledge through adjusting practice as last stage of experiential cycle. If learning satisfactory, new understanding results in different and more effective action.

The use of a structure helps students to begin to develop their reflective abilities. Table 8.2 shows a relatively straightforward example that can be used by students to guide reflective accounts. These can be used in discussion with their mentor, link lecturer or personal tutor to help apply theory to practice and enhance the quality of care that students are able to provide. Reflection should be used to underpin and consolidate learning in the context of all areas of professional activity and several authors have discussed in detail the use of reflection in practice (Johns, 2009; Taylor, 2006).

Skills in reflection continue to develop through one's professional career. Kember described a higher level of reflection as follows:

TABLE 8.2 *A Structure for Student Reflection*

1	Situation or experience	Describe what happened and the sequence of events that occurred
2	Causation	What were the factors that caused this experience?
3	Background	What background factors influenced the situation?
4	Reflection	What was I trying to achieve and why did I intervene as I did? What were the consequences of my actions for: myself, the patient/family, for the people I work with? How did I feel about this experience when it was happening? How did the patient respond and feel about it, and what did he/she say? What factors and/or knowledge influenced my decisions and actions?
5	Alternative Actions	Where other approaches were possible choices? What would results of those other choices have been?
6	Learning	Now, how do I feel about this experience? Could I have dealt better with the situation? What have I learned from this experience? What can I identify that I need to learn?

- Reflection operates at a number of levels; the highest level of critical reflection necessitates a change to deep-seated, and often unconscious, beliefs and leads to new belief structures.
- Reflection leads to new perspectives.
- More critical reflection, involving perspective transformation, is likely to take some time so there will be significant periods between initial observation and final conclusions (Kember, 2001: 174).

Throughout their programme students are expected to demonstrate increased sophistication in reflection. In addition to the issues already discussed, reflection offers the opportunity for thinking 'outside the box' and developing creative ideas to enhance care.

CRITICAL CREATIVE THINKING

A professional nurse has to make decisions based on critical and creative thinking and, thus, these must be addressed in pre-registration programmes. In principle, critical and creative are opposite approaches to thinking but in many ways they are complementary. Standing (2010) emphasises the importance of both modes of thinking in critical practice while drawing on evidence from various sources. Indeed some authors have incorporated creativity into the description of a critical thinker, for example, Ignatavicius identified the following characteristics of critical thinkers:

outcome driven, open to new ideas, flexible, willing to change, innovative, creative, analytical, communicators, assertive, caring, energetic, risk takers, knowledgeable, resourceful, observant, intuitive, and 'out of the box' thinkers. (cited by Popil, 2011: 2a)

Critical Thinking

The first issue is to clarify what is meant by critical thinking and this has been addressed by numerous authors (cited by Billings and Halstead, 2009). A definition of a critical thinker agreed through a Delphi Study of scholars, educators and experts in the area, is shown in Box 8.1.This corresponds with a logical approach applied in problem-solving, using clinical judgement and clinical decision-making.

Box 8.1 The Ideal Critical Thinker (Facione, cited by Billings and Halstead, 2009: 238)

The ideal critical thinker is **habitually inquisitive**, well-informed, **trustful** of reason, **open-minded**, **flexible**, **fair-minded** in evaluation, **honest** in facing personal biases, **prudent** in making judgements, willing to **reconsider**, **clear** about issues, **orderly** in complex matters, **diligent** in seeking relevant information, **reasonable** in the selection of criteria, **focused** in inquiry, and **persistent** in seeking results which are as precise as the subject and the circumstances of inquiry permit.

These activities require the critical thinking skills identified in Daniels et al. (2010) shown in Box 8.2 and used in carrying out patient assessments and care planning. Each nurse educator needs to be thinking about how to assist the development of these abilities.

Box 8.2 Critical Thinking

- Interpretation: requires categorisation, decoding sentences, clarifying meanings
- Analysis: ideas examined, arguments identified and analysed
- Inference: query evidence, consider alternatives, draw conclusions from the evidence
- Explanation: state results clearly, justify procedures used, present arguments to support results
- Evaluation: assess claims made from results, assess quality of arguments
- Self-regulation: critical examination and amendment of conclusions (if necessary)

The learning experience has to be challenging and lead the student towards learning and using critical thinking, supported by positive feedback from the facilitator and peer support. Planning such experiences involves six steps (Billings and Halstead, 2009):

- determining the learning outcomes for the session;
- creating an anticipatory set that will stimulate student involvement (i.e. requires active participation, is relevant to the student, is relevant to the class);
- selecting teaching and learning strategies that involve active participation;
- deciding how to implement strategies;
- designing closure to the session;
- determining the assessment strategies to be used (formative and summative).

Facione (cited by Standing, 2010) described in everyday language the necessary steps involved in problem-solving. Figure 8.2 draws on this work and demonstrates how students can develop their abilities, enhanced through active learning, facilitated by the lecturer.

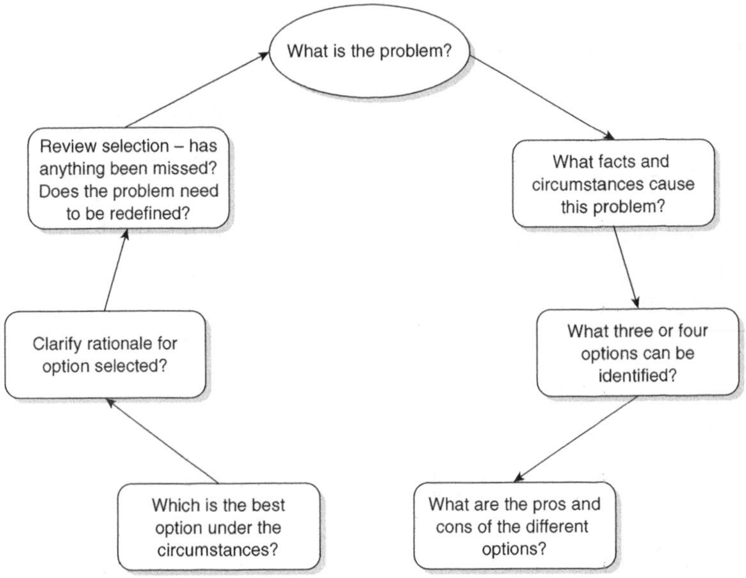

FIGURE 8.2 *Effective Thinking and Problem-Solving Cycle*

Burnard (2002) presents guidelines for the teacher to encourage development of critical thinkers, as shown in Table 8.3, but which are also similar to approaches for stimulating creative thinking.

Some approaches which can be used to facilitate critical thinking development if they are planned and implemented appropriately have been suggested (Billings and Halstead, 2009):

TABLE 8.3 *Development of Critical Thinking (Burnard, 2002)*

1	Affirm critical thinkers' self-worth	They challenge current thinking and need to feel their ideas are important; they need encouragement
2	Listen attentively to critical thinkers	Listening carefully to the students' new ideas will also challenge the lecturer's ideas and will expand the frame of reference for both
3	Be a critical teacher	Facilitator acts as a catalyst by encouraging students to question and to develop their own ideas. Facilitator shows: *'competence, courage, risk-taking, humility and political clarity'*
4	Model critical ability	*'Facilitator stays open to new ideas ... open to learning from the students'*
5	Learn to shut up!	Students need space to be able to talk to express their new ideas
6	Be conversational	Normal speech in which students are treated as equals encourages students to feel relaxed and to contribute to discussion

- Reflection has already been discussed as helping students to relate theoretical knowledge to other contexts.
- Mind or concept-mapping requires students to make links between different topics and areas of study.
- The use of case studies for problem or enquiry-based learning has been shown to '*encourage the development of critical thinking skills, ... help with problem solving, analysis, and problem identification*'. (Popil, 2011: 206)

The least useful teaching method for developing critical thinking is the lecture.

Creative Thinking

Critical thinking is enhanced by integrating it with creative thinking. Creativity involves thinking in unusual ways, using imagination, integrating differing ideas and coming up with new ideas or unique solutions to problems. In the context of nursing, creativity will enable the nurse to think of imaginative approaches

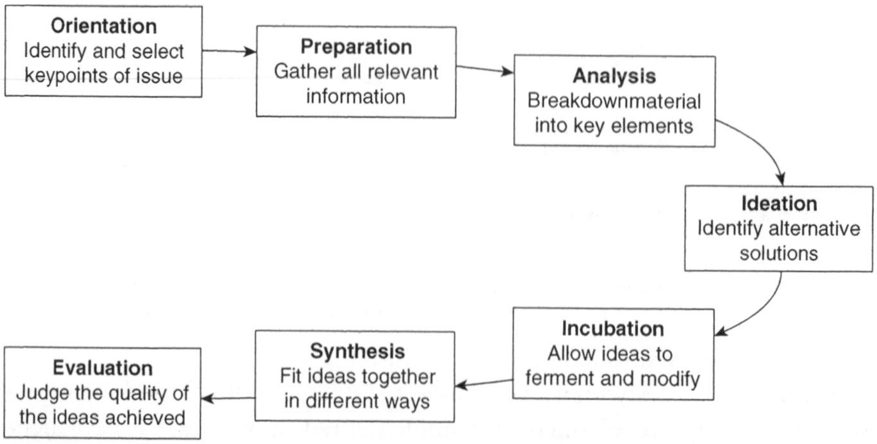

FIGURE 8.3 *Aspects of Creative Thinking (Based on Osborn's Seven-Step Model (Standing, 2010)*

to caring for individual patients or to develop a new intervention or way of working which is more economical, uses resources more efficiently, enhances the functioning of the multiprofessional team or has a better outcome.

Different models of creative thinking are a mixture of analysis and imagination (Jackson and Ellis in Standing, 2010) and are made up of similar activities. One of these models has the seven stages shown in Figure 8.3.

Adair suggests a simpler model:

- Preparation: all the necessary information is collected and analysed, and possible solutions identified;
- Incubation: mental work on subject continues subconsciously with parts of the problem separately and recombining;
- Insight: 'Eureka'. A new idea is generated, often when doing something unrelated;
- Validation: the new idea, insight, intuition, hunch or solution needs to be thoroughly tested (Adair, 2007: 82).

It is necessary to think about how to promote creativity. De Bono has written numerous publications related to creativity, including *Lateral Thinking* (De Bono, 1990), which focuses on the development of different ways of looking at a situation. He contrasts vertical thinking with lateral thinking. Vertical thinking follows the most obvious and best route towards the answer to the problem, it is analytical and sequential and characterised by the black hat thinking discussed below. Lateral thinking on the other hand goes off at tangents to find any possible routes toward a range of different answers. Table 8.4 clarifies the differences between these two types of thinking.

TABLE 8.4 *Modes of Thinking* (Adair, 2007)

Vertical thinking	**Lateral thinking**
Works within known parameters	Explores in unlikely directions
Chooses directions which follow from current situation	Selects directions which appear unlikely or irrelevant
Focuses on relevance to topic	Enjoys unexpected interventions
Looks for what is correct	Looks for what is different
Follows expected pathway	Is creative

De Bono suggests a number of techniques to trigger a change in the pattern of thinking. He describes these in detail with activities to develop ability in using them, such as: generating alternatives, challenging assumptions, accepting suspending judgement, evaluation, reversal, brainstorming etc.

Brainstorming is a useful approach for enabling a group to produce a wide range of ideas for further consideration. Marriner-Tomey (2009) suggests that the problem being considered should be relatively specific and straightforward: a more complex issue can be divided up into sections which can be considered separately. A group for brainstorming should be a size which will not intimidate participants (somewhere between 6 and 15 people) and the session should last about 30 to 45 minutes. Following appointment of a chair and note-taker, the ground rules are clarified, the issue to be considered is introduced and everybody is encouraged to suggest ideas which are listed on a flip-chart. Ground rules include:

- suspend judgement: all ideas are accepted without criticism or evaluation;
- welcome free-wheeling: let unusual ideas come forth;
- strive for quantity: the more ideas the better;
- combine and improve: see if ideas can be built on, or new ideas stimulated;
- do not edit: ideas should simply be stated and recorded. (Adair, 2007: 69)

Only after all ideas have been listed, should they be grouped and reviewed, and decisions made about the way forward.

This approach can also be used by curriculum development teams to generate innovative ideas. Whether it is used with students or staff it is important to ensure that it is done in an environment that will:

- support creativity and innovation;
- see risk taking as acceptable;
- provide employers with access to sources of knowledge;
- encourage new ideas and ways of doing things;
- allow a free flow of information;
- reward innovation;
- support good ideas. (Standing, 2010: 74).

PROBLEM-SOLVING AND DECISION-MAKING

Models of decision-making

Using clinical judgement in making decisions about care is one of the most important skills which students have to develop and demonstrate in practice under the supervision of the mentor. Students need to understand the range of options and the different factors which influence the situation, including relevant ethical issues. The importance of ethics in the curriculum has already been considered, but now students have to learn to take the ethical perspective into account in making clinical and other decisions.

The basic 7-stage problem-solving process is described by Marquis and Huston (2012) and shown alongside a simpler 5-stage decision-making process (Adair, 2007) in Table 8.5. It is clear that they are essentially the same. Having identified the issue and suggested a range of options, then

TABLE 8.5 *Decision-Making and Problem-Solving Process (Marquis and Huston, 2012: 7; Adair, 2007: 25)*

1	Identify the problem	1	Define the objective
2	Gather data to analyse the causes and consequences of the problem	2	Collect relevant information
3	Explore alternative solutions	3	Generate feasible options
4	Evaluate the alternatives		
5	Select the appropriate solution	4	Make the decision
6	Implement the solution	5	Implement and evaluation
7	Evaluate the results		

decisions need to be made. The Lobster Pot approach illustrated in Figure 8.4 can be used to sift down from the many possibilities initially produced through feasible options and eventually to the selected choice.

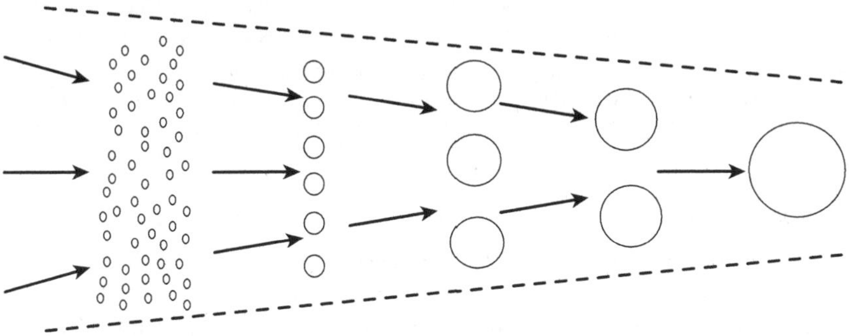

FIGURE 8.4 *The Lobster Pot Model of Decision-Making (Adair, 2007: 29)*

One approach in small group work that staff or students can use to differentiate between options has been suggested by De Bono (2000). The process involves the figurative use of six thinking hats (white, red, black, yellow, green and blue), each with a different focus, which can be called upon as needed to carry discussion forward. These can be used by individual students or by groups in project work, with the hat allocated specifying the role to be played at the specific time. Any or all members of the group can be asked for thinking as characterised by the colour of the hat; no one takes on the use of a hat for the whole time, everyone will use several hats at different times. Table 8.6 briefly describes the attributes of the different colours. An individual may be very good at black hat thinking (that is, *negative, logical, cautious and critical*) and be asked to put the yellow hat on (figuratively) and see what they can come up with by demonstrating an *optimistic and positive logical view* of the topic. Similarly, all members of the group may be asked to use red hat thinking to bring out *feelings, hunches and intuition,* or the green hat (*creativity*) to stimulate new ideas. The person acting as chair uses the blue

TABLE 8.6 *De Bono's (1986) Six Thinking Hats (from De Bono, 2000)*

Hat	Characteristics	Use
White	*Neutral*	Gathers information, decides what additional facts, figures and information is needed and how to get them. Does not evaluate. May result in parallel or contrasting information.
Red	*Feelings hunches and intuition*	Expression of feelings without need for explanation or apology. Hunches and intuition are based on experience and can be valuable in introducing ideas without explanation or empirical support.
Black	*Negative, logical, cautious and critical*	This is the critical hat. It introduces the problems and difficulties associated with a proposal. It is a very important hat as it recognises potential risks. However, needs to be counterbalanced.
Yellow	*Optimistic and positive logical view*	Counterbalances the black hat. Identifies all the possible benefits that may arise. Based on exploration and positive speculation but should aim to justify positions stated, and involves judgement.
Green	*Creativity*	Proposes new ideas. Considers options and alternatives. May submit modifications to ideas already considered. Can achieve 'out of the blue' ideas or use techniques for lateral thinking to promote creativity.
Blue	*Thinking overview or process control*	Used largely by chair and held for whole meeting although others may contribute to this thinking. Sets out purpose(s) of meeting and guides strategy for meeting. Asks for outcomes, conclusions, summaries.

hat (*thinking overview or process control*) but others can also be asked to contribute blue hat thinking in, for example, deciding where the group goes next.

In many ways this sounds an odd way to function, very different from the argumentative approach which often develops in a meeting. Using the hats in sequence to structure the meeting will ensure that the issue is looked at from all angles. Because it is the perspective of the particular hat which is being presented, people can give honest opinions without offending others. When the facts, feelings and intuition, critical views, optimistic views, creativity and control are all clearly identified and examined, then decisions may become self-evident. De Bono reports many instances of significant time savings in meetings and in making decisions when using this approach, with children and senior executives, and states that *'The Six Thinking Hats method may well be the most important change in human thinking for the past twenty-three hundred years'* (De Bono, 2000: ix). It is an approach which could be used in Problem-Based Learning (PBL) discussed earlier (Chapter 5).

CHAPTER SUMMARY

This chapter has considered some of the intellectual skills needed by students to make the necessary judgements about patient needs and the appropriate interventions. As qualified nurses they will need the same skills as they continue to develop throughout their careers, and have to make relevant decisions in whichever position they find themselves.

9 METHODS OF LEARNING AND TEACHING IN THE UNIVERSITY CONTEXT

INTRODUCTION

This chapter moves on to consider teaching and learning methods used primarily, although not exclusively, within the context of university-based teaching and learning and taking into account the various approaches that may be used within the curriculum. At different times the lecturer may be acting as a teacher imparting information or as a facilitator of student learning using very different skills. The aim is that lecturers will be able to select appropriate methods to achieve the necessary learning and the relevant outcomes.

Certain teaching methods are largely associated with traditional curricula, but most methods can be used within differing educational approaches. For example, a lecture is a core part of traditional programmes but can also be a resource within a more problem-based approach to learning. Many HEIs will have a large group of nursing students, for example 100 to 300 or more, and will need to choose teaching and interaction methods which the School can use effectively and efficiently with such large groups.

THE LECTURE

Billings and Halstead define the lecture as: a *'Teacher presentation of content to students, usually accompanied by some type of visual aid or handout'* (2009: 246).

This used to be, and probably still is, one of the most common methods used to transmit knowledge in nursing education. The planning and delivery of lectures is a core skill for all nurse educators and has the major advantage of being able to transmit a large amount of content quickly. It is a method that is particularly important with large groups of students.

Use and Planning of Lectures

Normally the teacher is the person who controls the content and delivery of a lecture. The contrast to this is in problem-based learning when a lecture may be requested by a student group specifically as a resource for the learning that the student team/group has determined it needs.

Lectures cannot provide all the knowledge that students need and should not regurgitate the content that is readily available in the selected textbook. Exley and Dennick have identified lectures as useful in the following situations:

- for communicating enthusiasm for the topic and motivating students to further study;
- for providing a structure or framework for learning about the topic;
- for tailoring material to the students' needs, examining relevant evidence from various sources and resolving conflicting evidence, clarifying complex or confusing topics;
- for providing current information including introducing recent, perhaps unpublished, research relevant to the topic;
- when using another different format is not viable (Exley and Dennick 2004a: 8).

However, Bligh (1998) summarises the detailed research evidence for the use and misuse of lectures, thus facilitating evidence-based educational practice:

- lectures are as effective as other methods to teach facts, but not more effective; (11)
- most lectures are not as effective as discussion methods for the promotion of thought; (13)
- lectures are relatively ineffective:
  - to teach values associated with subject matter, (17)
  - to inspire interest in a subject, (19)
  - for personal and social adjustment, (21)

  and thus changing attitudes should not normally be the major objective of a lecture; (17)
- lectures are relatively ineffective to teach behavioural skills. (22)

A lecture is an efficient method of teaching those aspects for which it is effective as one lecturer can teach many students at the same time. Fry et al. (2009) provide guidance on structuring a lecture to enhance its effectiveness (see Box 9.1).

Box 9.1 Effective Lectures (Fry et al., 2009)

- Creating and maintaining interest
  - Be enthusiastic and prepared
  - Use learning outcomes to clarify what they should be learning
  - Link to current news or activity, authentic problem or scenario, students' interests
  - Use examples and students' experiences to illustrate points
- Good structure and organisation with beginning, middle and end, using
  - Signposts to clarify structure and direction, links to previous or future lectures and between different parts of the lecture, highlight and emphasise key points
  - Vary demands on students: i.e. varying between lecturing and requiring different forms of active participation
  - Selected use of visual materials, web links, other artefacts, appropriate use of PowerPoint (see Chapter 12)
  - Limit length of periods of verbal presentation, with not too much content
  - Handouts: e.g. with gaps for students to add own notes, use of concept maps
- Student engagement
  - Encourage student participation using variety of activities, such as buzz-groups, worksheets, small group discussion fed back to all, peer-marked mini-tests (see Table 9.1)

Within an environment in which research is highly valued, and in many universities is still the main criterion for promotion, it is a strong temptation to use lectures for teaching even though the evidence cited above indicates that it may not always achieve the specified outcomes. It is important to recognise the shortcomings of lectures in promoting learning (see Box 9.2) but also to know how to adapt and utilise this method as effectively as possible.

Box 9.2 Disadvantages of Lectures (adapted from Quinn and Hughes, 2007)

- Lecturer control of the activity.
- Lectures do not cater for individual student needs.
- Pace of lecture does not suit all students.
- Lecturer's bias may be evident.
- Students hear material second-hand instead of from primary sources.
- Tendency towards student passivity during the lecture.
- Students' attention may wane.
- Students do not have to think during the lecture.

It is difficult to retain students' interest for the whole of a lecture of 50 minutes (the most usual length in HE) or more and it is not unknown for listeners to doze off during a less than scintillating lecture. The evidence supports the recommendation that a lecture should not last more than 20 to 30 minutes (Bligh, 1998) without using some different methods to stimulate the students and retain an appropriate level of alertness.

Student Involvement

Of considerable importance is incorporating a range of activities which will stimulate students' interest and encourage participation and interaction with the material being transmitted, thus facilitating understanding and retention. The range of activities which can be incorporated into a lecture will vary with the size of the student group and the arrangement of the lecture room. The least flexible arrangement is the large, tiered lecture theatre so beloved of many universities. Table 9.1 shows a number of stimuli and activities which vary what students hear, see or do, resulting in stimulation of attention, and which can be incorporated into a lecture. The first of these illustrates the role of lecturer as performer and, while some academic staff will have higher dramatic abilities than others, all should at least be able to present their material accurately, clearly, audibly and with variation in tone.

Some of these techniques can be used with any size of group, while some are only useful with smaller class sizes of up to about 50. Buzz groups of two to six members can be used for short discussions even within large classes of several hundred by getting students to talk to their immediate neighbours (up to three) and turn around to include those immediately behind (up to six). These are often used for short periods of

TABLE 9.1 *Stimuli and Activities within Lectures (from Exley and Dennick, 2004a; Fry et al., 2009; Bligh, 1998)*

Variation in what students hear	Lecturer varies pitch and intensity, speed of delivery and pauses to reduce monotony
	Sound bites and audio-recordings can illustrate points and add interest e.g. an interview with a patient
	Music can be used to illustrate points or to give students a break in a long lecture
Variation in what students see	Guest lecturers bring specialist expertise to a class but must be well briefed to ensure appropriate delivery which expands students' understanding. Input needs to be related to total module outcomes
	Visual aids such as flip charts, overhead transparencies, slide projectors etc., can be used, with PowerPoint probably now the commonest. Different AV-aids will alter the dynamics of the teaching session
	Demonstrations of structures or skills use models or samples as illustration
	Video-clips can be used to illustrate a particular activity or context
	Body language of the lecturer demonstrates interest or boredom with the topic
Variation in what students do	Give question or problem for individual thought and then small group sharing
	Present material (video/internet/demonstration) with instructions on what to look for
	Brief multiple choice question test - peer marking
	Problem solving in small group
	Discussion of research design or interpretation of findings
	Invent examples relevant to lecture topic and share with others
	Consider advantages and disadvantages of procedure or theory, then compare with lecturer's ideas
	Question and answer session (questions can be submitted in advance)

a few minutes, a couple of times during a lecture, when students carry out the specified activity. Such short (or longer) discussions, whether incorporated within a lecture or as the basic mode for the session, enhance learning and interaction with other students, as well as giving the lecturer a breathing space. They have value in developing relationships between students and lecturers, as well as promoting learning in various ways, as shown in Table 9.2.

Difficulties in Lecturing

Edwards et al. (2001) use case studies and reflection to consider a number of issues which can test both new and more experienced lecturers. The major issues affecting relatively inexperienced lecturers are performance anxiety and disruptive students. Figure 9.1 shows a concept map linking

TABLE 9.2 *Value of Discussion Techniques (from Bligh, 1998)*

Clarification:	Students may help to clarify concepts to each other, or the lecturer can do so when inadequate understanding is revealed
Feedback:	Lecturers receive feedback on their teaching
Consolidation of understanding:	Applying material taught or relating different parts of the lecture requires active thinking and aids understanding
Use concepts and terminology:	Using concepts and demonstrating the relationship between them aids comprehension
Practice specific types of thought:	Students can be given a task to analyse, synthesise or evaluate material considered in the lecture
Teaching relevance:	A task that uses the material taught but requires students to demonstrate application
Release tensions:	Listening to a lecture thoughtfully requires concentration and generates tension. A short break for a different activity will aid release of tension
Respite for anxious lectures:	Buzz groups give an anxious lecturer time to think and amend their planned lecture if necessary
Confidence for reticent students:	In small groups shy students are more likely to contribute to discussion and be listened to, aiding development of confidence
Building supportive relationships:	Working in small groups helps students to get to know others and develop friendships

causes of anxiety with approaches which can be used to help alleviate the difficulties through thorough preparation.

One of the issues that causes difficulties for lecturers is managing disruptions from, for example, students arriving late, using mobile phones during lectures, texting or chatting with neighbours, or even falling asleep (although in this case the student is not necessarily disruptive). A useful approach to minimising this is to work with the student group at the beginning to set ground rules for expected behaviour to pre-empt problems and ensure that one student cannot disrupt the lecture for others. A good relationship with students in which the lecturer is open and honest, and explains why particular approaches and actions are being used, is helpful in maintaining trust with students and promoting peer pressure to reduce disruption.

Experienced colleagues may be able to help with advice on how to deal with the occasional student who still causes difficulties. Discussion with the student's personal tutor (studies adviser) may be useful and may result in a joint meeting with the individual. If continued disruption occurs, most UK Schools of Nursing have a Fitness for Practice Committee to which such students can be referred for consideration of their behaviour as suitable or not in someone preparing to join the profession of nursing.

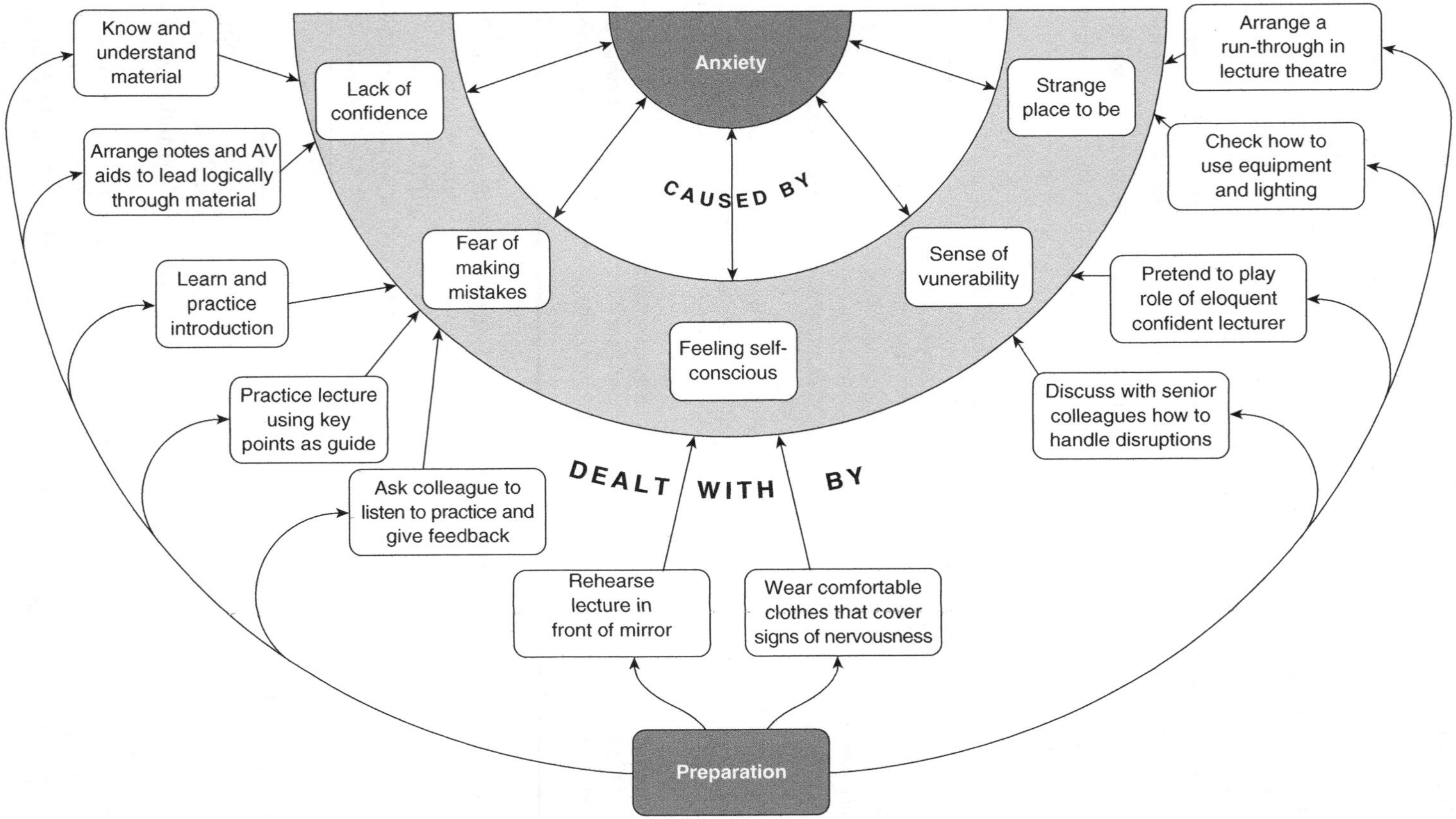

FIGURE 9.1 *Managing Anxiety through Preparation (derived from Exley and Dennick, 2004a)*

SMALL GROUP TEACHING (SGT)

As previously indicated, in contrast to lectures, small group teaching methods are useful for promoting thought and critical thinking, attitudes and psychomotor skills as well as the qualities identified as the aims of SGT (see Table 9.3). These qualities are the hallmark of a professional nurse and are essential outcomes of a pre-registration nursing programme. It is an approach that draws on the principles of adult learning (Knowles et al., 2011), however, both lecturers and students need to learn how to use SGT effectively to achieve the anticipated outcomes. Problem-based learning and its variants are founded on small group working, but also have potential for use in other educational approaches.

TABLE 9.3 *Aims of Small Group Teaching (Exley and Dennick, 2004b)*

Development of intellectual understanding and abilities	Clarifying concepts, theories, interrelationships and connections; thinking and problem-solving
Development of communication skills	Giving explanations, listening, questioning, presenting and defending a thesis, giving feedback
Personal growth	Testing values and attitudes, developing self-esteem and self-confidence
Professional growth	Acceptance of standards, values and ethics of the profession; use of models of nursing
Support for independence	Accepting personal responsibility for progress and direction of own learning
Development of group working skills	Group management skills, group roles - leadership, planning and organisation, support, setting tasks, monitoring progress
Reflective practice	Learning from successes and failures, develop understanding and planning future learning

Within small groups a wide range of different approaches can be used, which can provide many advantages over lectures. Table 9.4 summarises a range of these approaches and also includes SGT approaches that can be used in large groups. Small group working can use various methods of organisation to combine the value of SGT with the economies of scale related to teaching large numbers of students at one time:

- *Buzz groups*: As discussed above.
- ⋆*Snowballing* or *pyramiding*: Individuals consider a question, they join up in pairs and share ideas; these combine into groups of fours who negotiate a response, then into eights and so on to the sharing of ideas and answers across the whole group.
- ⋆*Cross-over groups*: Four individuals work together, then two swop with another group and share and further extend their response.

  [⋆ In both these approaches students can find themselves going over the same material again. Requiring groups in later steps to consider an issue related to but developing from the earlier stages minimises boredom.]

TABLE 9.4 *Approaches to Small Group Teaching (adapted from Quinn and Hughes, 2007; Exley and Dennick, 2004b)*

Categories	Examples	Group size	Notes
Tutor-led or facilitated SGT	Tutorials	4–12	Can be one-to-one, or 3–4 students with one lecturer, or controlled discussion led by lecturer or appropriate expert. Purpose related to size. Can also relate to personal tuition (or studies adviser) role of academic.
	Seminars	10–25	One or a few students present paper which is the basis for discussion within the group. Other students should prepare to be able to contribute. Can be used as assessed work.
	BPL groups	8–12	(Or other enquiry-based learning group.) Students work as group to analyse problem scenario, identify what they need to learn, and arrange learning process within group. Lecturer acts as facilitator.
Student-led SGT	Tutor-less tutorials	4–8	The lecturer determines the focus of the session, provides the framework, structure and resources. The student groups meet without a lecturer to carry out useful collaborative work.
	Learning sets	4–8	Learning sets act as a 'support and challenge' group, acting as resource to other members, aiding individuals to work through reflection. Used extensively in action learning when small groups work through repeated action learning cycles of: reflecting, learning, planning, action.
	Self-help groups	4–8	Small groups of students organise themselves to work together and help each other understand and learn. Also known as study groups or student support groups.
Virtual SGT	Virtual tutorials	4–12	Discussed in Chapter 10.
	Email discussions	4 upwards	
SGT in large groups	Syndicate work	10–100	Large class with overall task divided into small groups of about six students each. Each group given specific part of the overall task on which to work and report back.
	Problem classes	10–50	Students work in small groups on specified problems. Could be useful in nursing for developing skills in drug calculations, fluid balance, nutritional assessments, etc.
	Group practicals	10–100	Working on psychomotor skill development in small groups. Discussed in Chapter 10.
	Workshops	10–40	Extended SGT session (½ or full day) working towards achievement of set of outcomes through range of stimulating and relevant activities. Preparation for programme important, including breaks and plenary sessions for reports on progress.

- *Fish-bowling*: A small group of say eight students can be involved in discussion or problem-solving or role-play watched by a larger group around the outside. At intervals the larger group is invited to comment or make suggestions.
- *Syndicate working:* Small groups of students are given issues to research or work-sheets to complete, or write on post-its and position them on the wall or board to demonstrate ideas and their relationships. At the end of the session, they can give feedback to the whole class, or all students can view the post-it arrangements.

Planning SGT

Arranging SGT occurs within the structure and aims and objectives of the overall curriculum and the outcomes expected from the session need to be clearly identified (Biggs and Tang, 2007). The structure of the session needs to include preliminary work to make it easier for the group to work together. This will include introduction and ice-breaking, clarifying the role of the tutor and students, setting the ground rules, specifying the time available, specifying the tasks to be completed, and identifying who will carry out any necessary roles. Preparation also needs to include ensuring a suitable venue, arranging the room to facilitate interaction, and acquiring any resources which may be needed.

The tasks to be carried out relate to the content of Table 9.4, which considers different discussion techniques, and Table 9.2, which identifies the potential benefits for students and staff. Some specific techniques that can be used to promote thinking include:

- *Brainstorming*: Stimulates generation of new ideas and lateral thinking. In stage 1 many ideas are proposed, nothing is rejected. In stage 2, ideas are grouped, deleted, interrelationships identified and priorities specified.
- *Mind-mapping/concept-mapping*: Central idea or concept placed in the middle with related items surrounding the central concept, with lines to show relationships between the differing items (Figure 9.1 is an example). This helps to clarify relationships and facilitate understanding, but it takes time to develop skills in this approach.
- *SWOT analysis*: Analysis of proposal under headings of Strengths, Weaknesses, Opportunities, Threats. It is particularly useful in considering change management. Following small group work, a plenary session is held to identify appropriate actions.
- *Case studies/problems/case scenarios*: This is an in-depth analysis of a real-life situation to apply theoretical knowledge and develop problem-solving skills.
- *Role-play*: Students are briefed to play the roles of individuals in different situation relevant to practice. Following the role-play the debriefing analyses the situation and facilitates critical thinking about practice.

- *Simulations*: Real life clinical situations are imitated with mock patients (or animated models) and students playing the role of professionals. It enables students to confront clinical situations, analyse and carry out appropriate care within a safe environment (see Chapter 11).
- *Issue-centred discussion*: A small group has an open discussion on a specified topic and feeds conclusions back to the whole group in plenary session.
- *Problem-based learning*: As discussed in Chapter 5.

(Billings and Halstead, 2009; Exley and Dennick, 2004b; Fry et al. 2009)

Group Functioning (Race, 2005; Exley and Dennick, 2004b)

The importance of preparation for SGT by the lecturer has been indicated above, but preparing students for participation in group work is also important. They will be able to contribute more effectively if they understand how groups develop and can recognise the stages in this development, and understand the roles undertaken by group members. Belbin (2010) identified a number of roles that team members tend to assume, as shown in Table 9.5. Recognising the importance of the contribution made

TABLE 9.5 *Team Role Characteristics (Belbin, 2010)*

Role Type	Description	Weaknesses
Intellectual Roles	*Plant*: is creative and imaginative, presents new ideas	Ignores details, may not communicate well
	Monitor Evaluator: analyses and judges options	May be too critical, may lack ability to motivate others
	Specialist: provides specialist knowledge and skills, single-minded	Overlooks 'big picture', narrowly focused contribution
Organisational Roles	*Co-ordinator*: good chair, clarifies goals promotes decision-making, delegates well	May be seen as manipulative, delegates personal work
	Resource Investigator: develops contacts, explores opportunities, communicative	Overoptimistic, may lose interest after first enthusiasm
	Team worker: co-operative, diplomatic, perceptive, listens, averts friction,	Indecisive, can be easily influenced
Action Roles	*Shaper*: challenging, dynamic, drive and courage to overcome obstacles	May provoke others, may hurt feelings of others
	Implementer: disciplined, reliable, efficient, turns ideas into practical action	May be inflexible, slow to respond to new opportunities
	Completer Finisher: conscientious, looks for errors and omissions, finishes on time	Has difficulty with delegation, may focus on small details

by each role to the overall group functioning will help each individual to use their own skills towards the whole. The Six Hats approach (De Bono, 2000) in the previous chapter (see Table 8.6) may also be useful.

Quinn and Hughes (2007) also cite the work by Tuckman who described four phases of group development in reaching full effectiveness, and the final stage after completion. He identified these phases as follows:

- *Forming:* In the early stages of the group everyone wants to be accepted and so tends to avoid controversy. Thus meetings are comfortable but not very productive.
- *Storming:* As important topics begin to be tackled, disagreements arise and confrontations can occur, either about roles and responsibilities or the work being undertaken. Conflict is likely to mean that the issues are beginning to be identified.
- *Norming:* Conflicts have been resolved and everyone recognises the skills and experiences of others. They are prepared to listen to each other and to change their ideas. The group is functioning effectively, but is also resistant to change in case it reverts to the previous stage.
- *Performing:* In this phase the group has high morale, is working smoothly and well with flexibility and interdependence. Not all groups reach this level of function in which everyone is comfortable and their energies are directed towards the task.
- *Adjourning:* The task is completed and the members have to disengage from an enjoyable and fruitful activity, with pride in their achievement.

Some groups do not function as well as they ought and some thought is necessary about approaches to promote group functioning. The key point is good preparation, initiation and monitoring, so that students know each other and what they are meant to be doing, and are undertaking tasks appropriate to the group. The role of the facilitator is important in promoting group functioning; the key aspects of this role are teaching students how to function in a group and facilitating the development and agreement of ground rules. An example of ground rules for SGT which focus on respect, contribution and outcomes is shown in Figure 9.2.

Group working involves debate and discussion which can result in the development of conflict and hostility within a group. Some degree of conflict can be of value as students are challenged to defend their assumptions, and are forced to review their own values and understanding in moving towards agreement in the group. Resolution of the conflict can result in a deeper understanding of the subject. To minimise the risk of dysfunctional

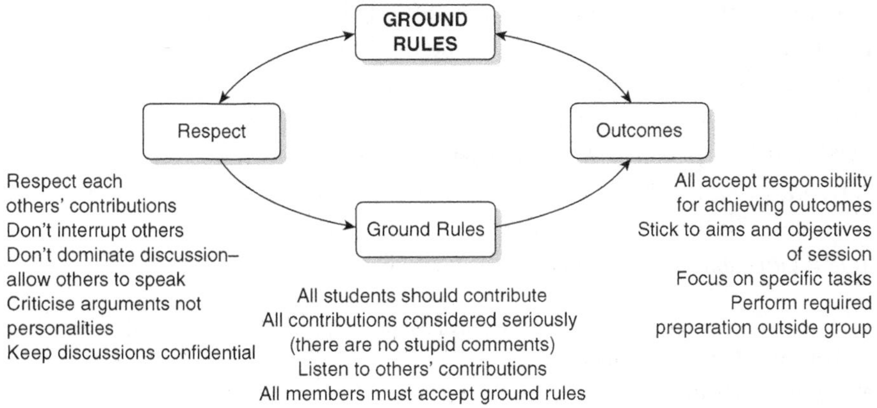

FIGURE 9.2 *Ground Rules for Small Group Teaching (Exley and Dennick, 2004b)*

hostility arising, the ground rules should emphasise that ideas and arguments are challenged – not people and their personalities.

Another key issue is managing the contribution of a group member who may dominate the discussion, or one who does not participate, or is completely cynical about the activity. Emphasising the ground rules and using peer pressure are important, but organising the group into small subgroups, valuing everyone's contribution, sometimes calling on a named individual to contribute can also contribute to managing these situations. An individual student may sometimes need to be counselled on the importance of group contributions to achieve the specified goals.

FACILITATION

As discussed in Chapter 5, problem-based learning and its variants involve small groups or teams of students working together with a facilitator to decide what they need to learn and arrange to access resources to acquire that knowledge or skills. The qualities and mode of functioning of the facilitator is crucial. As discussed in Chapter 2, Rogers identified *genuineness, acceptance and empathy* as essential for effective facilitation (Rogers and Freiberg, 1994). Encouragement of students who demonstrate creativity and critical thinking is crucial in supporting the development of these qualities in the professional nurse.

Over many years Heron has developed theoretical understanding and practical application of a model of facilitation for use in group situations, including in education, which involves learning through '*experience, action and practice … dealing with more external and technical skills, such as nursing and medical skills, … and with the theoretical knowledge that underpins such skills*' (Heron, 1999: 2). He identified six dimensions of facilitation which can be related to the functions of the stages of group working discussed above and a '*facilitative question*' in relation to each dimension:

- *Planning: How shall the group acquire its objectives and its programme?* This is the goal orientated aspect of facilitation.
- *Meaning: How shall meaning be given to and found in the experiences and actions of group members?* This cognitive aspect is about ensuring understanding of what is going on.
- *Confronting: How shall the group's consciousness be raised about* what it needs to face and how they may resist and avoid issues?
- *Feeling: How shall the life of feeling and emotion within the group be managed?*
- *Structuring: How can the groups' learning be structured?* What methods of learning will be used?
- *Valuing*: *How can … a climate of personal value, integrity and respect be created?* The important element here is creating a supportive environment in which students can be genuine and empowered. (Heron, 1999: 6–7).

The facilitator needs to be able to distinguish between the activities within the group which relate to each dimension, although they must be interrelated in application to form a coherent whole. The different dimensions of facilitation are expected to elicit different aspects of group activity and learning. The other key aspect of facilitation is the way in which each of these dimensions will be dealt with in relation to the decision-making. The mode applied will determine who will make the decisions in relation to each dimension and the aim is that the group of students will move through the three modes of facilitation:

- Hierarchical: the facilitator is making the decisions and guiding the learning through taking full responsibility for the decision-making about all the dimensions of learning.
- Cooperative: decision-making is becoming a collaborative activity between the facilitator and the group. The role of the facilitator is to guide the student group to become more self-directed in their decision-making about their learning.

- Autonomous: student group has developed to direct their own activities and make decisions about their learning needs and how these should be met. The facilitator has helped create conditions in which students are able to be self-directed in learning.

The knowledge and skills required for facilitation are very different from those needed for more traditional teaching approaches. Academic staff moving towards this form of working may need to arrange for some support from Staff Development to develop the necessary competencies.

DEVELOPMENT OF SCENARIOS

Clinical scenarios (commonly known as problems in PBL) may be used in pure or hybrid Problem-Based Learning as a major focus for student learning, or as an example which illustrates and applies material which has been taught in lectures. In the context of a pure PBL curriculum, these scenarios must lead students to identification of concepts and achievement of knowledge and understanding which meet all the standards specified by the Statutory Body. In hybrid PBL or other use of scenarios in learning, it is necessary to be clear what outcomes are expected from the group activity, and how these contribute to the overall module and curriculum outcomes.

Stanton and McCaffrey (in Barrett and Moore, 2011) discuss PBL as using *'real world problems as a context for students to learn critical thinking skills and problem solving skills and to acquire knowledge of the essential concepts of the course'* (Watson, cited in Barrett and Moore, 2011: 36). The key elements are that the scenario fully engages the students, stimulates their interest in learning, and guides them towards achieving the planned learning. Features identified as important in achieving effective problems are summarised in Figure 9.3 and ensure the scenarios are realistic, are structured to promote learning based on previous knowledge, and will stimulate group working. The careful use of ill-structured scenarios to provide additional intellectual challenge for students can be valuable.

In a PBL programme the learning outcomes to be achieved with each scenario need to be plotted against the outcomes for the module and

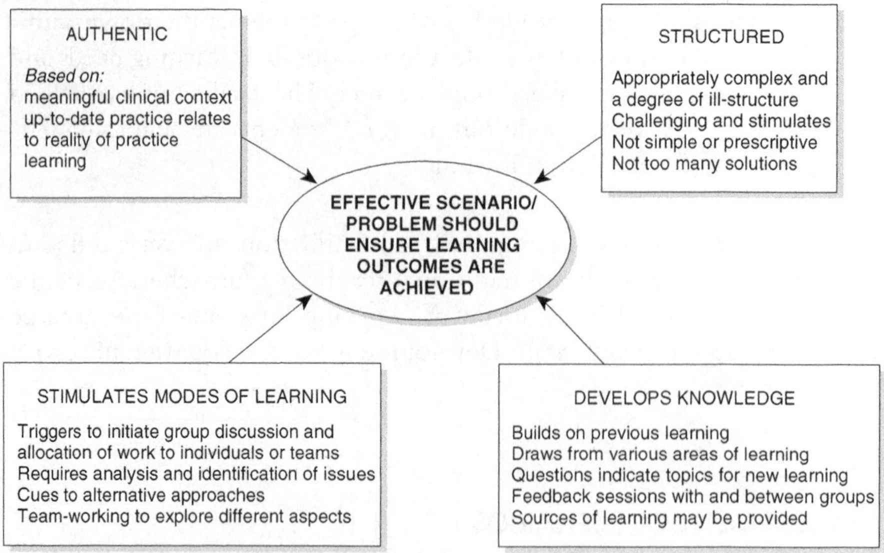

FIGURE 9.3 *Summary of the Key Features of Effective Problems (Barrett and Moore, 2011)*

programme. As students progress, the expected outcomes for each scenario must reflect the higher academic level to be achieved and the increasing depth and breadth of knowledge applied (Wilkie and Burns, 2003).

In developing the scenarios for any use, Korin and Wilkerson (in Barrett and Moore, 2011) discuss how problems can be brought to life by using video clips or role-play of, for example, a nurse admitting a patient and hearing about how the patient became ill. Jackson and Buining (in Barrett and Moore, 2011) discuss the use of design thinking in developing PBL scenarios which will promote imagination and creativity. Design thinking does not follow the logical, analytical pathway common in health sciences but is a process of exploration with extensive questioning. It has some similarities with brainstorming in that numerous ideas are generated and then choices are made from amongst them.

CHAPTER SUMMARY

This chapter has considered the selection of teaching methods used in the university context. Developing skills in using lectures has received considerable attention as the single most common teaching method used in HE but, while this method is valuable as a stimulus or to provide structure for learning, its value for developing critical thinking skills is limited. The importance of using methods which stimulate the development of critical thinking has been emphasised. While development of one's abilities as a facilitator of learning through small group work requires commitment and effort from the lecturer the outcomes for learning can be more effective. However, developing effective small group work requires support from within the School, along with recognition that preparation for such approaches takes time although time is later saved in promoting learning.

10 SKILLS AND COMPETENCE DEVELOPMENT FOR PERSON-CENTRED CARE

INTRODUCTION

Nursing is a practice discipline and the qualified professional must be able to apply the knowledge gained in demonstrating skill and competence in providing care. Opportunities to develop the values, skills and competencies required by a registered nurse have to be planned with care and are the major focus in this chapter. While the three elements are separated for purposes of discussion here, in reality they are integrated in the provision of person-centred care. This aspect of the course requires a major input from clinical practice: 50% of the programme (2300 hours) is practice learning with a maximum of 300 hours of this simulation based.

The values associated with person-centred care (PCN) are essential if high quality care is to be provided, and these are the most difficult to incorporate in the planning of a programme. They include care and compassion – which (with communication) is the first of the Essential Skills Clusters specified by the NMC (2010a). These are crucial attributes of a nurse and are often considered to be present or not as exemplified by the phrase 'she's a born nurse' and are characteristics sought for at selection. Although these values are demonstrated partly through communication, this is considered with other skills.

The word 'skills' is being used in this book to refer to separate tasks and aspects of care such as psychomotor or communications skills, which can be taught and practised in an artificial situation and then applied, refined and adapted to the individual in the practice setting. The development of intellectual skills has been discussed earlier. The range of skills involved in nursing can be classified in various ways but here we are considering the development of the groups of skills as follows:

- communication skills;
- personal care skills;
- fundamental clinical skills;
- technical clinical skills;
- leadership and entrepreneurial skills.

Competence is defined as '*the combination of skills, knowledge and attitudes, values and technical abilities that underpin safe and effective nursing practice and interventions*' (NMC, 2010a: 11). Within the NMC Competency Framework four domains of practice are identified: professional values; communication and interpersonal skills; nursing practice and decision-making; leadership, management and team-working (Figure 2.4), with a number of competencies in each domain. The six themes previously identified in this book (see Figure 2.5) can also act as a framework. However, to be competent means '*having the necessary ability or knowledge to do something successfully*' (OED, 2006) and the graduate nurse must be able to perform the totality of the expected role, by integrating the theory learnt with the skills acquired and the values instilled in order to practice high quality person-centred care. Approaches to facilitating the development of competence are discussed later in this chapter.

Selection of Skills and Competencies

One consideration in the selection of skills and competencies to be achieved is the type of clinical practice for which students are being prepared. There are two major developments in health care to be taken into account. The first is the increase in community-based care with considerable chronic illness management by nurses, more acute care in the community and a major focus on public health. Secondly, hospitals now contain an increasing proportion of critically and severely ill patients and perform growing numbers of day procedures. These and other changes in practice have considerable implications for the education of nurses.

In the UK, the four fields of practice (adult/general, children, mental health and learning disability) include many of the same skills and competencies but also incorporate those specific to the field of practice.

Taking account of the field of practice which is the focus of the programme, an analysis of the pattern of competencies required is helpful in ensuring that students learn the necessary skills for them to optimise their achievments in practice learning situations. They need to be able to contribute to patient care and to develop their ability to adapt skills to individual patients' requirements. Table 10.1 outlines the types of skills required across all fields of practice. In addition, each field has skills specific to its own area.

TABLE 10.1 *Outline of Types of Skills Applicable Across all Fields of Practice*

Communication skills (Burnard, 2002; Dickson et al., 1997)	Interpersonal skills: initiating interaction, questioning, reflecting, giving information, completing interaction
	Authoritative interventions: prescriptive, informative, confronting
	Facilitative interventions: cathartic, catalytic, supportive
	Other communication skills as appropriate to field of practice and context of care
Personal care skills	Promotes self-care when appropriate
	Uses skills to promote hygiene and comfort, positioning and maintaining mobility, eating and drinking, supporting elimination
Fundamental clinical skills	Patient assessment and observation
	Ensures patient safety, including through infection control
	Specimen collection and testing
	Simple wound care
	First aid
Technical clinical skills	Drug administration, orally and by injection
	Other technical skills as appropriate to field of practice and context of care
Leadership and entrepreneurial skills	Problem-solving and decision-making skills
	Organising, delegating and supervising care provision
	Record-keeping and clinical incident reporting
	Risk analysis, analysis of need for change and project planning
	Development of standards and guidelines

VALUES IN PERSON-CENTRED CARE

Values and beliefs were discussed in Chapter 2. Applied values are central to the practice of nursing and are demonstrated through **how** one provides care and are the main focus in person-centred care.

> There is no doubt that it (caring) is the factor which raises nursing from being simply a series of technical skills. (Grindle, 2000: 329)

The values expected of a nurse which demonstrate caring can be described as follows:

- Applies ethical principles throughout practice and maintains confidentiality.
- Maintains dignity, privacy and respect for individuals and values and accepts cultural and spiritual diversity.
- Demonstrates warmth, sensitivity and kindness, uses touch appropriately, and recognises and responds appropriately to emotional responses.

Person-Centred Nursing (PCN) (McCormack and McCance, 2010)

The PCN framework is shown in Figure 10.1 and demonstrates the sort of person-centred outcomes the majority of nurses would hope to achieve

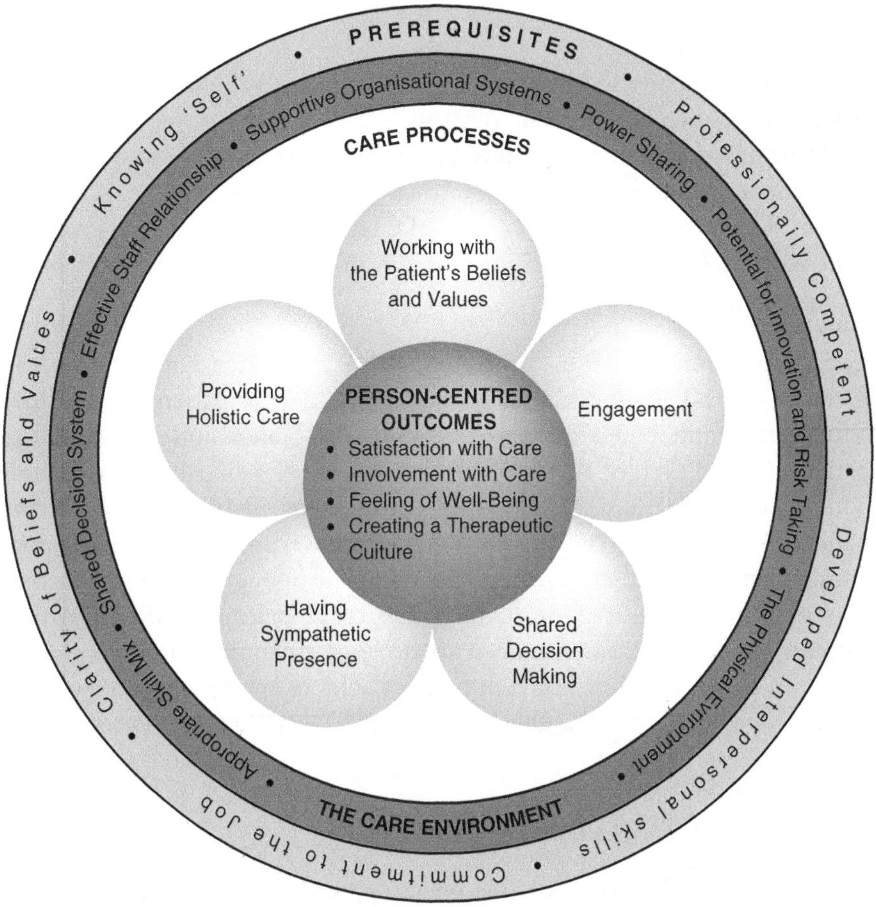

FIGURE 10.1 *The PCN Framework (McCormack and McCance, 2010: 34)*

through the prerequisites, managing the care environment and implementing the care processes. The care processes specified provide a structure to discuss the relevant values.

Working with Patients' Beliefs and Values

Valuing a person's individuality is central to providing PCN and to do this it is essential to get to know the patient, their values and what they understand about what is happening to them. Individuals are the result of their history and relationships and, for nurses to understand their patients in a way that enables PCN, they need to spend time getting to know them. Using a biographical or life stories approach to assessment has been proposed as useful, particularly with older people; knowing about their earlier experiences helps the nurse to understand their current behaviour and provide care that values their individuality (Clarke, 2000).

Shared Decision-Making

Based on the recognised importance of beliefs and values discussed above, shared decision-making is an obvious and necessary development. The nurse brings expertise to the interaction and negotiates as an equal with the patient, while making it clear that the final decision lies with the patient. The aim is to achieve a clinically effective outcome that is consonant with the patient's wishes and manageable within their lifestyle.

Engagement

Engagement refers to the 'connectedness' of the nurse with the patient, focusing on the unique interaction with the specific patient at that particular time, and based on understanding the beliefs and values of the patient. One difficulty that is identified is that of being blind to ethical considerations because of the total engagement involvement with the patient. However, three levels of engagement can be identified: total engagement, partial disengagement and complete disengagement, the second two of which permit a more objective consideration of the situation through reflection. Students need to develop an understanding of these stances and how to move between them to achieve an appropriate outcome acceptable to the patient and achieving satisfactory therapeutic results.

Having Sympathetic Presence

This has been defined by McCormack as

> an engagement that recognises the uniqueness and value of the individual, by appropriately responding to cues that maximise coping resources through the recognition of agendas in daily life. (cited by McCormack and McCance, 2010: 100)

This is comparable to the authentic concern (Christiansen, 2009) discussed below. It can be compared with the concept of empathy meaning *'the ability to understand and share the feelings of another'* (OED, 2006), which is frequently considered as important in nursing. Sympathy is often understood as *'feelings of pity and sorrow for someone else's misfortune'* but perhaps more relevant here, it is also defined as *'understanding between people, common feeling'* (OED, 2006). Whether one can fully understand someone else is arguable and 'sympathetic presence' is possibly a more accurate term although empathy is also used.

Providing Holistic Care

This incorporates the physical and technical, as well as psychological, sociocultural and spiritual, aspects of care in which patients want the nurse to be professionally competent. It acts as the route through which the previous care processes are utilised and only in combination with these can be fully effective in achieving the person-centred outcomes shown in Figure 10.1. Achievement of the skills and competencies for this aspect of PCN is discussed later in this chapter.

Identifying and Developing Values for PCN

Within the pre-registration nursing programme it is important to enhance and develop the ability to express the values discussed above in the care of patients and interaction with families. But, how does one achieve this? Media reports have not always been complimentary about the quality of caring provided by nurses and other healthcare professionals, although it is difficult to imagine anyone entering the nursing profession who does not want to help people. Nevertheless, it is essential that the teaching team consider how they can enhance and encourage qualities that are present and promote the individual's abilities in applying them in providing PCN.

A qualitative study by Christiansen (2009) examined manifestations of *'authentic concern'* in Norwegian nursing students' relationships with patients in which body movement, voice and style expressed their attitude towards their patients. This does mean that students must be involved and able to recognise and understand the patient's experience and feelings; an involvement which may result in an emotional response in the student requiring support from mentor or peers. Students also have to *'cultivate a personal style in correlation to expectations of the nurse's role'* (Christiansen, 2009: 432). To present authentic concern to their patients, students need to develop their own *'dramaturgical awareness'* (Goffman cited by

Christiansen, 2009) through which they become aware of how they are presenting themselves, in order to be able to demonstrate their compassion and empathy.

It is often stated that caring can only be taught at the bedside with real patients but more than this is needed. The challenge is to find ways in which 'the patient' can be brought into the classroom to help students recognise and value these attributes. Patient involvement in teaching and developing teaching materials was discussed in Chapter 3.

Grindle (2000) has examined the use of the arts in nursing education to promote care, compassion and empathy (and by extension, the values for PCN) through emphasising the human aspects of nursing, matching the ideas considered in the Caring Curriculum (Bevis and Watson, 2000). Examples of literature, poetry, drama, advertisements, music, songs, paintings and photography, both serious and humorous, were used in the preparation of Nurse Tutor students who were then able to incorporate these within their own teaching of student nurses.

> The high imagery nature of the arts seems to generate more reflection over time ... further enhancing and developing the degree of learning. (They) have the capacity to convey to the students the need for the various components of caring – competence, respect, compassion, empathy and insight. (Grindle, 2000: 327)

In addition, student nurses reported an increased capacity to understand, learn and remember material presented in this way, illustrated in Box 10.1.

Box 10.1 Student Nurse's Comment on Arts in Teaching Nursing (Grindle, 2000: 291)

A student nurse's response to reading The Death of Ivan Ilyich by Tolstoy (cited by Grindle):

... nurses and doctors should be aware of the (feelings of) isolation and 'impending doom' that accompanies the sick role. The lesson I learned from the book is ...

(a) *patient's need to know about the disease,*
(b) *what it's doing to that individual socially, personally ...*
(c) *(the need to understand) pain and ways to deal with it effectively,*
(d) *(the need to) discuss the dying process so that the patient can let go with dignity.*

Students tend to remember from this mode of learning; a student nurse in the study commented on the impact of poetry on memory:

> ... I would remember those poems ... you would remember how someone feels in a situation where they felt so alone ... then there is the child who had asthma, and again, I haven't been able to look up the notes on this, but I can recall it fairly quickly. So that is the kind of impact – fairly quick recall of those classes. (Grindle, 2000: 281)

TEACHING SKILLS

A number of authors (cited in Exley and Dennick, 2004b) have described frameworks for psychomotor skill development, three of which are shown in Table 10.2. Simpson in particular gives a detailed description of stages of the process through which students progress.

A number of approaches can be used to develop students' abilities in carrying out skills:

- teaching about the importance of the different skills;
- role modelling by academic staff and mentors;
- role play and discussion.

TABLE 10.2 *Frameworks For Psychomotor Skills Development (cited in Exley and Dennick, 2004b)*

Author	Stages	
Simpson (1966: 112)	Level 1:	*perception* – identifies need to perform skill
	Level 2:	*set* – learner ready to act
	Level 3:	*guided response* – skill performed after demonstration
	Level 4:	*mechanism* – skill has started to become habitual
	Level 5:	*complex overt response* – accurate and efficient performance
	Level 6:	*adaptation* – skill internalized and can be adapted
	Level 7:	*origination* – creative development of new skills
Fitts and Posner (1967: 113)	Cognitive phase:	skill being learned
	Associative phase:	performance becoming skilled
	Autonomous phase:	skill automatic, carried out without thinking about it
Miller (1990: 113)	Knows about:	knowledge about skill, not yet practising it
	Knows how:	knows how to do skill and is practising it
	Shows how:	basic competence under controlled conditions
	Does:	competent and independent practitioner in working conditions

While these three approaches are usually used in this order, often they will all be used in development of a specific skill and some will be integrated and used together. These are implemented within the university context followed by practice under supervision in the real world of clinical practice. Reflection and discussion are relevant to learning individual skills but are of greater importance and are discussed later in relation to competence development. Box 10.2 demonstrates a basic system for teaching psychomotor skills through which students enhance their understanding and smooth performance with feedback from the teacher.

Box 10.2 System for Teaching Psychomotor Skills

1. Short introduction to the when and why the skill is used, preparation of the patient, any other key issues about particular skill
2. Silent demonstration of complete skill in real time, including equipment and patient preparation for procedure and after care, clearing away, and leaving patient comfortable
3. Skill demonstrated again with detailed commentary which explains principles and rationale for different aspects of the procedure, including a focus on patient safety and comfort. Students may ask questions
4. Instructor may carry out procedure again following students' instructions and asking instructions to ensure students' understanding of the procedure and its uses
5. Students then practice the procedure individually or in groups with feedback from each other and the instructor

Teaching about the Importance of the Different Skills

As discussed in Chapter 9, lectures are not effective for teaching skills. However, short lectures in association with, or just prior to, demonstration do have a role to play in providing knowledge about the rationale for the use of particular skills within a wider learning context. Adults need to know why they need to learn something before they will commit to putting the necessary effort into learning (Knowles et al., 2011), and this applies to skills as well as knowledge. Thus this is an essential aspect of skills teaching. However, the use of a PowerPoint presentation in skills teaching can result in a passive response from students: PowerPoint equates to lecture, and lecture can equate to switching off. A short talk or briefing is more appropriate.

Role Modelling by Academic Staff and Mentors

Social Learning Theory (Bandura, 1986) indicates that students tend to model their behaviour on what they see demonstrated by those they respect; in this context these are their university lecturers and their clinical mentors. Thus lecturers who show respect for their students and demonstrate compassion with professionalism when students have difficulties provide a model of the type of behaviour expected in professional practice.

In relation to psychomotor skills teaching, modelling (or demonstration) is an important part of the process. To support modelling, the use of imagery can facilitate learning of some skills, using the PETTLEP model to improve the level of performance in motor skills through the following components:

- Physical: the position and equipment used;
- Environment: identical to the environment where the skill would usually take place;
- Task: the task being imaged;
- Timing: the imagery being completed at the same speed as actual execution of the task;
- Learning: adapting the imagery as skill proficiency is gained;
- Emotion: emotions associated with completion of the task;
- Perspective: can be either internal (first person) or external (third person).

The use of this approach has been shown to significantly enhance performance in measuring blood pressure but not in carrying out aseptic techniques (Wright et al., 2008) supporting the premise that it is useful in learning skills with a strong motor component, but less so in those requiring recall and adaptation. Further research is needed in this area.

Simulation, the use of videos and other technological approaches useful in relation to teaching are discussed in Chapter 11.

Role Play and Discussion

This approach can be used in developing various types of skills in nursing. The differentiation between role play and simulation is blurred as one merges into the other. Various forms of role play and simulation are used in relation to developing personal care skills, fundamental clinical skills, technical clinical skills and also leadership and entrepreneurial skills.

Role play usually involves the students playing different roles in an unscripted situation watched by others in the student group. Each player is briefed for their own role and they all work through the situation, using their own words within the character they have been briefed on. Following completion of the role play which typically lasts 15 to 20 minutes, discussion focuses on clarifying reasons for actions and words displayed, alternative approaches that could have been used within the situation, and feelings elicited within the players and the observers. This can be a valuable way of increasing students' understanding of how patients may feel in different situations. Video recording role play can allow all participants to review the interaction again and enhance their learning. Communication skills training (CST) (Dickson et al., 1997) is a specific form of role play useful in developing interpersonal interaction skills including communication, teaching, and leadership and entrepreneurial skills. The following chapter builds on this section in considering simulation with and without using technological support.

DEVELOPING COMPETENCE

While some limited degree of competence can be developed in a simulated situation, it can only be acquired and demonstrated fully within the real situation of practice in clinical contexts. The support provided during practice learning is essential for developing competence in the role of a nurse.

The importance of experience with reflection for learning has been discussed earlier in this chapter and is central to developing competence in the role of a nurse. One of the major factors in practice learning is becoming able to make the correct decision for the appropriate use of skills, to combine and integrate different skills for use together (for example communication skills with empathy while carrying out clinical skills), and to be able to predict and prepare for future events.

Key elements in promoting development of competence are: preparation for the clinical setting; practice learning context; learning activities in the clinical setting; and the support, supervision and feedback from qualified professionals. Stuart (2007) emphasises the close interrelationship between assessment, supervision and support in clinical practice but in this book, assessment of skills and competence is dealt with in a later chapter.

Preparation for the Clinical Setting

In a sense the whole pre-registration programme is preparation for working in the clinical setting. However, a number of issues need consideration shortly before students commence a practice learning module to enable them to obtain maximum benefit from the experience. Obviously it is important that students know what they are meant to be achieving, so it is important to examine the outcomes for the particular practice learning experience. They also need to have learnt the necessary skills and knowledge for the clinical environment to which they are allocated. Using scenarios to present clinical problems, and requiring students to use clinical judgement in PBL in order to deal with the situation, helps to build critical thinking skills and prepare them for the reality of clinical practice (Forbes et al., 2001). This can include working within the interprofessional team (of nursing and medical students) in a simulated admission ward and evaluating performance on:

- collaborative teamworking;
- effective leadership;
- ability of the team to prioritise the workload, and
- competence in clinical performance. (Ker et al., 2003)

Students also need to be quite clear about 'supernumerary status' in which they are primarily present in a clinical area to learn to be a nurse, not to meet the needs of patients, although they will only become skilled professionals through the practice of giving care. On a busy clinical unit it is very easy for students to become bound up in the practicalities of nursing patients and, while there may be emergencies when this is necessary, they have to understand that they are there primarily in a learning role. If the service role becomes routine, they should discuss the situation with the appropriate clinical or university staff member. The roles of the different staff involved in supporting practice learning are discussed later.

One of the most important aspects of preparation is consideration of values and role. The application in the clinical context of the ethical and professional principles previously studied and the NMC (2010b) *Guidance on Professional Conduct for Nursing and Midwifery Students* are reviewed. The care processes for PCN as discussed above need to be emphasised.

Particularly before their first clinical experience, students need to learn how to use their time effectively for learning in the clinical setting. Based on assumptions about adult learning, Sharples (2009) provides a useful guide for students covering such topics as:

- how to learn as an adult and be motivated to overcome difficulties encountered during practice learning;
- understanding the role of their mentor and how to work effectively and accept feedback from him or her;

- understanding different learning styles and the importance of using all of these for different types of activities;
- preparing for clinical practice to reduce anxiety and make the most of the learning opportunities;
- being a self-regulated learner who takes responsibility for identifying and negotiating opportunities for learning in clinical practice and applying the different styles of learning to the stages of the experiential learning cycles (see Figure 8.1).

It is important that students understand the limitations of their knowledge and skills but also that they should recognise their strengths. Beckett et al. (2007) found that students were aware of their limitations but did not recognise the importance of their relationship skills and their understanding of ethical principles in practice. They perceived the emphasis as being on technical ability but needed support to see the value of the contribution they could make and were making to care, partly because of their limited experience and fresh view of the situation. It is important that students know what to do if they see practice which does not meet the standards they expect. Their mentor and practice education facilitator are the first people to discuss it with but if they do not feel that their concerns are being taken seriously, they need to know that they will be listened to sympathetically by their link lecturer or personal tutor. If appropriate they will need to be supported through any further action taken by the employer and the NMC.

Practice Learning Contexts

During the programme each student will be allocated to a number of different settings. Placements are planned to enable the achievement of the expected behaviours at the different stages of the programme as specified by the NMC and to acquire the approved course outcomes and competencies required by the NMC for registration.

Within the placement allocations students must have the opportunity to achieve the following:

- become proficient in the necessary range of skills;
- become comfortable and able to demonstrate development in the processes which contribute to PCN;
- understand the major contexts of care within their field of practice, including institutional and community care;
- contribute to decision-making at a level appropriate to their stage of education;
- recognise the importance of health promotion in all areas of nursing;
- develop the ability to manage their own and, later in the programme, others' workloads;
- achieve development through the stages of the programme as specified by the NMC (2010a).

Practice learning experiences can be arranged in differing ways but need to take account of the changes occurring in practice. Thus, community experience is important along with a variety of hospital experience to develop the necessary skills and competence for acute care. Some programmes are now aiming to arrange for half of the total practice learning time to be spent in community settings.

Students prefer longer rather than shorter placements and short allocations of less than seven weeks are often found by students to be stressful and sometimes of limited value (Warne et al., 2010). However, particularly in adult nursing, there are a considerable number of different settings in which nursing takes place and it is not possible to provide lengthy allocations in all the different areas. A 'hub-and-spoke' arrangement can be used, through which each student is allocated for a substantial period, perhaps 12 to 16 weeks or longer, to a particular clinical area in which PCN will be possible and they will be able to achieve a number of the specified outcomes. From this setting they can visit other relevant settings for short 'taster' experiences. The mentor for that student will arrange visits or short periods of experience in relevant settings and time with specialist nurses or other health or social care professionals (see Figure 10.2). These will enable each student to gain a good understanding of the breadth and depth of care available. The

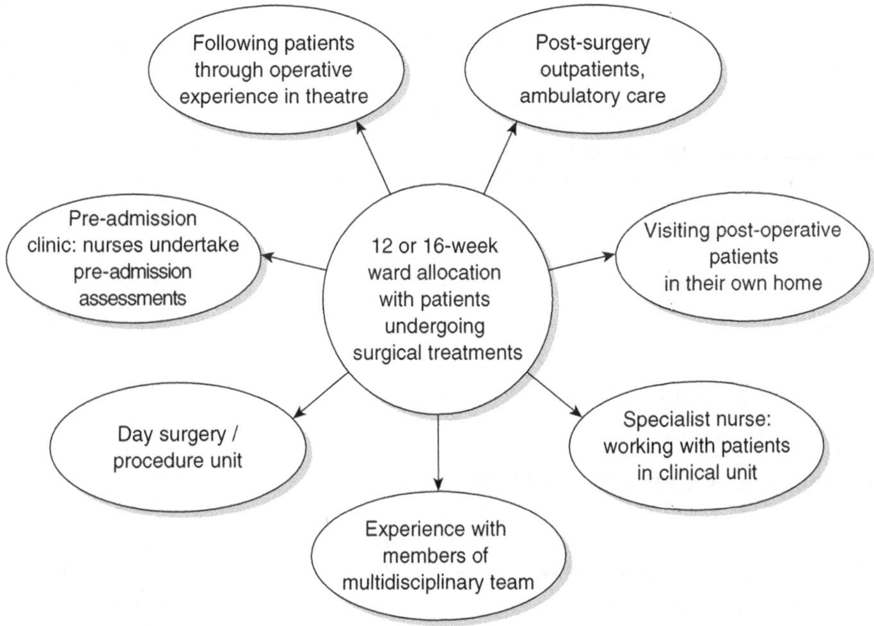

FIGURE 10.2 *Example of 'Hub and Spoke' Practice Learning*

'hub' based mentor will provide stability for the student, demonstrate the relationship of the 'spoke' experiences to the main focus of the overall experience and help to set them within the broader context of nursing.

Pre-registration students may undertake up to six months (not more than 17.5%) of the programme in an international setting and this may be:

- a period of theoretical and/or practice learning of not more than four weeks, which may include direct care but which is not summatively assessed, or;
- a period longer than four weeks of theoretical and/or practice learning which may include direct care that is summatively assessed and contributes to the overall achievement of programme outcomes. (NMC, 2011a: 1)

The contribution of international experience to the overall outcomes of the programme must be clearly defined and, if over four weeks in length, the experience must meet all the NMC (2010a) Standards. It is essential that a suitable person is available to provide necessary support and supervision, and that students are fully prepared as specified by the NMC (2011a). There is considerable work involved in arranging these, but such experiences can greatly enhance students' understanding of the breadth and depth of nursing in different cultures and healthcare systems.

In the UK, pre-registration nursing education programmes must include a period of 12 weeks practice learning towards the end of the programme, to enable students to consolidate their learning and demonstrate an acceptable level of competence. This enables mentors and sign-off mentors to be confident in their decision to confirm that the outcomes necessary for registration have been met (Chapter 13). Equally important for students is the development of confidence in their own ability to perform at the level expected of a registered nurse. Until relatively recently this experience has been undertaken in institutional settings, but with the increased emphasis on community care, this may now be undertaken in the community. Students undertaking such experience were permitted to visit patients on their own when their mentor considered them ready. The value of such experience was demonstrated in a small qualitative study (Anderson and Kiger, 2008), the results of which are summarised in Figure 10.3.

Learning Activities in the Practice Setting

In the UK, the HEIs work in partnership with the service providers to deliver nurse education programmes and they are jointly responsible for ensuring that suitable learning opportunities are provided. The HEI is required to carry out regular audits with the clinical manager to ensure that the environment and opportunities are suitable for practice learning. Almost all activities can provide learning opportunities for the motivated

FIGURE 10.3 *Themes from Students Undertaking Community Final Placement (Anderson and Kiger, 2008: 446)*

student with an enthusiastic mentor. The use of a learning contract at the beginning of placement clarifies the objectives, what the student needs to learn within the placement, and how they will be achieved, and is signed by student and mentor. Within the principles of adult learning, the student may identify areas of particular interest which they wish to learn about, in addition to those specified for the placement. An example of the type of form used is shown in Figure 10.4. As the student proceeds through the practice learning experience, notes are kept on progress in achievement.

Action plans are developed when a student is not progressing as well as anticipated. While these seem similar to learning contracts, the difference lies in how they are used. The learning contract is essentially learning focused while the action plan (Figure 10.5) is focused on assessment of achievement. All areas where the student is not achieving as expected are identified and if they are not achieved the student will not have met the outcomes for the placement. Within the new NMC (2010a) Standards, these are formative assessments, except at the end of the specific stage of the programme, but are indicative of student development.

Overall the mentor is responsible for ensuring that the student is exposed to opportunities to meet the learning outcomes for the particular clinical experience. Mentors arrange experience so that students build up the requisite skills and competence through their time in practice, starting with relatively straightforward situations and progressing to more complex ones. Mentors also provide feedback and encourage reflection on the practice undertaken.

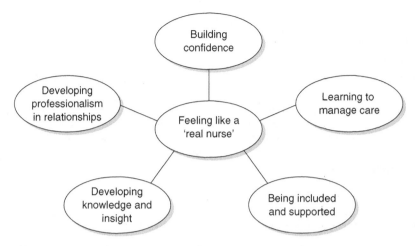

LEARNING CONTRACT				
Name of student:			Cohort:	
Placement:			Mentor's name:	
Learning needs	Objectives	Resources and strategies	Target date	Evidence
What do I want to learn? – topic area	What do I want to have achieved at the end of my learning? – specific objectives	How will I learn, and who will help me? – learning strategies	Date of achieving learning	How will I know I have achieved my intended learning?
Pre-contract Signature of student:			Date:	
Mentor's signature: Date:				
Name of link lecturer/practice educator: Name of personal tutor:				
Comments on achievement of contract objectives: Signature of student:			Date:	
Mentor's signature:			Date:	

FIGURE 10.4 *An Example of a Learning Contract (Gopee, 2008: 27)*

ACTION PLAN		**Mentee's name:**		**Mentor's name:**	
Mentee's learning needs	Specific objectives to be achieved	Who will help mentee achieve the objectives and how?	Other resources required	Achieve by dates	Evidence of achievement of objectives
AGREEMENT OF ACTION PLAN Mentor's signature		Date:	Mentee's signature		Date:
ACHIEVEMENT OF OBJECTIVES Mentor's signature		Date:			

FIGURE 10.5 *An Example Of An Action Plan (Gopee, 2008: 165)*

Mentors will also facilitate students in contributing to the work of the multidisciplinary team and developing their knowledge of the role of the different team members. Understanding the contribution to health and wellbeing of, for example, physiotherapists, social workers and others enables students to collaborate effectively with different members of the team. Students can also learn specific skills to apply in giving care, such as learning from the Speech and Language Therapist how to feed someone who has had a stroke. In addition, time spent with specialist nurses also helps students to recognise the scope of nursing practice.

A number of different staff groups are involved with practice-based education, contributing in different ways to students' development in achieving the necessary skills and competencies and applying theory into practice. A collaborative partnership in which all understand everyone else's role and work to facilitate student learning is essential to enable students to obtain maximum benefit from their clinical experience.

Interaction between peers can also contribute to learning. Other students can play an important role in helping their peers to adjust to a new clinical setting and to deal with the sometimes distressing situations they encounter. While their mentors are crucial in supporting students, their peers can often empathise more readily with their feelings and provide insights into their situation from the position of another student. While undertaking a particular practice learning placement, and indeed during theoretically-focused sections of the curriculum, students may form small learning groups which meet at regular intervals to share experiences, discuss progress in relations to learning outcomes, identify opportunities for learning and generally support each other. Of particular value is teaching and support provided by more senior students to help new students fit into the clinical setting.

CHAPTER SUMMARY

The focus of nursing education is to prepare nurses able to provide high quality person-centred care. Reinforcement of the values, development of the skills and integration of these with the requisite knowledge into the competence required of a qualified nurse is the key aim of nursing education. The use of different approaches to practice learning and the ways in which this can be arranged in the clinical setting have been discussed. Issues to be considered in relation to the selection of appropriate placements have been considered. While all the issues considered in this book are important in different ways, the content of this chapter is central to the enterprise of educating nurses.

11 TECHNOLOGY IN NURSING EDUCATION

INTRODUCTION

This chapter deals with issues related to technology, which is now playing an important role in nursing and in nursing education. In planning a curriculum the resources required need to be identified and the team needs to work out how to use their current facilities most effectively, while also identifying additional technological requirements (within the budget available). Information about resources needs to be included within the course document. Figure 11.1 identifies a range of ways in which technology impinges on nursing students. These include the clinical and management aspects of care, as well as academic uses, and skills and competence development. Nursing practice is using computerised information systems for care planning, patient results management, discharge planning, duty rosters and a range of other activities. To use these effectively, students have to become competent in nursing informatics.

Four ways in which information technology (IT) can enhance initial and continuing education for healthcare professionals are:

- Transmission of quality content;
- Support of lifelong learning;
- Flexibility of access;
- Improved communication networks. (Haigh, 2004: 548)

Increasing the use of online learning materials has extended the opportunities for learning to take place at the student's choice of time and place.

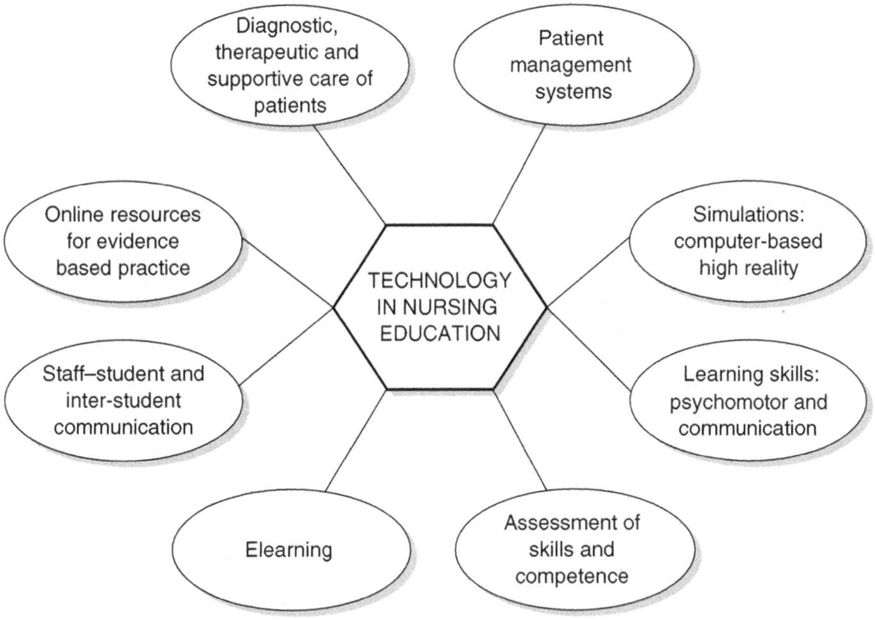

FIGURE 11.1 *Technology in Nursing Education*

In addition, within nursing education we have moved a long way from the early practical rooms where injection technique was practised using oranges, through a period when many of these rooms were removed because clinical skills were expected to be taught with patients in the clinical environment, to nursing skills laboratories where skills and competencies can be learnt initially in a safe environment. Nursing skills have become a central focus in pre-registration programmes, integrated with the other aspects of the programme, and the nursing skills laboratories are becoming increasingly important with, in many HEIs, students having access to the facilities for individual or small group practice whenever they wish. The nursing skills laboratories vary considerably in the sophistication of their layout and equipment. Some of these have substantial amounts of highly sophisticated simulation equipment while others achieve comparable results with less complex (and less expensive) resources. Effective use of these approaches involves the application of educational principles supported by the technology (Twomey, 2004). Technologically-based innovations for assessment have also been developed.

The use of these new resources can help to provide high quality and consistent opportunities for learning for students within the current situation of large student numbers and cuts in funding for HE. It also provides opportunities for Continuing Professional Development (CPD) for qualified nurses in practice that might otherwise have been inaccessible. However, academic staff need preparation and support to use these facilities effectively.

COMPETENCE IN INFORMATICS

The importance of competence in using computers has grown as IT systems are introduced into healthcare for patient management, and the intra- and internet are increasingly used for inter-professional communication. Moreover, evidence-based practice necessitates access to appropriate evidence online. In HE, IT competence is also essential in order to access the learning resources available. In addition, many universities now have a Virtual Learning Environment (VLE) which aims to assist students in the management of their learning. However, students need to develop the necessary skills to operate such systems. On entering university, most students have the basic skills of word-processing, email and accessing the web but many need further preparation in IT use for academic and professional purposes throughout their programme. A Canadian study (Jetté, 2010) of nursing students finishing their college-based education found that all responding students used a computer, while almost all used email and the web at home and 50% had undertaken a word-processing course. However, the numbers who had had training in using PowerPoint, searching databases, using computerised nursing or clinical information or clinical-administration systems dropped significantly (30% and less).

IT in Education

At an early stage additional preparation in IT is needed both to deal with various issues which are of concern to staff, and to develop other skills which will enable students to study effectively, including:

- ethical and safe use of the web;
- limitations of the web and evaluation of websites;
- how to access databases and carry out a literature search;
- to understand plagiarism as an academic crime, to clarify what it is, how to avoid it, and the range of penalties which may be applied.

Some of these issues, particularly using databases and plagiarism, will need revisiting at later stages in the programme as students move towards undertaking dissertations. They will also need to learn to use other IT resources including effective use of PowerPoint for presentations, although they also need to understand its limitations. PowerPoint tends to reduce material to an easily-presented format, lacking analysis; it can show outlines but detail needs to be supported with handouts (Tufte, 2003).

In many universities students are given an email address as a major means of communication with staff and other students. This is particularly useful when students are dispersed while on clinical placements. In many HEIs it is made clear that staff will only reply to emails using the university provided email address.

Virtual Learning Environment

It is stated that '*a VLE should make it possible for a course designer to present to students, through a single, consistent, and intuitive interface, all the components required for a course of education or training' (Wikipedia, 2011).* Most universities now have a VLE, a web-based learning environment which enables all students to access the resources, support and communication mechanisms that they need. Each institution will develop their own website which will provide administrative, educational and social materials through a range of tools. An example of tools available on one VLE (University of Ulster, 2011a) is shown in Box 11.1. Online discussions or chat rooms may or may not be included on the web home page, which can be customised to suit the individual student.

Box 11.1 Example of Tools in a VLE (University of Ulster, 2011a)

Announcements	Calendar
My Courses	My Organisations
My Tasks	User Directory
My Grades	Personal Information
Training and Support Available	Address Book
Send Email	

VLEs can vary in scope. Many universities have a system which will deal with all aspects of the student's programme – all modules/courses are dealt with through the one system. However, they can be more restricted in scope, as demonstrated by Edwards et al. (2008) who describe a VLE for undergraduate students which focuses specifically on working with older people.

IT in the Health Context

Depending on the IT distribution and use within the health services, students will also need to learn about the clinical and administrative systems in use. The stage in the course at which this is introduced will depend on the point at which they will be coming into contact with these systems in practice. The management component of the programme in particular should focus on the administrative programmes in use. However, while students need to learn about and recognise the systems in practice, in many health service organisations they are not permitted access to them. As equal partners in nursing education, these organisations need to facilitate the preparation of students for all aspects of their role as registered nurses including use of the IT administrative systems.

IT resources can also be extremely useful for professional development and there are now many resources available, including online educational programmes about different areas of practice and professional issues, and resources for helping to maintain a professional portfolio. One example is the Development Framework developed by the Northern Ireland Practice and Education Council for Nursing and Midwifery (NIPEC, 2011) which provides a broad range of professional development resources for Registered nurses and midwives. It provides resources in five areas:

- an online professional portfolio which can be developed and maintained on the website;
- competence assessment tools which enable nurses to identify their own learning needs;
- learning activities of varying types and sources to which individuals can gain access;
- career planning resources for the present or future job;
- a guide to help development of new roles.

In addition, there is a student section of the website developed in partnership with the three universities in Northern Ireland. Students can be introduced to this during the first semester and use it throughout their educational programme. This incorporates information in three main areas:

- electronic portfolio: where students can prepare their own portfolio to record their achievements and reflections as evidence of their development as they progress through their programme. Access can be permitted for those involved in their assessment to selected aspects of their portfolio to provide evidence of their learning;
- learning activities: helps the student to identify their own learning style and explore opportunities for learning through information about a wide range of different learning activities;

- career planning: provides information about different career paths to help students begin thinking about their strengths and what jobs may be suitable for them in the future.

From all sections the student can gain access to information about reflection and can store their own reflections. Following qualification, on entry of their PIN graduates can transfer their materials to the main section of the Development Framework for Registered Nurses and continue to maintain their portfolio. NIPEC guarantees the confidentiality of the individual's materials.

PREPARATION FOR PRACTICE

Introduction

Technology can assist in the learning of clinical skills and the development of competence in management of clinical situations in simulated environments within the HEI. Students need to understand the principles of the equipment in use within clinical settings and, with the help of their mentors, to become competent in managing the apparatus in practice. Some of this equipment will be introduced within the HEI as part of preparation for practice.

A number of approaches using technology can help to achieve accuracy and sensitivity in the performance of psychomotor skills, to enhance awareness of clinical situations and facilitate development of clinical judgement. These include the use of videoclips, web-based simulations to produce a virtual environment, and simulated patients using varying levels of sophistication. Most schools of nursing have skills laboratories to facilitate this learning.

Principles of Simulation

The NMC Standards now permit 300 hours of simulation for practice learning within the 2300 hours of required practice learning (NMC 2010a). A simulation has been defined as:

> a mock up of a real situation that allows students to learn or practise their skills, abilities and behaviours without putting anyone at risk. The situation is carefully managed so that the experience is meaningful. The observer will gain enough information to provide the student with valuable feedback for future use where appropriate. (NAMS cited by NMC, 2010c)

While limited simulations has been used for many years, the facilities now available allow much more realistic situations to be used in skill and competence development. Jeffries (2007) has described simulations along a continuum in relation to the extent to which they resemble reality, as indicated in Figure 11.2. Role play comes at the lower end with electronic mannequins which demonstrate high biological reality at the higher end. However, high biological reality does not necessarily correspond with high social and psychological reality. These are dependent on the contribution of the teaching staff in planning and the quality of the role play of the participants in the scenario.

Low Reality ↓	Case studies Role play	⋯▶ to educate about patient situations ⋯▶ to immerse in clinical situation
Moderate Reality ↓	Training models e.g. IV arms	⋯▶ to practise psychomotor skills
Fairly High Reality ↓	Computer-based clinical scenario	⋯▶ practising problem-solving and clinical decision-making
High Reality	High fidelity mannequin with adjustable signs and symptoms	⋯▶ practising patient observation and clinical decision-making in response to changing conditions

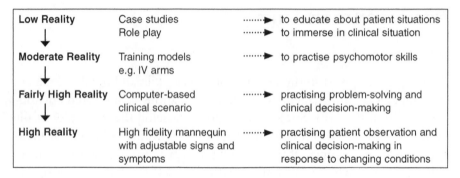

FIGURE 11.2 *Continuum of Reality in Using Simulations (Jeffries, 2007)*

Many academic staff are creative in developing scenarios and methods for facilitating learning using simulation. In some simulations, senior students can contribute to the design of scenarios as part of PBL. A framework which identifies the key elements to be considered provides a guide for the development of simulation scenarios (see Figure 11.3).

Using the framework shown, simulations must be carefully planned to be effective. Initially, the overall objectives must be determined depending on the stage of students in their programme, the availability of facilities including staff expertise, and the anticipated contribution to the programme outcomes. The details of the simulation need to take into account the level of overall fidelity of the simulation and how it will be managed to incorporate problem-solving and enhance student learning. The management of the debriefing is an important issue as it facilitates learning through integration of experience and reflection.

Evaluation considers the quality of learning in relation to acquisition of knowledge and skills, but also the appropriateness of decisions made using critical thinking and problem-solving, and student satisfaction with this mode of learning.

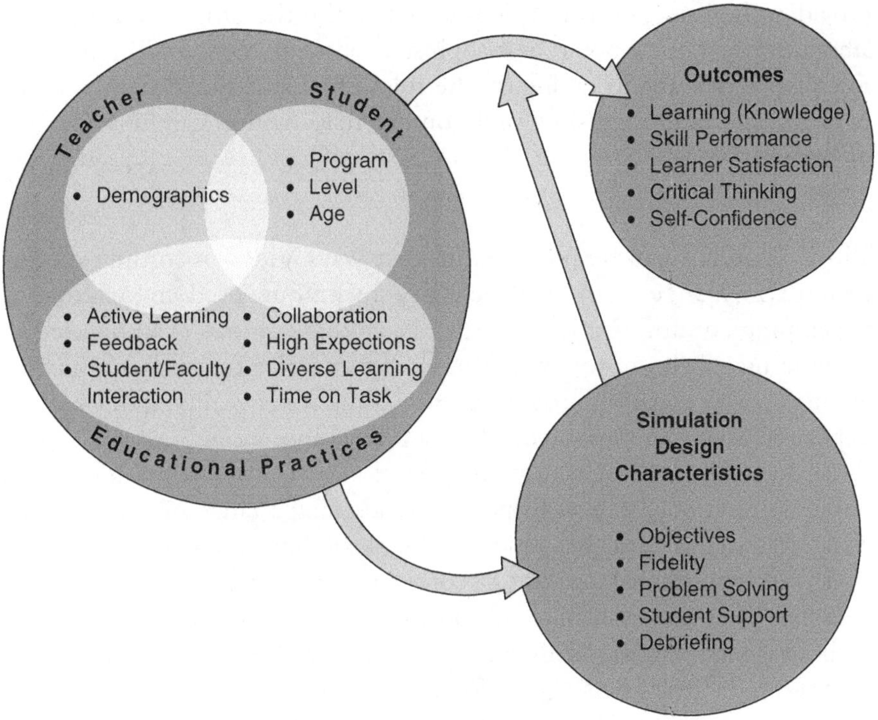

FIGURE 11.3 *The Nursing Education Simulation Framework*

Source: Jeffries, P.R. (2007) *Simulation in Nursing Education: From Conceptualization to Evaluation*. Reproduced with the permission of the National League of Nursing, New York.

Resources

Clinical Skills Laboratory

The clinical skills laboratory is usually a simulated ward environment, although some HEs also have a simulated home setting. These are an important resource for staff to model skills and for students to practise the skills they are learning. When feasible, video-taping the performance of skills (as in Communication Skills Teaching (CST) below) helps students enhance their level of competence (Emerson, 2007). For students to see the detail of the presentation and to receive adequate supervision during practice the group size needs to be relatively small, commonly about 25 to 30 – it is therefore expensive in terms of staff time with the large student groups now common.

The skills laboratory can include a number of very expensive electronic mannequins which can be programmed to exhibit varying signs and symptoms, enabling different clinical scenarios to be presented and requiring students to demonstrate clinical judgement and decision-making. The disadvantage of these is that, unless the teacher organises it through introducing effective role play, there is low social fidelity and the complexity of providing holistic care is not demonstrated. On the other hand the skills laboratory may incorporate less sophisticated equipment and be used for role play with students taking on the roles of patient, nurse, family members etc. and practising skills and competencies within carefully planned scenarios.

Video Materials

Video materials can be used in different ways. Video-recording of student performance with feedback is a technique used in relation to developing communication skills, and a similar approach can be used in developing psychomotor skills. Video clips can also be used as inserts in lectures or in elearning programmes to bring some reality about patient experiences to the knowledge-focused teaching.

To deal with lack of reality, Kelly et al. (2009) investigated the use of online instructional videos as models for learning a range of clinical skills. They found that students enjoyed the flexibility and self-management aspects of using these, but did not consider that this replaced the lecturer's demonstration and availability for answering questions. The use of videos with an online workbook linking theory to practice, and supported by a pocket-sized *Clinical Skills Quick Reference Guide* within practice, has been a valuable resource for first year student nurse learning (Carlisle and Scott, 2011). Similarly, short (2–3 minute) video clips showing different ways of dealing with difficult situations were produced. They were available for students to revisit as they wished in combination with lectures, with the aim of enhancing self-efficacy in such situations. Although not a controlled study, these video clips resulted in a significant enhancement of self-efficacy over time (McConville and Lane, 2006) and provided effective support in learning.

Skills Development

Psychomotor Skills

Psychomotor skill development is frequently carried out within a nursing skills laboratory with the most common mode of use being '*teacher demonstration, followed by student repetition and practice until the students become confident and competent … (which) facilitates self-paced learning*' (Wellard and Heggen, 2010: 41). They are generally recognised as being a safe environment in which students can practise and develop their clinical skills. They are most commonly modelled on acute care settings, so are of limited (but some) use in preparation for mental health and learning disability fields of practice. Jeffries et al. have compared using a skills laboratory for lecturer-directed skills learning with an interactive self-directed learning system in which pairs of students work around learning stations where they follow the guidelines to practise the particular skill, learn the content from interactive media, and discuss study questions and research evidence presented. The four dimensions they examined were:

- General principles: underlying principles that need to be known when performing a selected nursing skill;
- Process/mechanics: the actual procedure for performing the skill;
- Client teaching: information the client must have prior to, during or after the procedure;
- Critical thinking: simulated events, questions, or situations presented that place the students in real-life situations requiring students to synthesize and apply the information they have learnt. (Jeffries et al. 2002: 15)

There were no significant differences between the groups in knowledge or ability to carry out the skill, but the self-directed learning group were significantly more satisfied with their learning.

Communication Skills Teaching (CST)

CST is a valuable technique to help students develop their communication skills. The most suitable accommodation is a specifically developed interpersonal skills training suite of several pairs of recording and playback rooms with closed-circuit television (CCTV). The recording rooms contain some furniture which can be arranged to suit various scenarios and contain microphones and remote controlled cameras with the TV monitors, video recorders and controls in the recording rooms (Dickson et al., 1997). However, CST can be carried out in any room large enough to allow several subgroups to participate.

CST involves role playing of interaction to practice a particular aspect of communication and consists of three stages: sensitisation, practice and feedback. Table 11.1 shows the micro-skills to be developed and then the clinical communication contexts and, later in the programme, leadership and management scenarios into which the micro-skills are integrated. Scenarios related to differing skill sets are developed. Approaches to teaching some of the different types of communication skills are discussed in detail by Burnard (2002).

TABLE 11.1 *Communication Skills and their Application (Dickson et al., 1997)*

Basic communication micro-skills	Non-verbal communication Questioning Listening and attending Reflecting, reinforcing and encouraging Information-giving and explaining Initiating and terminating interactions
Clinical communication combining micro-skills	Taking nursing history Providing comfort and reassurance Patient teaching Giving bad news Preparing a patient for discharge Pre-operative preparation Communicating with elderly people and stroke patients Helping families communicate with critically ill members
Leadership and management skills	Communicating with other members of the healthcare team Dealing with complaints Organising nursing teams Giving report Giving and receiving supervision Managing team meetings

The three stages of CST are summarised here but discussed in detail by Dickson et al. (1997):

- *Stage 1: sensitisation.* This is an essential stage in CST in which students learn about the process of CST, recognise their own skill level, understand the range of micro-skills they will be developing and the skill sets they will be learning to use in clinical contexts. Box 11.2 indicates some of the approaches that can be used in this stage of CST. The key element is that students recognise the importance of developing their communication skills to a high level of performance through thoughtful practice.

Box 11.2 Approaches to Sensitisation in CST (Dickson et al., 1997)

- Short lecture/discussions, possibly including buzz groups.
- Handouts and readings to identify relevant psychological and sociological terms.
- Relational exercises which portray elements of the communication process.
- Discriminating skills used in 'live' modelling by the lecturer, video recordings, audiotapes or written transcripts to form the focus for discussion.
- Modelling an experienced therapist (nurse) talking with a client (patient) demonstrating the target skills during the communication.
- Focusing students' attention on the relevant skills.
- Retention encouraged by visualisation or using imagery.

- *Stage 2: practice.* This stage enables students to learn to use communication skills through simulation using role play. A staff member, other nursing student, drama student, willing patients or trained individuals play the patient role, and individual students practise the micro-skills and later the integrated professional skills. The use of CCTV is particularly valuable to enable students to recognise the difference between what they think they are doing and what they are actually doing. They have the opportunity to perform the professional role for which they are preparing, and to gain confidence in their ability to communicate effectively. When in the clinical situation students continue to practise their communication skills with real patients with different problems and conditions.
- *Stage 3: feedback.* This is the final essential stage in CST having been shown to be necessary for improving performance (Baker, Daniels and Greeley cited by Dickson et al., 1997). Feedback can be considered theoretically as providing motivation, reinforcement or information, but practically is likely to be a mix of all three. The role of the lecturer is important in helping students to become comfortable with both giving and receiving feedback in discussion with peers and lecturer.

TABLE 11.2 *Feedback Characteristics (Dickson et al., 1997)*

Extrinsic vs intrinsic	Intrinsic feedback is internal to the interaction itself and is responded to in order to achieve the necessary goals. It is important that students develop the ability to recognise and respond to intrinsic feedback. However, extrinsic feedback is an effective method of promoting skills learning but needs to be gradually removed as performance develops.
Results vs performance	Value of results or performance depends on student's performance. Feedback on both often provided, with lecturer facilitating comparison of performance with the model previously shown.
Concurrent vs terminal	In most CST sessions, feedback is provided at the end. However, feedback can be provided via an earpiece during the intervention, particularly in training of therapists.
Immediate vs delayed	Delay in providing feedback should be kept to a minimum, although the use of video replay allows some delay up to 24 hours while still being effective.
Positive vs negative	*'feedback is more effective when it contains a moderate amount of positive feedback with a selected and limited amount of negative feedback'* (Brinko, cited by Dickson et al., 1997). When negative feedback is necessary, it should be: • sandwiched between positive information; • self-referenced (i.e. to the student's performance) rather than norm-referenced; • 1st or 3rd person, not referring to 'your performance'; • factually not emotionally based; • include positive alternatives; • sensitive to self-esteem of student. Feedback should be constructive
Descriptive vs prescriptive	Descriptive feedback needs experienced students able to recognise what should have been done. Encouraging reflection may be all that is required to enhance performance. Prescriptive feedback includes more evaluation of performance when information about what should have been included is needed.

Some of the feedback characteristics found to be of value are shown in Table 11.2. The most important achievement is for the student to recognise and respond to self-feedback when they have reached a level of understanding and sensitivity to be able to evaluate their own performance accurately and continue to improve.

SIMULATION

There are various ways of simulating events. These include: computer based events; using sophisticated mannequins programmed to demonstrate physiological changes; less sophisticated simulations using scenarios with students playing different roles; external events involving other organisations.

In a review of the literature on simulation in nursing education, Sanford (2010) identified a number of advantages and disadvantages of using simulation. The advantages identified from several studies cited by Sanford were:

- the ability to experience a crisis situation before meeting it in clinical practice;
- being able to evaluate and reflect on the activities in a safe environment;
- artificially creating situations which students may not otherwise meet;
- enhancing the effective use of overcrowded, hard-to-get clinical sites.

Students report that simulation exercises add a welcome variety to their learning experiences and provide an opportunity for them to think and feel in the manner required in practice, but at a slower pace. This allows them to experience how theory underpins practice and to envisage how they will respond when the actual demand is made on them in a practice setting.

Sanford (2010) reported that students said simulation:

- was a bridge between classroom teaching and skills learned in the lab;
- provided realism in the scenario;
- was superior to reading about a particular disease or condition;
- provided depth of experience;
- improved their self-confidence;
- allowed them to understand the gravity of what could happen in practice when a patient is unwell, and enhanced awareness of e.g. allergies and medications;
- helped them learn to work as team members and to collaborate with one another.

Application of Simulations

Simulating aspects of the practice setting when teaching clinical skills, communication and decision-making processes allows students to practise in a safe learning environment. There are numerous examples where this approach has been found to be of value, but others where limited benefit has been found. Some examples are given below of simulation at different stages in the programme.

- Simulation has been used with students in the first year to teach patient safety practices, specifically hand washing and patient identification although with limited sustained improvement (Gantt and Webb-Corbett, 2010). However, it is recommended that continued practice with simulation can enable these skills to become second nature.
- Second year students worked through simulation practice of assessment, planning and implementation of patient care, including administration of medications, which was followed by debriefing and time for additional learning. On repeating a comparable simulation, the number of medication errors was significantly reduced compared to a control group. Students were '*thrilled for this experience as it helped them identify their knowledge gaps and provided them with a safe opportunity to learn without potentially harming their client*' (Sears et al., 2010: 55).
- Learning about managing cross-infections either through study groups considering a scenario with or without a teacher, or by simulation. The simulation experience '*made the students more aware of how complex each scenario was, and they experienced many aspects they had not thought of*' (Mikkelsen et al., 2008: 669). It was stated that the increased staff time found to be required in this study would make it difficult to use this approach widely in the curriculum. However, not all authors agree with this.

Simulations are particularly beneficial when students need to integrate their knowledge and skills in complex situations such as assessment and planning care for the acutely ill or deteriorating patient. Some examples given below demonstrate the application of the principles of simulation. Medium to high simulation practice was used with students near the end of their programme in preparing for the complexity of their management assessment, followed by a questionnaire to evaluate the experience (McCaughey and Traynor, 2010). Results under five main headings demonstrated the value of simulation through the effects on:

- students' perception of clinical effectiveness: the majority considered that abilities to provide holistic care for patients, and patient safety would be enhanced.
- students' perception of their professional development: well over 90% of the students reported they were '*able to identify areas for improvement in their practice and learn from their mistakes*' (831).
- helping to link theory to practice: simulations were regarded as very helpful in preparing for practice, although some students commented on lack of simulation authenticity.
- perceived preparation for management assessment in year 3 undergraduate nursing students: students' skills for their management assessment were enhanced, although anxiety was also increased.
- student preparation for their role as a registered nurse: '*Simulation was an extremely useful teaching example to highlight the challenges faced in clinical practice*' (831).

The value of this study is in the '*prospective benefit of increased competence and safe practice of practitioners following exposure to simulation*' (McCaughey and Traynor, 2010: 831).

A series of low reality simulations involving role play and debriefing including reflection can be used to help students develop their understanding of mental health issues and approaches (see Box 11.3). With ingenuity and care large parts of the curriculum can be covered in this way.

Box 11.3 Simulation of a Mental Health Nursing Visit

Background: Peter, aged 45 years, is married to Jose, 43 years. Their eldest son John (19) was diagnosed with autism aged 5. John has experienced a first episode of psychosis in recent weeks and spent time as an inpatient. He has been discharged to the care of a community psychiatric nurse.

Situation: The community psychiatric nurse makes an appointment to meet the family for the first time and wishes to discuss with John the importance of concordance with medication. During the visit Jose gets very emotional about her son having a mental illness and starts to cry. John remains agitated and states that he continues to hear voices in his head.

Students play all the roles in the scenario, which can be extended to include some or all of the adolescent children and the son with learning disability, general practitioner, consultant psychiatrist.

Debriefing: The mental health nursing students explore the different perspectives and develop their understanding of how a diagnosis of mental illness affects the patient and all members of the family. They apply their knowledge of psychological therapies and approaches in considering appropriate interventions.

Cardiopulmonary resuscitation (CPR) is a skill many students are nervous about doing in clinical practice and simulation provides an opportunity to work as a team in identifying early risk factors and managing cardiac and/or respiratory arrest in a non-threatening environment. This is an experience which cannot be guaranteed in practice learning experience and is usually taught and assessed through simulation. This is often carried out on a developmental basis with students developing in competence throughout the programme.

An example of a simulation with final year students, which is applied to competence development incorporating clinical skills but also leadership and management skills associated with chaotic and unpredictable situations, is carried out in the University of Ulster pre-registration programme for Disaster Relief Nursing (see Box 11.4). This involves both adult and mental health nursing students and is carried out in collaboration with the British Red Cross. Related to this area of work, students also report considerable learning from the experience of participation as casualties in major incident simulations involving the emergency services.

Box 11.4 Simulation in Disaster Relief Nursing

Third year students on the BSc Hons in Nursing participate in a Disaster Response exercise simulating emergency response after terrorist attacks. Casualties are brought to a front-line healthcare facility consisting of a casualty clearing station, a 10-bed emergency ward and a Survivor Reception Area. A Voluntary Ambulance Service is provided by British Red Cross, Order of Malta and St John Ambulance to transport casualties. Social services and police provide staff for the Survivor Reception Area.

Up to 30 undergraduate nurses, from the University of Ulster, staff the casualty clearing station, emergency ward and provide nursing support to Ambulance Services and Survivor Reception. They manage these facilities across a 12-hour period and communicate with other simulated agencies, i.e. local hospitals, military, police and ambulance in the assessment and management of mass casualty situations.

Adult and mental health nursing students participate using their different areas of expertise to care for casualties with physical injuries and psychological trauma. Year 2 nursing students from the University of Ulster act as casualties and family members. They are able to provide invaluable feedback on experiences of being victims of a disaster.

Virtual Environment

This is an example of adaptive media in which computers *'alter their state in response to the user's actions'* (Laurillard, 2002). In the nursing context this can be a computer-based simulation of a ward in which students can respond to the model presented by feeding in their decisions about ward management or care of individual patients. The simulation changes enable students to see the consequences of their actions. Feedback on performance and discussion within the groups will help their understanding and develop competence.

Possible Disadvantages of Simulation

The major disadvantages of simulations are related to the lack of evidence to support its use, the cost of high reality simulation equipment and the demands on academic staff of the time involved in developing scenarios and planning the teaching sessions. There is limited evidence that high reality simulation is more effective in promoting learning than less sophisticated approaches. Cant and Cooper (2010), in a systematic review of simulation-based learning in nursing education, found that in one study this approach was superior to lectures in promoting knowledge. However, there was little variation between the efficacy of simulation learning methods and other interactive approaches such as clinical seminars, videotaped simulations or case study presentation. Factors which were used in studies found to enhance learning are shown in Table 11.3 and can all be used in moderate and lower fidelity simulations. There is anecdotal evidence that if even moderate reality simulation exercises are planned carefully and the scenarios are clinically current, valuable learning can be achieved without excessive staff or technological resources. The essential factor is the linking of experience with reflection.

TABLE 11.3 *Simulation Components Used by Effective Studies (Cant and Cooper, 2010: 12)*

Physical environment	Manikins in applicable clinical setting with equipment orientation
Curriculum-based scenarios	Clinical care scenarios based upon curricula, incorporating best practice guidelines
Academic support	Academic staff throughout the simulation
3-step simulation process	Stepped learning process based on (i) briefing, (ii) simulation and (iii) debriefing
Exposure	Repeated simulation exposure in individual or teamwork settings

ONLINE LEARNING

A major use of technology in education is providing learning materials through computers used in various ways including:

- PowerPoint presentations and handouts made available to students online;
- a course delivered totally online with electronic communication between teacher and students which can enable those at a distance to access a university course;
- blended learning with elearning materials studied in combination with face-to-face learning activities.

PowerPoint Presentations (PPPs) and Handouts Online

Many universities now expect PowerPoint presentations and handouts to be placed online in advance of lectures to help disabled students to prepare for lectures. However, these materials are probably the most common aids used with lectures and the unlooked for side-effect of this strategy is that many students download these materials and then do not bother to attend the lecture. The challenge for academic staff is to prepare materials which guide preparation for face-to-face teaching and also encourage attendance. Some short preparatory reading followed by questions to be considered, gaps to be completed or issues to be identified which will be addressed in class may mitigate this lack of attendance

There is considerable variability in how PPPs and handouts are used and in the preparation of lecturers to use them effectively. The approach for promoting successful learning is to consider lecture, PPPs and handouts as an integrated package with each element making a different contribution (see Figure 11.4). The mechanics of using PowerPoint is easily acquired and Box 11.5 provides some guidance in preparation of the PowerPoint materials to be presented.

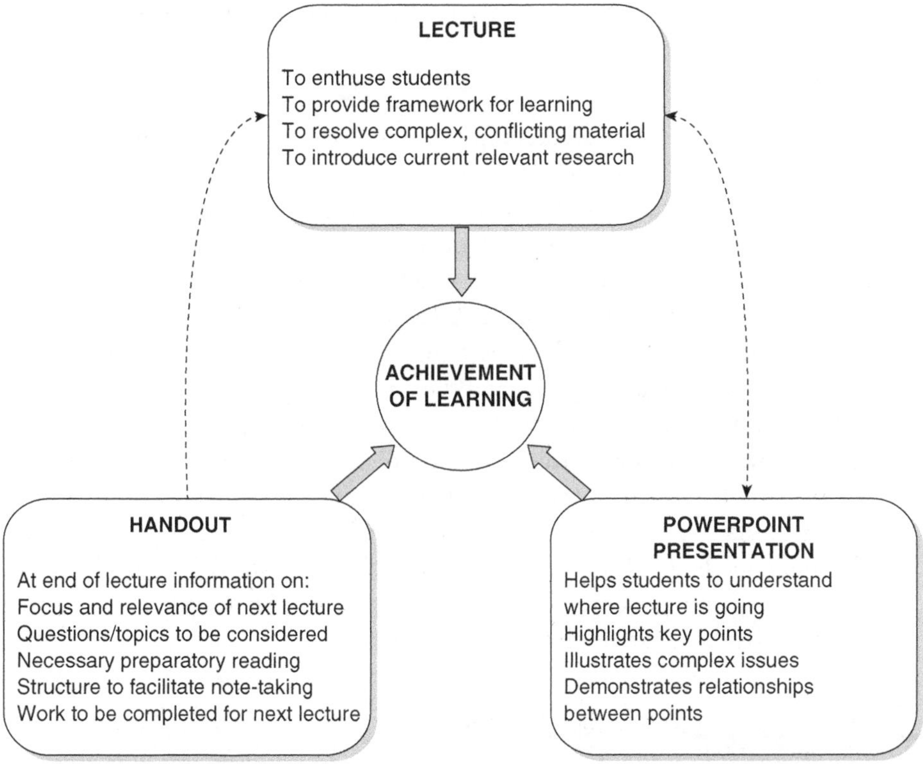

FIGURE 11.4 *Lectures, Powerpoint Presentations and Handouts In Promoting Learning*

Box 11.5 USING POWERPOINT

Points to consider in preparation of presentation:

Think about how you are going to use PPPs within lecture

Do not read out loud what is on screen – talk about the content indicated

Do not put too many words on screen: about 6–8 lines of text, 8 words per line

Selected use of images can be helpful

CHECK VISIBILITY FROM BACK OF LECTURE THEATRE

Do not use too many slides – about 1 per minute

Use animations only when necessary to illustrate difficult concepts

Requiring academic staff to place these materials online in advance of the lecture is largely to meet the needs of students with visual or hearing disabilities. Following the advice in Box 11.5 may mean that these needs are not met and other approaches will be needed. Arranging to make video-recordings to be available online after the lecture may deal with this issue, and advice from student support can offer other guidance as necessary.

Elearning

Twomey (2004) discusses theoretical issues underpinning online learning (elearning) and proposes that the most appropriate approach is a constructivist one in which the teacher is the facilitator for students to achieve an understanding of the topic themselves. A problem-solving approach in which students are involved in discussion and collaborative achievement of knowledge and understanding is suggested. However, much elearning material is based on standard instructional approaches and the particular approach used needs to fit the academic's particular teaching style and the aim of the course being delivered.

Developing elearning materials to promote effective learning is complex and requires application of thinking and time. Clark and Mayer's (2008) book brings together much of the relevant empirical research and from this they have identified a number of principles which should underpin developing elearning (see Table 11.4). Within the book, guidelines for different approaches to elearning are presented based on these principles to act as a valuable resource for those developing such materials.

TABLE 11.4 *Principles for Elearning Development Based on Empirical Research (Clark and Mayer, 2008)*

Multimedia principle	Use words and graphics rather than words alone
Contiguity principle	Align words to corresponding graphics
Modality principle	Present words as audio narration, rather than on-screen text
Redundancy principle	Explain visuals with words in audio or text: not both
Coherence principle	The addition of material just because it is interesting can detract from learning
Personalisation principle	Use conversational style and virtual coaches
Segmenting principle	Break a continuous lesson into bite-size segments
Pretraining principle	Ensure that learners know the names and characteristics of key concepts

Fully Online Learning

Elearning may be used alone for students studying at a distance – in nursing, these are most likely to be qualified nurses undertaking CPD. Achieving online the group interaction, shared identity and mutual support which is frequently a characteristic of the normal university experience is a challenge to be met by those teaching online, and methods that can be used are discussed by Macdonald (2008). These can include online discussion groups which can be synchronous (that is, all members of the discussion group are participating at the same time) or asynchronous, or chat rooms. An asynchronous discussion is run over a set period of time, for example two weeks, when a site is set aside for discussion on a specified topic and individuals can add their contribution to the discussion at a time which suits them. This is particularly valuable when running international courses. The e-tutor monitors the discussion, identifies themes arising in discussion and contributes new ideas to keep the discussion going (known as 'threading').

Blended Learning

Blended learning is when elearning is combined with activities in face-to-face learning which build on previous learning and provide the foundation for future work. In developing blended learning the elearning and different face-to-face activities have to be planned to help students achieve the specified learning outcomes. The face-to-face part of blended learning can involve any of the methods of teaching and learning discussed in previous chapters. A number of different types of activity can be combined with the elearning to provide an interesting programme including: small group work of various types, the occasional specialist lecture to inspire and introduce new ideas, and skills development simulation sessions.

ASSESSMENT

Simulations have the potential to contribute to assessment of skills and competence through using Objective Structured Clinical Examinations (OSCEs – discussed in Chapter 13). In addition, they can be extremely valuable in formative assessment of student performance in relation to patient care, particularly in situations where clinical experience is limited and mentors may be unable to carry out assessment of some abilities in the practice situation.

One example of this is in children's nursing where the focus is on family involvement in care – students may have difficulty in obtaining as much practice and mentor feedback as needed and may lack confidence when qualified. Simulation enables the opportunity to practise and gain feedback that is needed (Brimble, 2008).

Another example relates to an area of concern in nursing practice, that of identifying a deteriorating patient. Cooper et al. (2010) used simulated environments to assess final year students' knowledge, skills and situation awareness when caring for a deteriorating patient. The study identified generally satisfactory knowledge, but significant deficiencies in applying this in managing the deteriorating patient. As the patient's condition worsened, the student nurses became more anxious, were less likely to undertake the essential vital signs measurements, and failed to call for help. Nevertheless, the researchers suggested that such high reality simulations repeated frequently have the potential to impact on practice.

LECTURER SUPPORT

Staff Preparation

Academic staff involved in teaching skills and competencies in preparation for clinical experience are now almost certain to have access to highly technological equipment, but what is not certain is how well they have been prepared for its use. In a small study, Dowie and Phillips (2011) found that 90% of respondents were using high fidelity simulation in teaching but only 40% of them said that they felt confident in doing so and only 35% said they had been sufficiently prepared. All considered that high fidelity simulation was a valuable aspect of teaching but the preparation of the scenarios to be used was problematic.

Three major aspects of preparation need attention. Firstly, operating the equipment and how to use it in teaching need attention. Relatively few nurse teachers have received formal preparation in the use of simulation, particularly high fidelity use. Such preparation should be incorporated into the Post-Graduate Certificates in Education for nurses, midwives and specialist community public health nurses for those aiming for a teaching qualification recorded by the NMC. In addition, there are undoubtedly many academic staff who would benefit from workshops to develop their skills in this area.

The second issue is the preparation of clinically accurate, evidence-based and relevant scenarios to enable students to learn the situation awareness, clinical judgement and decision-making appropriate to the clinical context. A number of staff felt lacking in confidence to undertake this as they rarely spent time in the clinical environment. It is important that they are allowed time to spend in practice and that clinicians are involved in developing the scenarios for student education. New academic staff have an important contribution to make with recent relevant experience to contribute to scenario development and working within the team to ensure that all appropriate learning outcomes are achieved.

Thirdly, many lecturers who wish to develop their modules to include elearning have no understanding of how to start. It is recommended *'before you try to do it, be an elearner yourself'* (Race, 2005: 191). Some universities offer short online courses for academic staff to learn to be e-tutors. Such courses are expected to be completed before staff commence working with elearning, and they introduce many of the tools that can be used with students.

Legal Issues

Staff involved in web-based learning must also become aware of the legal issues involved (Haigh, 2010), including:

- Who owns educational materials prepared by a lecturer employed by an HEI? Copyright on educational materials is normally held by the institution as work prepared as part of employment belongs to the employer. However, a lecturer's work is flexible in place and time, and may be undertaken on equipment owned by the lecturer. Many HEIs operate a mixed system in which authors are permitted to use their materials for teaching and publications, but the institution retains ownership of the course of study. It is sensible to find out the situation in one's own place of employment.
- Who owns materials being incorporated into educational materials? It is necessary to find out who owns the copyright of the original publication or website that materials are taken from and to obtain permission to use substantial amounts of copyright material. However, what amount is substantial is not specified. Advice can be sought from specialist library or information services staff.
- Confidentiality must be considered. Materials which relate to individuals must be used with care to guard their anonymity. If video clips involving patients are being considered for use, permission in writing must be obtained before inclusion.

Continuing developments in the area mean that ongoing development of staff is also necessary. An interest group of staff in different institutions who share ideas and discuss innovations in their teaching through regular meetings and online communication can benefit everyone. It is helpful if some identified experts are available within the School to support other staff.

CHAPTER SUMMARY

This chapter has considered a constantly evolving theme and doubtless there are other technological approaches being used to facilitate learning. Some of the ways in which technological developments can enhance access to learning through a range of methods are presented here. However, it is worth reiterating that with imagination and effort, the lower reality approaches can be as effective in promoting learning as the high reality equipment. In addition to the benefits for student learning, these technologically based developments may facilitate staff in balancing their range of activities. Although development of these new approaches takes time, the longer term use of them for facilitating learning may minimise staff time.

12 ASSESSMENT OF KNOWLEDGE AND INTELLECTUAL SKILLS

INTRODUCTION

Assessment is an extremely important aspect of education for professional practice, but is also one of the most complex aspects to be mastered (if that is possible). Its importance is emphasised by Brown et al.:

> Assessment defines what students regard as important, how they spend their time and how they come to see themselves as students and then as graduates. Students take their cues from what is assessed rather than from what lecturers assert is important. (1997: 7)

Thus, *'assessment for learning is placed at the centre of subject and programme design'* from the earliest stages of curriculum development (Boud and Associates, 2010).

Academic assessment has changed in response to the recent radical alterations that have occurred in HE in the UK, although in many cases without real thought about the effect of such changes. There has been a dramatic rise in the proportion of young adults entering higher education, with an increase in the variability in student motivation and academic ability. Staff numbers have not increased in parallel and staff student ratios (SSRs) are reported as becoming radically worse (Bryan and Clegg, 2006). However, in relation to the cost centres for nursing and paramedical studies any consistency in movement in staff–student ratios between 2001/02 and 2009/10 cannot be readily identified. Some

HEIs show an improvement in SSRs while others have worsened and others have varied throughout the nine years reported (HEIDI, 2011). However, it is not clear how these figures are being calculated or how they relate to teaching and class size; the reliability of these figures is questionable. Nevertheless, many academic staff subjectively feel that the pressures of work have increased.

Most UK universities allocate work by class contact hours and a significant increase in class sizes has resulted, with some staff members now teaching classes of several hundred students, with 'tutorials' for 25 or 30 students at a time. However, the resulting assessment load is rarely taken into account when distributing the overall workload.

Assessment approaches have usually been modified to achieve a marking workload that reduces the time investment to a manageable level. As assessment influences student learning, this is an important issue with potentially damaging results. An exception is the Open University where assessment is seen as the driving force for each module of study, with staff appointed to undertake this activity, which will motivate distance learners to undertake the expected work. It is estimated that students on some standard undergraduate courses undertake about 2% of the assessment undertaken by an Open University degree student (Bryan and Clegg, 2006).

Because assessment leads learning, the selection and management of assessment becomes one of the most important issues in course planning and delivery. Figure 12.1 illustrates six principles of assessment for learning which together will promote learning. Table 12.1 identifies the different ways in which assessment supports learning through the type of assessment, and the characteristics and student response to feedback.

The focus of this chapter is assessment of the more theoretical and intellectually focused content of the programme taught mainly within the university, although many issues discussed are equally relevant in relation to assessment of students' clinical competence. Some of the positive results of assessment to enhance learning are:

- encourage intrinsic motivation
- build learner confidence
- give learners a sense of ownership and control
- provide detailed feedback
- enhance learners' strategic awareness
- encourage collaboration between students. (Broadfoot, 2007: 126).

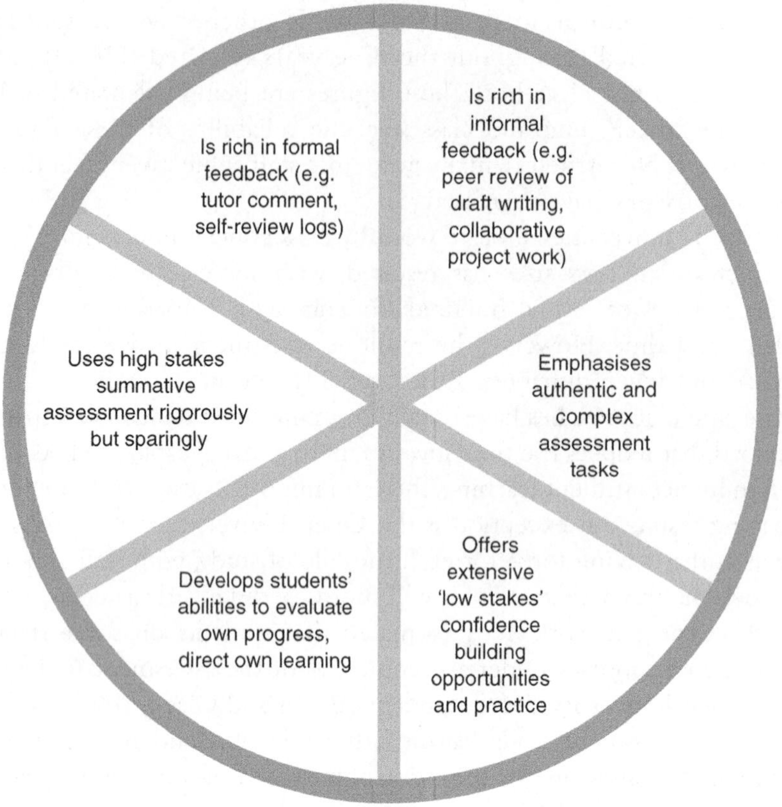

FIGURE 12.1 *Six Principles of Assessment for Learning*

The complexities of assessment are considerable and this chapter aims to provide some guidance through these.

WHAT ASSESSMENT DOES

Assessment is usually discussed in terms of formative and summative or assessment **for** learning and assessment **of** learning (Broadfoot, 2007). However, this is a somewhat artificial distinction as most students focus their learning on what is required for assessment. The assessment requirements of a programme determine what students learn, thus the distinction between formative and summative becomes of limited relevance. Nevertheless it is useful for the lecturer to be clear about the intentions of the two.

TABLE 12.1 *Assessment Supporting Learning*

Conditions	**Rationale**	**Aiming to:**
Quantity and distribution of student effort	Assessed tasks capture sufficient study time and effort	Ensure students study sufficiently out of class and prevent them getting away with relatively little study
	These tasks distribute student effort evenly across topics and weeks	Ensure evenness of effort and minimise 'question spotting' and lack of attendance at later classes
Quality and level of student effort	These tasks engage students in productive learning activity	Encourage students to take a deep approach to and engage with learning
	Assessment communicates clear and high expectations to students	Explicate goals that students can understand and that demonstrate high expectations
Quantity and timing of feedback	Sufficient feedback is provided, both often enough and in enough detail	Provide enough detailed feedback to orientate students to required standards early
	The feedback is provided often enough to be useful to students	Provide feedback to help students to become self-assessing. Methods have to balance frequency with other factors
Quality of feedback	Feedback focuses on learning rather than on marks or students themselves	Encourage students to read feedback, which is more likely without marks provided
	Feedback is linked to the purpose of the assignment and to criteria	Enhance impact of feedback through emphasis on goals, criteria and standards
	Feedback is understandable to students, depending on their level of sophistication	Help students understand feedback through classroom discussion of feedback and how to use it in improving quality of work
Student response to feedback	Feedback is received by students and attended to	Emphasise importance of feedback by speed of return and class discussion of key issues
	Feedback is acted upon by students to improve their work or their learning	Enhance use of feedback by making some of it generic, using feedback on drafts or stages of work to be submitted

The intention of formative assessment is to provide students with feedback on their performance to enable them to develop their intellectual skills and to learn what is expected of them as they progress. It is particularly important at the beginning of a programme when students are making the transition into higher education: most institutions provide students with the opportunity to undertake some written work early in the first semester as a diagnostic tool.

Summative assessment in nursing programmes has two main aims: first is to judge whether the student meets the necessary level of knowledge, skills and attitudes to receive the professional qualification, and second is to determine the level of the academic award. An important part of the first is carried out in the clinical environment, but both theoretical and clinically-based assessment are a part of determining achievement of the qualities necessary to provide high quality care evidenced through the professional qualification AND the level of the academic award. The feedback provided on summative work aims to enhance future performance, thus providing a formative dimension.

PRINCIPLES OF ASSESSMENT

Because assessment is central to learning, it plays an essential part in maintaining academic standards and should meet the following principles to maintain standards, derived largely from the University of Ulster (2010b) Assessment Handbook.

- *Validity*: There are various types of validity including construct, predictive and others. However, the one that most concerns us here is the extent to which assessment reflects the learning outcomes being judged. In relation to the programme as a whole, the course team should prepare a schedule of assessment which clearly identifies how all the outcomes and constructs for the programme will be assessed.
- *Fairness*: Assessment must assess the outcomes of the module, be free of bias, be readily understood by all students, give students with disabilities an equal chance, and result in a reasonable student workload.
- *Equity*: Assessment should be comparable for modules of the same academic level and credit weighting. This assists in reviewing the workload of the total assessment package. The external examiner has an important role in commenting on this.
- *Reliability*: Reliability in marking aims to ensure similar marks are awarded for comparable work. With a large student cohort and thus a number of staff involved in marking this is not always easy to achieve and is discussed later in this chapter.
- *Rigour*: Assessment has to examine the intellectual demands appropriate to the academic level of each module which students complete during their programme (outlined in Box 3.2). Levels 4, 5 and 6 are equivalent to years 1, 2 and 3 of an honours degree in England, Wales and Northern Ireland (QAA, 2008a). Some countries (for example, Scotland, Republic of Ireland) use the same, or similar, descriptors but designate different level numbers. The specified university procedures must be carried out.

- *Discrimination*: Assessment must allow differences between the performance of students to be recognised and rewarded with appropriate marks.
- *Explicitness*: All relevant information must be clear and easily accessed by all students and staff.
- *Practicality*: Having emphasised the importance of assessment in encouraging learning, there is the potential that academic staff will find themselves with a very large marking workload. Assessment needs to be planned to obtain the necessary valid information with a manageable workload.
- *Authenticity:* The extent to which what is being assessed relates to the real world of practice.

WHAT IS BEING ASSESSED

'Authentic assessment' is identified as important in helping students to learn (Boud and Falchikow, 2007). It relates to real life situations. In the context of nursing it will include activities based on patient-focused scenarios such as presentations about patient care related decision-making or other issues, or requiring preparation of portfolios including reflection on students' own practice.

The following areas were identified as relevant for assessment in secondary schools in 1992

- Written expression, knowledge retention, organization of material, appropriate selection
- Practical, knowledge application, oral, investigative skills
- Personal and social skills, communication and relationships, working in groups, initiative, responsibility, self-reliance, leadership
- Motivation and commitment, perseverance, self-confidence, constructive acceptance of failure. (Hargreaves, cited by Broadfoot, 2007: 9)

These appear equally applicable to nursing education today, particularly in relation to the generic skills to be achieved and applied in the professional context.

The assessment schedule for the programme must include assessment of all course outcomes and all NMC specified outcomes. However, beyond that, universities vary in their requirements. Some require every module to be assessed separately, and all required module outcomes to be assessed (although some bonus outcomes may be included in the module outline and do not have to be assessed). How they are assessed is identified in the course document. Other institutions may allow outcomes from different modules to be assessed jointly but the necessity of ensuring that all outcomes are achieved remains. This includes not just knowledge but application of knowledge through problem-solving, decision-making, critical thinking etc. within the professional context. Outcomes to be assessed also include the skills and attitudes required in a nurse.

Overall programme outcomes should be mapped against modules and assessment activity to ensure that all outcomes have been achieved and assessed.

METHODS OF ASSESSMENT

The leading role of assessment in determining learning (Gibbs in Bryan and Clegg, 2006) makes paramount the organisation of assessment to ensure (or at least encourage) students to learn those parts of the curriculum essential for safe professional practice.

There are two main groups of assessment approaches – examination and coursework. While there may be some overlap between activities undertaken within these, they differ in several ways. A subset of coursework is assessment of small group learning of various types, including problem-based learning.

Examinations

The NMC (2010a) states that within the pre-registration programme there must be *'at least one unseen invigilated examination in the assessment process'* (82).

In general, examinations are undertaken under controlled conditions with invigilators tasked to prevent cheating. There are some variations in written examination type:

- *Unseen*: In this case the paper is seen for the first time at the examination. Except when clearly specified as part of the examination conditions, students do not have access to literature or other resources.
- *Open-book*: Here, students are allowed to look up information in a book(s) during the examination. It has been suggested that this reduces anxiety and reflects real life when information often has to be looked up. An alternative is to provide all students with a pack of materials to use during the examination. A variant is when students are given a question and allowed access to the University Library and other resources for a specified period (for example, 6 hours) before handing in the answer. This is only possible when numbers are small enough that all students will be able to gain access to the relevant materials in the time available.

- *Pre-viewed*: Topics or questions are provided in advance to permit students to prepare and they write their answer under examination conditions. They may be allowed to take limited notes into the examination. Students vary in their response to this approach; many perform well, but some become highly anxious.
- *Restricted choice*: One of the problems with examinations is that students may 'spot the questions' and restrict revision to those topics they expect to appear. This form of examination aims to minimise this behaviour. It may include a compulsory question or set of short questions, before a selection from which to choose. Another version is that students are given a paper in advance with, for example, eight questions and told that three of these will comprise the examination paper and they will have to answer all three questions.

Table 12.2 indicates some of the types of questions which can be incorporated into examinations depending on the outcomes to be assessed. The case study type of question in particular enables a degree of authenticity to be achieved.

Setting examination papers is not easy for inexperienced lecturers. Questions need to be worded clearly, concisely and achieve the expected answers to the questions set. Questioning needs to be appropriate for the academic level of the module, provide opportunities for good students to demonstrate their ability, and enable students to answer in the time available. The course team should review papers to minimise ambiguities in wording, check that the syllabus is adequately covered, module assessments do not overlap and ensure that the same questions are not being used in resit papers or in succeeding years. The marking guide for each question should also be agreed by the course team.

Coursework

The importance of organising assessment to motivate learning means that the schedule of assessment should mirror the outcomes of the programme, that is outcome assessment. The range of professionally focused and generic outcomes in a nursing programme requires thought and creativity in meeting the necessary complexity in assessment.

In addition, while examinations are undertaken by each individual at a specific time and place, coursework is carried out at a time and place of the student's choosing. It may be undertaken individually or in small groups, which can be part of the organisation of teaching or informal study groups set up by students. It can involve a wide range of different types of activity some of which are shown in Table 12.3, but which are limited only by the imagination of the teacher.

TABLE 12.2 *Assessment Through Examination*

Essay type questions	Usually 2 to 5 questions in three hours. Students provide answers in their own words allowing assessment of knowledge and ability to organise material and to demonstrate relationships between different areas of content. Permits considerable variability in the type of questions and creativity in the answers.
Short answer questions	Numerous short answers presented with or without choice in those to be answered. Tends to assess knowledge but, with thought and effort, can require some problem-solving or application of knowledge. Answers can incorporate notes or diagrams. Time allowed per question tends to vary between about 10 and 20 minutes.
Case study approaches	Scenario presented with specific questions to be answered. Additional material is provided throughout the examination with additional questions to be addressed. Structured to be clinically authentic when they have to be able to respond as the situation evolves and use clinical judgement in answering.
Concept/mind mapping	Rarely a core aspect of an examination but can assist students in identifying concepts and organising relationships. Can be helpful in initial structuring of answers.
Interpretive questions	Introductory material such as a paragraph, table, chart etc. is presented and students have to interpret or make a judgement about it.
Objective tests	Frequently used to test knowledge but can also be devised to assess application of knowledge. Advantage of rapid, reliable, easy marking; disadvantage of tending to encourage superficial learning.
Multiple choice	Consists of: the stem - problem or statement the key - correct answer distracters - at least three incorrect responses students select correct answer
Matching items	Consists of two lists (column A and column B). Student is required to match items from column A with correct responses in column B
True-false	Student identifies each of a number of statements as true or false. Guesswork offers 50% chance of correct answer
Assertion-reason	Two statements, an assertion and a reason. Student has to decide whether (a) assertion is true and (b) whether reason is correct explanation
Short answer (missing word)	Statement with one or more words missing. Student is expected to insert missing word(s)
Multiple completion	Selection of more than one correct answer from a list of several options.
Ordered response	The student has to place items in correct order

In preparing coursework for submission, students are expected to access and use relevant literature, and to reference it correctly. At early undergraduate level the use of secondary sources is usually acceptable but for final year dissertations and postgraduate work primary sources are expected to be used whenever possible.

TABLE 12.3 *Assessment Through Coursework*

Essay	As in Table 12.4. In coursework essays students are expected to access, find and cite correctly, relevant primary sources to support arguments.
Portfolio	A collection of student work to demonstrate achievement of specified outcomes, either paper or electronic based. May include a critical review of the progress demonstrated within the portfolio. Shows a broad sample of work, but requires considerable lecturer time for marking and giving feedback.
Poster	Used by individual or small groups of students to illustrate learning from groupwork or project. Enables learning to be shared with others.
Presentation/seminar	Single or a few students prepare a presentation on a selected topic or based on group work and, following presentation to discussion group, answer questions and lead discussion.
Oral examination	Used mainly for research degrees (MPhil, PhD). However, sometimes used with undergraduate students at borderline of a class of degree to determine final result, or to confirm results of a project or when plagiarism is suspected.

Essays

It is essential that students understand the implications of the type of coursework set and the expectations associated with words used, whether in examination or coursework. Table 12.4 clarifies the intention of wording frequently used.

Alternatives to essays can be used including such activities as writing an article for a academic or a professional journal, preparing a book review, presenting a case for introduction of an innovation in care, or others depending on the imagination of the lecturer.

As students have time to prepare coursework, the level of presentation expected is considerably higher than in examinations. Students are expected to demonstrate relevant use of literature in presenting a well-reasoned argument with appropriate conclusions. They should demonstrate relevant links between different aspects of the paper, show critical analysis and the ability to synthesise concepts and evaluate conclusions. Imagination and creativity are welcomed. The work submitted should be well structured, with clear, accurate (and preferably concise and elegant) use of English including correct grammar and punctuation, with accurate referencing in the system specified by the School.

Dissertations

In many HEIs students taking honours degrees complete a dissertation, *'a substantial report on a major project'* (University of Ulster, 2010b: 40), as part of their final year work. This will be at level 6 and may be 4000 to 6000

TABLE 12.4 *Types of Essay Questions (Habeshaw et al., 1998)*

Discuss/Comment on (statement) Write an essay on	These may be difficult for students to determine what is wanted. Good students will be able to demonstrate creativity, analysis, synthesis and evaluation in relation to the topic, quotation or other stimulus statement. Weaker students may have difficulty in selecting and organising material appropriately.
Describe/Give an account of	These words give clearer guidance on the expectations in the essay. The first two expect a relatively straightforward, well-organised description of the topic with a concluding summary of the key points.
Compare/Contrast/Explain	These three terms require a more sophisticated presentation in which similarities and differences are identified and described, contradictions identified, with a considered conclusion.
Assess/Analyse/Evaluate	These are at a higher intellectual level than those above. They require demonstration of the higher level skills of critical analysis, synthesis and evaluation, provide opportunity for creativity and conclude with a reasoned conclusion.
Role play essay	Students are expected to carry out a task from the position of a specified role. This approaches the 'authentic assessment' previously discussed.
Structured essay	The content required is made clear by structuring the topic into several statements or sub-questions. Such essays assess specific knowledge or techniques but not what the student thinks is important.
Interpretation of evidence	Students are given a set of data, asked to interpret what the data reveal, and then asked to comment or answer specific questions drawing on the data.
Note-form essay	Tends to focus on recall of information or test simple understanding. Less suitable for assessing analysis, synthesis or creativity.
Hypothesis formation	Can be combined with other activities (e.g. data interpretation) in asking students to identify possible relationships between factors.

words in length. HEIs will have different requirements for the dissertation but it may be one of several types of work, such as:

- a small research project;
- a research proposal;
- a systematic review of the literature;
- development of clinical guidelines;
- an audit;
- a proposal for introduction of an innovation into clinical practice.

The time required to obtain ethical approval to carry out a clinically-based research project (which most nursing students would wish) makes this very difficult to organise within the time available so this option is now being implemented infrequently at undergraduate level.

Students often find this the most challenging piece of work in their degree because they:

- have difficulty in identifying the topic and setting parameters to make it manageable in the time available;
- have never prepared anything of this length;
- are unsure about the standard required;
- are nervous about carrying out an empirical study (if this is required).

Dissertations are usually prepared with academic supervision, during which students receive some formative assessment. However, to ensure equity it is important to provide guidelines for academics on the amount and type of feedback to be given during dissertation preparation. Academic staff have very mixed experience in supervision of academic work; those with a PhD may be supervising doctoral students, while others will only have been supervised themselves as undergraduates. In most circumstances each member of staff in the supervision team will have several students to supervise and will need to manage this potentially very demanding aspect of their workload. Some of the issues considered in supervision guidelines include:

- individual supervision or group supervision sessions;
- number, timing and length of supervision sessions;
- aspects of the dissertation to be discussed;
- when, how much and what written work will be submitted for supervisor's feedback;
- limits on written comments provided.

Marking of dissertations takes substantial time and effort and most institutions state that

> Dissertations should be second marked. Where there is wide discrepancy in the two marks and a compromise cannot be reached a third marker may be involved. (University of Ulster, 2010b: 41)

Interpretations of 'wide discrepancy' usually range from a difference between markers greater than 5 to 10 % marks (depending on the School) and are dealt with as follows:

- for a difference of this size and below, the mean mark is taken and rounded up;
- a greater difference (which is more likely to occur with an inexperienced marker) is usually resolved by discussion and clarification of how criteria have been applied by the assessors;

- a third experienced marker will become involved to resolve any remaining discrepancies and the result will usually be the agreed mark.

Only in exceptional circumstances does the external examiner become involved in determining the mark awarded .

An example of an assessment schedule for a dissertation consisting of a research proposal is shown in Table 12.5; other assessment schedules are developed for other types of work. Assessment of dissertations sometimes involves an oral examination, although this is now used less frequently with the very large student groups. However, this may still be used with students

TABLE 12.5 *Assessment Schedule for Dissertation*

I confirm that the work submitted has been produced through my own efforts. Student Signature:

ASPECT OF PRESENTATION	**COMMENTS**	**MARKS**
Summary		
Clarity		
Appropriate detail		/ 5
Literature Review		
Justification for study		
Appropriateness and level of analysis of literature reviewed		
Logical development of content and structure (beginning, middle, end)		
Research question developed from literature		/ 30
Methodology		
Aims/hypotheses		
Proposed design		
Population/sample		
Methods of data collection		
Robustness of data collection methods		
Data analysis		
Pilot study		
Procedure for main study		
Ethical considerations		
Appendices		/ 40
Planning for research		
Potential value of study		
Time scale		
Resources		/ 15
References		/ 5
Presentation of proposal		
Including use of English		/ 5
Total Mark		**/ 100**
Moderation		
AGREED MARK		**/ 100**

at the borderline of a class for a degree, or when there is any question about plagiarism.

Assessment of Small Group Learning

A number of the generic and professional outcomes that students on nursing programmes are expected to achieve are developed through group work, Problem-Based Learning or other collaborative activity. Recognising the importance of assessment in guiding learning, it is necessary to assess the skills and competencies of small group working, as well as what is learnt. In Table 12.6 some common aspects of group work and approaches to assessment which may be used are identified. In assessing group work, a number of different assessors can be involved.

TABLE 12.6 *Examples Of Assessment In Small Group Teaching And Learning (Exley And Dennick, 2004b)*

What is being assessed?	Possible assessment methods	Marking
Knowledge and understanding, written communication skills	Individual written assignment based on the topic of the group activity and learning in group work Essay on topic with a remote link to group work Contribution by individual of section of group project report	Tutor marked May involve peer marking with tutor moderation
Presentation skills	Preparation of poster of group work conclusion Group mark awarded may be same for all or group may decide allocation of marks between group members depending on contribution	Tutor and peers marking % of overall mark limited
Oral presentation skills and leading discussion	Presentation by individual or several group members, each individuals contribution assessed Criteria for allocation mark agreed by group with tutor before presentation Percentage of overall mark limited	Tutor and peers marking % of overall mark limited
Team/Group working and individual contribution	Review of preparatory notes, recorded observation, contribution record Peer group considers contribution of members and agrees distribution of marks awarded	Tutor assessed Peer marking % of overall mark limited
Student development	Professional portfolio, reflective log/journal Links with student academic record	Personal tutor

The collaborative approach to learning can also be applied to assessment with the tutor, peers and individual students all participating in judging the quality of work completed. Involving all members of the group in assessment helps to resolve the issue of who carried out how much of the work. The skills developed in SGT (particularly PBL) include problem-solving, team working, self-directed learning, and communication skills and are essential for continuing professional development throughout one's professional career (Savin-Baden and Major, 2004). Marcangelo et al. (in Hammick and Reid, 2010) discuss self and peer assessment of work presented, as well as the functioning of the group itself, and emphasise the importance of preparation for participation in assessment. Figure 12.2 indicates the different aspects of preparation to enable students to develop their abilities for self-assessment. Learning about knowledge, reflection and emotional aspects all feed into these skills which are then refined and developed through regular debriefing.

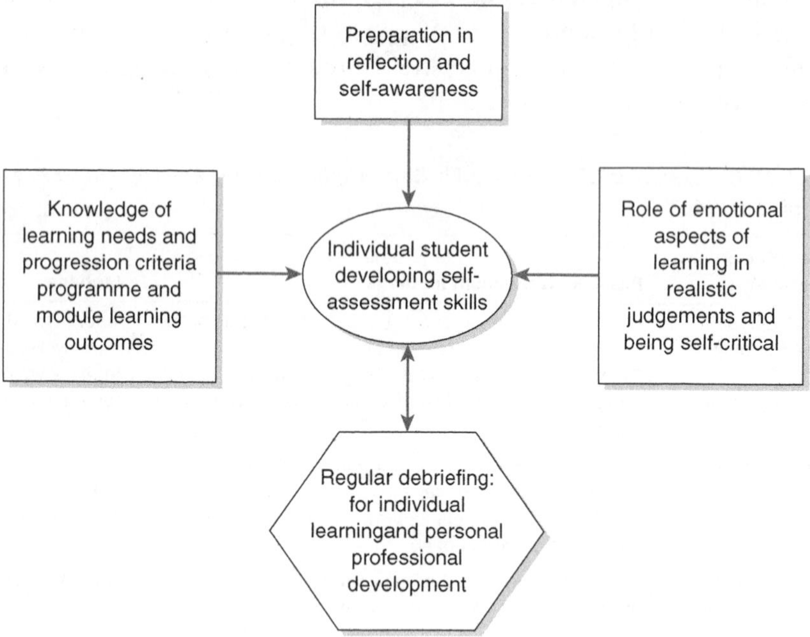

FIGURE 12.2 *Preparation for Self-Assessment*

In managing peer assessment, ground rules need to be agreed and preparation of those involved is essential. There are two aspects of peer assessment: marking the work presented and assessing the contribution of each member to the functioning of the group. Members of the peer group need to acquire appropriate attributes to contribute effectively to assessment of work presented, such as:

- Knowledge: of how to assess, including the criteria to be used, how to judge performance and what feedback is needed.
- Skills: making accurate judgements and giving feedback. Accepting the emotional aspects of assessing peers.

- Attitudes: fairness and equity; not colluding with others in group to give unearned high grades (Marcangelo et al. in Hammick and Reid, 2010).

When peers mark each other's work using the criteria set and agreed, it helps students to develop their own abilities in self-assessment. The development of criteria for marking coursework is discussed below and is similar to that used for self assessment. Criteria for assessing how individuals functioned within the group also have to be agreed and one example is shown in Table 12.7.

TABLE 12.7 *Assessment Criteria for Group Working*

Criteria	5	4	3	2	1	Criteria
Regular attendance at group meetings						Poor/non-attendance at team meetings
Active contribution to the discussion						Finds it difficult to contribute
Works amicably with other members of the team						Has difficulty working with others
Shows excellent ability to plan and complete own work						Has not yet shown they can organise their own work
Is good at solving problems						Has difficulty in suggesting solutions
Responds well to advice						Resents criticism and is reluctant to accept advice

One of the key issues in determining summative assessment marks is the contribution of the lecturer's assessment and peer assessment of the work presented, and peer assessment of the contribution of each member to the functioning of the group. The allocation of marks will be determined in advance so that all concerned are aware of their responsibilities, with the lecturer carrying the overall responsibility for the fairness and appropriate level of the marking. Peer assessment usually counts as a limited percentage of the total such as 20 or 30%.

There are a number of alternatives for allocating marks, including:

- The same mark is allocated to each individual within the group by the lecturer, reflecting the quality of the submission or presentation.
- A mark is allocated by the lecturer for the work completed by the group as a whole multiplied by the number of students within the group; this total is allocated to individual students by the group, reflecting the contribution made by each.
- The proportion of marks allocated in different ways is specified, for example:

- o Lecturer's mark on assessment of quality of the work – 70% of total (as the expert in the field) and allocated equally between members;
- o Peers' mark on assessment of quality of the work – 20% of total based on criteria previously agreed and allocated evenly between members;
- o Peers' mark on contribution to group functioning – 10% reflecting how the group recognises each member's contribution.

- Peer assessment can be used as formative assessment only.

The course team will need to consider advantages and disadvantages of the different approaches, select the one that best meets their needs and ensure that all staff and students understand the principles and practice of the method selected.

MARKING

Marking has two key elements – awarding a grade or mark, and providing feedback to enable students to learn; feedback is discussed below. In summative assessment, the marking of students' work has two functions:

- to award a grade or mark which, with other work as specified in the regulations, will determine the level of academic award, i.e. pass or fail, or class of degree;
- in the context of nursing, to determine whether the student meets the necessary standards to be permitted to enter the profession.

These two purposes tend to reflect the use of norm versus criterion referencing:

- In norm referencing, the work is marked and rank ordered with that of other students in the group. Cut-off points are established for pass/fail and for setting grade points above this. This approach is sometimes used in determining class of degree.
- Criterion referencing is when the work is compared with previously prepared criteria or standards. This is commonly used in assessment of clinical competence.

While these appear clearly different, in practice in HE a subtle blend of the two may be the reality. The process of preparation for marking discussed below will result in agreed criteria for cut-off points for grades or pass-fail, thus using a form of criterion-referencing within a (formally) norm-referenced approach.

Approaches to Marking

There are two main approaches to marking:

Impression Marking

This is based on the lecturer's overall impression of the work submitted and is fairly quick. This approach is sometimes used with a broad description of expectations for different grades (see Table 12.8) for marking honours degree work. Although intended for marking essays it can also be used for examinations. A useful approach for individual lecturers in using impression marking is to mark some (perhaps 10) scripts and allocate them to the different levels they represent to clarify the expectations for each grading level. All papers (including the first ten) are then marked and graded.

TABLE 12.8 *Proposed Guide for Marking Essays*

%	Overall description	Criteria
90>	Outstanding answer	Very rarely achieved. Demonstrates excellent use of literature and critical thinking; clear, succinct, well structured (preferably elegant) use of English
80s	Excellent answer	Rarely achieved. Demonstrates good use of literature and high level of critical thinking; clear, succinct, well structured (preferably elegant) use of English
70s	Very good answer	Demonstrates good use of literature and critical thinking; clear, succinct, well structured (preferably elegant) use of English
60s	Good answer	Demonstrates good use of literature and some critical thinking; satisfactory structure with clear and correct use of English
50s	Adequate answer	Demonstrates restricted use of literature and limited critical thinking; satisfactory structure with some errors in use of English
40s	Weak but just adequate answer	Shows some use of the literature and restricted understanding of the topic. Weak structure and some errors in grammar and spelling
30s	Poor answer	Demonstrates limited knowledge and understanding. Shows inadequate use of the literature and is poorly structured
20s	Very poor answer	Rarely achieved. Shows some limited understanding of the topic but muddled, poorly structured and with poor use of the literature
<20	Exceptionally poor answer	Very rarely achieved. Almost no relevance to the question and poorly organised

Analytical Marking

This is a system in which a detailed marking checklist is prepared and each examiner marks against the different categories. This system contributes to reliability, but takes longer than impression marking and preparing the checklist must be done with care. A checklist which specifies every item that should be mentioned ends up giving high marks to someone who simply mentions each item but a low mark to someone who demonstrates creativity and a high level of analytical and synthetic skills: such a checklist is not valid for marking degree work. Table 12.9 illustrates a marking checklist which enables reward of a high level of intellectual skills.

TABLE 12.9 *Example of Analytical Marking Scheme*

Discuss the use of a specified model of nursing for promoting self-care and enhancing the quality of life in older people and the scope and importance of the role of the nurse in this area of care. (3000 words)

Element	**Description**	**Marks (out of 100)**
Introduction	Demographic changes Growing demands on the health service Nursing and health promotion	10
Model of nursing	Value of using a model of nursing Rationale for selection of a particular model of nursing Description of model selected Application of model in assessment and planning care to promote self-care and enhance quality of life	30
Role of the nurse	Assessing patient strengths, weaknesses and resources Planning integrated care involving nursing and other health care professionals as appropriate and family Supervision of provision of care by non-professionals Liaison with social services and voluntary organisations to ensure external contacts Evaluation of efficacy of intervention	30
Conclusion	Summary of key points with clear statement of overall conclusion	5
Academic and intellectual skills	Selection of references to support theoretical and empirical arguments Logic and coherence of arguments and discussion Creativity Correct use of English, i.e. accurate spelling and punctuation, good sentence and paragraph construction Correct citing and listing of references	25

Preparation for Marking

Variation in the standard of marking can be reduced by training in which all staff examining that module mark the same sample of work representing a range of marking bands. The results are then reviewed and discussed in depth. An examination is usually just given a mark, and discussion about factors involved in awarding a mark within a particular class or band helps all examiners to recognise their own approaches and achieve comparability.

In marking coursework, the same approach is used but with the addition of considering the feedback given to students. All examiners are sensitised to the key elements expected in scripts being awarded different grades/classes.

Reliability in marking

Preparation for marking will contribute to reliability of marking as will the approaches below.

- *Double marking:* This aims to ensure that a similar standard of marking is applied across the work submitted by all students. Every student script is marked by two independent markers. This used to be the normal procedure within HE. It is an important part of induction of new lecturers to help them recognise appropriate standards by pairing them with an experienced staff member. However, the very large student groups now undertaking nurse education result in an unmanageable workload and true double marking is now less frequent.
- *Moderation:* This aims to achieve a similar standard of marking across the whole student group. A sample from each marking band from each examiner is reviewed. This sometimes identifies a marker who consistently gives marks higher or lower than colleagues and enables an adjustment factor to be applied to the batch marked by that examiner. More difficulty is caused when a marker is identified whose marking is inconsistent, in which case their whole batch will have to be re-marked.

Examination Marking

In examination marking, numerous factors can lead to results which do not properly reflect the ability of the student(s) (see Table 12.10).

TABLE 12.10 *Sources of Examination Error*

Student factors	Student anxiety and examination stress Home pressures and responsibilities resulting in inadequate study Some students do not use their time effectively - inadequate study in preparation for examination Poor examination technique Illness or unforeseen circumstances
Examination factors	Questions are ambiguous or confusing, so students do not provide the expected answer The paper may ask more than can comfortably be completed in the time Variation in question difficulty Guesswork may be used in multiple-choice papers
Marking process	Lack of procedures to ensure reliability of marking within a team Lack of clarity in standards expected at the particular level being assessed The 'halo' effect when knowledge of the previous answer (or the student) influences the mark given
Marker factors	Fatigue due to large marking load Variation in marker expectations for answers

Various approaches can be implemented at different stages of the examination process to minimise the effects of these.

- *Student factors:* The studies advisor (personal tutor) plays an important role in helping students to recognise their difficulties and identify the appropriate action. This may include giving advice on completing the necessary forms for consideration of exceptional circumstances or recommending approaching the University's student support services for assistance with examination technique, stress or anxiety.
- *Examination factors:* Care in setting papers and preparing marking schedules aims to eliminate these. The external examiner also plays a role.
- *Marking process and marker factors:* The halo effect, in which the marker's knowledge of a student influences the mark awarded, is reduced by anonymous marking (although it is sometimes possible to identify the writer). This is now the norm for examinations in most universities and for coursework in many HEIs.

FEEDBACK

Table 12.1 emphasises how assessment enables learning and reinforces the importance of high quality feedback, through ensuring that feedback meets the following criteria (Race et al., 2005, Chapter 27):

- *Timely:* Feedback received soon after completion of the work is much more effective than when it is received weeks or months later, when it seems irrelevant. Some universities set a time limit, such as three weeks, for provision of feedback from coursework. Such marks are provisional until after ratification at the examination board, and students must be informed of this.
- *Personal and individual:* Feedback should relate to each student's individual needs, although this is not easy when providing feedback to a large class.
- *Articulate:* Feedback should be written clearly with points readily understood.
- *Empowering:* Care in wording is needed when giving critical feedback to help students use it constructively.
- *Manageable:* For students, too much feedback may 'drown out' the major points made. Marking and giving feedback needs to be managed effectively and efficiently by staff.
- *Developmental:* Feedback should help students recognise what was good or weak and how to enhance performance.

However, most academic staff have experienced students not even collecting their marked coursework, let alone reading and acting upon feedback. So what approaches can we use to enhance the value to students of feedback? Box 12.1 provides some guidance on giving feedback. As most students focus on the mark received, requiring student involvement before giving the marks (see point 5) may encourage attention to feedback.

Box 12.1 Giving Students Feedback

1. Give short feedback points instead of ticks and crosses; they are more motivating and less negative.
2. Feedback should be realistic and honest; suggestions should be achievable and students should be told about problems.
3. Feedback should be legible; a typed list of points with codes to identify issues can be used, or it can be given by audiotape or email.
4. Giving feedback as soon as possible makes it more likely students will read and learn from it. A model answer with comments about points which cause difficulty can be given out when work is handed in and students can compare it with their own work.
5. Feedback without marks increases students' motivation to read it and learn from it; they can be asked to read feedback and identify the mark they believe they should get. They should give these marks in before getting their allocated mark. A significant discrepancy should be discussed with the individual student.
6. Discussion about the feedback with a class or groups of students helps them to realise they all make errors and can learn from each other.

As the major motivator for learning the volume of assessment necessary is an important issue. Approaches to reducing the load are discussed by Race et al. (2005), mainly revolving around using technology and pre-prepared marking schedules. Two additional approaches are:

- Involving students in peer marking, and ensuring that they understand the value they can gain from it. Using prepared criteria and working in small groups, each piece of work is marked anonymously by two students (with pairs changed for each script), or three if a discrepancy in marking occurs. The lecturer is responsible for moderating marking from the different groups.
- Using class time for self- or peer-marking of some work, before taking it in to record marks and check a random sample of marking.

FAILING STUDENTS

'Failing students' is an issue which has been discussed in some detail in relation to two meanings both of which are of concern to lecturers in nursing:

- students who fail to meet acceptable academic standards;
- institutions which are failing students. (Peelo and Wareham, 2002: 2)

These interact in contributing to 'wastage' or loss of students from higher education with implications for individuals, the institution and society at large. The move towards a mass higher education system has resulted in the proportion of the population moving into HE radically increasing, with lower entry qualifications and more mature students. A rise in wastage seems not unexpected, but

> Notwithstanding progress on recruitment, institutions should focus on retaining students, particularly those from disadvantaged backgrounds. Widening access to higher education must not lead to an increase in the number of people who fail to complete their courses. (Secretary of State for Education and Employment, 2000, cited by Peelo and Wareham, 2002: 28)

Thus it is important to understand failure, how it occurs, and approaches to reducing failure without dropping standards below an acceptable level.

What is meant by failure? To the student it can mean different things. It means that they have failed to achieve a pass mark in something – but the context and implications of this can vary considerably:

- Failure of a single piece of coursework or an examination within a module but:
  - permitted a resit of an examination or resubmission of coursework;
  - allowed compensation or condonement within the module. (*Compensation* is when the marks from more than one piece of work are averaged and, if an overall pass mark is achieved, this is carried forward as module mark. *Condonement* is when the student is permitted to carry a failed piece of work, as long as the overall mark for the year is satisfactory. Some HEIs do not permit condonement.)
- Failure of an overall module, but permitted a resit or resubmission, or even allowed compensation with other modules in the year or condonement for that module.
- Failed resits or resubmissions and not permitted to progress within the course.
- A student may also consider that they have failed when they decide that the course is wrong for them, even though formally they have achieved a pass.

Failure in clinical practice is discussed in the next chapter.

It is important to understand how students respond to a failed piece of work in order to be able to interact appropriately with them. A focus group study (Robshaw and Smith, 2004) of students who had failed an assignment identified four key themes:

- *Desire to succeed:* Motivation increased as students progressed through the programme. Shared goal setting with personal tutors was important.
- *Acceptance of personal failure:* This was felt more strongly with junior students and related to high expectations of clinical mentors. Senior students succeeding in practice recognised the potential implications of failure on registration as a nurse.

- *Recognition of personal attributes that are required for success:* The importance of hard work and prioritising the different aspects of their life was identified. There was some resentment about the demands of the course and effect on their life, but these were recognised as part of undertaking the programme.
- *Responsibility for both personal success and failure:* Mature and school-leaver students were aware of their own responsibility for passing or failing but identified that collaboration with their personal tutor in setting goals was essential.

The two factors that students felt would most help them to succeed were personal support and financial help. Academic support from the personal tutor, student services, peer support groups and others are all important and should be associated with collaborative goal setting and guidance on time management. In addition, guidance on financial management is needed.

University regulations usually permit a student to have a second attempt (and sometimes a third) to pass a module on several occasions throughout a programme. There may be some who are repeatedly failing as they progress although they may eventually complete all parts of their programme. Failing students have considerable implications for staff and the HEI in terms of time and cost of support needed from their studies adviser and from a range of support services provided by the institution.

PLAGIARISM

Plagiarism is one type of cheating and is considered a severe form of academic dishonesty. It is described by Turnitin (a search engine, cited by Quinn and Hughes, 2007) as an act of fraud and the following are all types of plagiarism:

- Submitting another person's work as your own;
- Copying words or ideas from another person without giving credit;
- Failing to put a quotation in quotation marks;
- Changing words but copying the sentence structure of a source without giving credit. (Quinn and Hughes, 2007: 334)

All HEIs have policies for dealing with plagiarism, starting with a written warning and progressing through stages to expulsion from the university. However, for nursing students, plagiarism is also a professional issue: if a student cheats in this way, they may, for example, falsify patient charts or drug records. The *Guidance on Professional Conduct for Nursing and Midwifery*

Students, under the principle of *'Be open and honest, act with integrity and uphold the reputation of your profession'*, states that students should:

- Be honest and trustworthy when completing all records and logs of your practice experience
- Not plagiarise or falsify coursework or clinical assessments. (NMC, 2010b: 17)

In most universities, nursing students who plagiarise or otherwise cheat in academically focused or clinically-based submissions are reported to the Fitness for Practice Committee of the University and may be discontinued from the programme. If permitted to continue, at the end of the programme the declaration of good health and good character, normally signed by the programme leader, with the statement of completion of the programme, may be returned to the NMC unsigned.

In recent years plagiarism has increased, with access to websites providing readily copied material, and some sites selling fully written essays. One effect of this appears to be an increase in formal examinations instead of coursework, even though in a nursing programme coursework is usually seen as more authentic.

Identifying and Minimising Plagiarism

In marking assessments it is important to identify plagiarism when it occurs. The University of Ulster (2010b) has identified possible indications of plagiarism shown in Box 12.2.

Box 12.2 Indications of Plagiarism

(a) The work is unduly sophisticated for a student in language and in content.
(b) There is a discrepancy between the plagiarised elements and what the student has written unaided in terms of level (and) use of language.
(c) The work may seem unfocused as it moves from paragraph to paragraph or sentence to sentence from diverse sources, or indeed different parts of the same source, without any clear linkages or movement. While a lack of organisation is certainly a feature of some work that has not been plagiarised, it is the combination of quite sophisticated sequences with a lack of focus that may denote plagiarism.
(d) Internet plagiarism may be spotted in certain cases through features such as Americanised spelling; through a change in script or formatting for downloaded sections; from the existence of linked sites; from reference to another country in the text as being the one in which the student is writing.
(e) The work is much better than that normally produced by the student. A difficult one this, since people do improve and the issue should not be

pre-judged. In a situation where examinations and much coursework are anonymous, this may also not become apparent until quite a late stage.

(f) Where internet plagiarism is suspected, an appropriate plagiarism search engine (e.g. Turnitin) may be used. Staff have also found that feeding a number of key words or phrases into a search engine has enabled them to locate the source.

Many universities subscribe to Turnitin, a plagiarism search engine which is available to staff and students allowing them to check their work before submission. Some Schools require students to include a Turnitin report with submitted coursework.

The seriousness of plagiarism makes it essential that students fully understand what it is and the potential implications. Early in their programme and with small instances of plagiarism, students may genuinely have omitted to reference material and need guidance rather than imposition of penalties.

Approaches to assessment will influence the opportunity for plagiarism and help to minimise it. Coursework that requires students to draw on recent developments and their own experience makes it more difficult to plagiarise. Bryan and Clegg discuss some approaches which focus on the *'extent to which an individual has increased skills and understanding'* (2006: 219) in which students must demonstrate how they have learnt and how different items of information link to their own experience. Some approaches are: *'oral examinations (*vivas*), debates, portfolios, skeleton drafts, reflective logs, teamwork projects'* etc. (2006: 219). Topics based on recent issues, using primary sources and requiring recent relevant references all reduce the potential for plagiarism. Requiring students to confirm that submissions are their own work, reinforces the importance of avoiding plagiarised work.

CHAPTER SUMMARY

The theme running through this chapter is that assessment determines learning and the principles underpinning assessment and a number of different methods are discussed. However, a programme is only successful for an individual student if he or she achieves the necessary standards to pass the assessment set to make judgements about the academic level achieved. Preparation for assessment and ensuring student understanding of the academic conventions, including not plagiarising other people's work, is necessary. Without effective feedback assessment is of limited value.

13 ASSESSMENT OF SKILLS AND COMPETENCE

INTRODUCTION

The NMC (2010a) *Standards for Pre-Registration Nursing Education* includes the first generic competence statement for entry to the register, which states that *'all nurses must act first and foremost to care for and safeguard the public'* (2010a: 12). In the same document the first of the Standards for Education is '*Safeguarding the Public*' (2010a: 49). These two statements underpin the supervision of students' activities during practice learning and emphasise the importance of assessment of skills and competence in practice, the focus of this chapter.

One issue of debate is around the academic level of clinical competence to be achieved. Pre-registration nursing programmes are now offered at degree level. Nevertheless, there is disagreement about whether students should be demonstrating practice at degree level and indeed about what degree-level practice is. This chapter looks at skills and competence. Many of the skills discussed in Chapter 10 can be reasonably assessed as pass or fail – i.e. does the student carry out all the stages of the procedure safely and correctly, or not? This approach tends to place the emphasis on skill development. However, this presents challenges in relation to confirming that students are demonstrating development and application of cognitive abilities at the appropriate academic level in their practice. It can be argued that competence includes critical thinking demonstrated through reflection, decision-making and integration of knowledge, skills and values in the planning and provision of care. These competencies involve the use of intellectual skills and can, therefore, be assessed at the different academic levels (4, 5 and 6) as students progress through their programme.

The development of skills and competence was discussed in Chapter 10. Stuart emphasises the importance of formative assessment in clinical practice in developing student competence and provides detailed guidance for mentors in preparing students who are '*fit to practice*'. The importance of '*having the courage to fail students when standards are not achieved*' (2007: ix) is emphasised.

In the programmes of nurse education now being implemented following the NMC (2010a) standards, competence is judged using continuous assessment – formative throughout each period of practice learning in all clinical contexts experienced, and summatively at:

- the first progression point;
- the second progression point; and
- the end of the programme.

ROLES IN ASSESSMENT

Assessment of clinical competence involves a number of different individuals through a student's programme and all qualified nurses have a role in the supervision, and thus preparation, of nursing students during their practice learning. The NMC (2008a) has specified roles for supporting students in learning and assessment in practice and additional roles have evolved in healthcare providers and education providers (Table 13.1).

The NMC (2010a) clearly identifies the mentor and, at the end of the programme the sign-off mentor, as responsible for the assessment of student competence throughout practice learning and at end of each stage of the programme. However, universities vary in the involvement of the link lecturer in this process. One of the major potential problems in relation to assessment of clinical competence is ensuring reliability. A number of approaches are used to endeavour to enhance this:

- development of an assessment schedule jointly by HEI staff and clinical staff;
- training of mentors to help them all to understand the assessment schedule and make judgements of performance in the same way;

- the involvement in clinical assessment of an experienced assessor working with a number of mentors in several clinical settings over a prolonged period of time to develop a shared understanding of level of performance expected. This may be the link lecturer from the HEI or someone from the practice setting such as a practice education facilitator.

TABLE 13.1 *Roles in Assessment of Clinical Competence*

Role	Specified by:	Responsibilities of role
Mentor	NMC: required	Responsible for assessment of performance at end of Stage 1 and Stage 2 pre-registration programmes.
Sign-off mentor	NMC: required	*Pre-registration students*: must make final assessment of practice and confirm that required proficiencies for entry to the register have been achieved. *Specialist practice students:* supported and assessed by sign-off mentors or practice teachers. *Midwifery students: supported and assessed by sign-off mentors*
Practice teacher	NMC: required	*Specialist community public health students:* supported and assessed by practice teachers.
Practice Education Facilitator Education Development Facilitator	Service provider: optional	Role titles and responsibilities may vary with different service providers. Role likely to include liaison with HEIs and support of mentors. With HEIs, ensures mentor updating and maintenance of local register. Other aspects may vary. May play role in ensuring assessments carried out as required.
Link Lecturer Academic in Practice	HEI: optional	University lecturer: takes responsibility for liaising with specific clinical areas. From some HEIs, they visit students regularly (e.g. fortnightly) to help apply theory to practice, and participate in clinical assessments, enhancing reliability. Facilitates students and mentors in action planning to enable students to meet outcomes. Focus on supporting failing students and their mentors as well as issues above.
Service users	HEI and service provider: optional	Mainly involved in formative assessment, particularly in relation to generic skills such as communication.

An important and developing role is that of the service user in (usually) formative assessment of student competence in a range of healthcare professions. Davies and Lunn (2009) involved volunteer patients in using a visual analogue scale with healthcare students to assess different aspects of communication. This formative assessment tool enabled novice students to perceive 80% improvement and experienced students 86.4% improvement in their own performance and to incorporate these assessments in their professional portfolios. The items specified are shown in Box 13.1 and are as relevant to nurses as to other healthcare students.

Box 13.1 Items of Communication Assessed with Healthcare Students (Davies and Lunn, 2009)

The statements concerned addressed how students:

1. introduced themselves to the patient;
2. maintained eye contact when talking to the patient;
3. gathered information from the patient;
4. used words that the patient can understand;
5. listened to what the patient has to say;
6. answered the patient's questions about their treatment;
7. involved the patient in decisions about their treatment;
8. cared about the patient as a person;
9. gave the patient his/her full attention;
10. displayed sensitivity when discussing the patient's medical history;
11. explained any verbal advice given to the patient; and
12. explained any written advice given to the patient.

The NMC (2010a: 82) states that *'programme providers must make it clear how service users and carers contribute to the assessment process'*. This appears to assume that they will have a role in assessment although there is no guidance provided on how this is to be implemented. There have been some instances of service user involvement in the assessment of mental health students but very little published in relation to adult nursing students. Stickley et al. (2010) identified four categories to include in an assessment tool to be used by service user assessors of student mental health nurses:

- attitude;
- communication skills;
- personal awareness;
- knowledge and development.

However, while there were benefits to be gained by students, there were also difficulties in including service users (particularly those with long-term mental illnesses) in assessment and it was recommended that they be involved as reviewers instead. The selection of reviewers should be carried out by mentors with agreement from the student, who can include the service user reviews within the portfolios as evidence of development.

THE ASSESSMENT

Assessment related to practice learning is complex. It involves judging the performance of skills and competence in clinical practice but also requires demonstration of decision-making and clinical judgement based on theoretical learning. The NMC requires that theory and practice are equally important in determining the final award but this can be interpreted in different ways. It is not essential that marks are awarded but an adequate level of competence must be demonstrated for the student to achieve the academic award which is recognised by the NMC for registration as a nurse.

There is ongoing debate about giving a pass/fail or a graded result for clinical performance and there are a number of difficulties with using a grading system for assessment of clinical competence, including:

- a tendency towards inflated grades/marks leading to upwards skewing of degree classifications;
- poor inter-rater reliability, with a very large number of mentors and a considerable number of link lecturers and others involved;
- development of descriptors which enable a reasonable degree of comparability across assessors.

While content validity can be assured through the use of expert panels it is difficult to ensure reliability in use of the assessment schedule. The use of more grades in a marking system increases the reliability of the scale (Cresswell, 1986) but a pass/fail grading system simplifies the assessment. The judgement to be made in clinical assessment may simply be whether the student is safe or unsafe in practice and a pass/fail decision on this basis has a reduced likelihood of awarding an incorrect result. However, if one of the purposes of assessment is to differentiate between the just adequate student and those who perform at a very high level, this aspect of validity is reduced. In addition, motivation to excel in practice may be lessened.

Assessment related to clinical practice is likely to involve a range of methods which can be used in different ways. Some are only about performance judged by the mentor. Others involve work that is submitted to be assessed for academic performance (such as a portfolio which includes reflection on practice and items demonstrating their achievement of specified outcomes) but also contributes to the assessor's judgement related to clinical competence.

SKILLS ASSESSMENT

In Chapter 10 the teaching of a range of skills was considered. It is now necessary to consider how the achievement of a safe and effective level of performance of these skills can be assessed. Some skills can be isolated and safe effective performance assessed individually. However, in clinical practice skills are applied as part of the totality of providing care, and performance of skills assessed as part of holistic care is also essential. A combination of methods can be used in assessment of skills.

Safe effective performance of individual skills can be assessed as being at a pass level within the environment of the nursing skills laboratory but students also need to demonstrate competent performance of the skill combined with the other relevant aspects of care, such as communication. For most skills this will be in the clinical context with patients requiring care which is observed by mentors and may be combined with the use of checklists, as in the example shown in Table 13.2.

TABLE 13.2 *Checklist for Assessing Wound Dressing*

Preparation	Checking patient's notes for previous treatment and wound condition
	Does wound dressing need to be changed?
	Selection of correct equipment and arranging trolley appropriately
	Clearing space for undertaking procedure, closing window
Patient comfort	Patient is asked if dressing can be performed now
	If agrees, patient is given information about procedure and what is to be done, given pain relief if necessary
	Privacy maintained both by use of curtains etc. and by covering patient appropriately
	Patient is positioned comfortably with adequate access to wound area
Infection control	Trolley and all equipment cleaned appropriately
	Hands washed before preparing equipment, after loosening soiled dressing, after completion of dressing
	Wound cleaned in way that prevents discharge being carried to clean area using non-touch technique, possibly clean hand-dirty hand technique
	Soiled materials and equipment deposited in polythene bags to prevent contact with clean objects
Care of wound	Appropriate solutions, dressings, ointments, tapes etc. selected according to condition of wound, previous treatment and prescription
	Wound cleaned from clean to dirty areas, from outside to inside, with materials that will not damage or stick to healing tissue
	Necessary procedures carried out correctly (e.g. suture removal)
	Clean, non-stick dressing applied and secured
Finalising procedure	Make patient comfortable again
	Answer any questions arising from procedure
	Clear soiled materials into appropriate disposal bags
	Place reusable materials in appropriate storage
	Report condition of wound to senior nurse and write in report

However, some skills can be assessed in a simulated setting, especially those which a student may not meet in practice such as CPR (Cardio-Pulmonary Resuscitation). The value of formative assessment of skills within a simulated setting can be enhanced by using video recording and reviewing each individual's performance. The key element is the feedback which is enhanced by use of the video, with students identifying a number of positive themes after using videos (Brimble, 2008) (see Box 13.2). Following a study focusing on identifying deteriorating patients, which used simulation and video-recording of student performance, Cooper et al. (2010) suggest that these approaches may be particularly valuable in nursing education. Objective structured clinical examinations (OSCEs) which use simulation are discussed below.

Box 13.2 Positive Aspects of Using Video-Recording (Brimble, 2008)

- Visual feedback as well as verbal
- Analyse and improve own practice
- Increases confidence
- Learn by watching others
- Feedback from peers as well as lecturers
- Objectivity
- Increased self-awareness
- Good teaching and learning methods

Most to least often mentioned by students ↓

Objective Structured Clinical Examinations (OSCEs)

OSCEs can be used for assessing (formatively or summatively) clinical skills or competencies in a simulated context, usually requiring integration of differing skills. They were originally used in medical education and are now applied in some nursing education programmes. OSCEs are planned as follows:

- *Objective:* All students undergo the same assessment with identical marking schemes used by all examiners. Marks are awarded for each item completed correctly.

- *Structured:* A number of different stations are set up, at each of which students are required to perform a different task, usually with a simulated (although sometimes real) patient and an examiner. The stations are planned to cover the content specified to test the relevant outcomes. The 'patient' is given very specific instructions to ensure that each student is faced with the same situation. Instructions for the students are provided at each station and are identical for each student.

- *Clinical:* The focus is on clinical skills and the application of theoretical knowledge to clinical situations.
- *Examination:* Tasks to be performed and questions asked are the same for every student, with marks allocated for correct performance or answers according to the designated detailed marking scheme.

OSCEs consist of a number of stations. Sometimes they are short (5–15 minutes), and are arranged as a circuit in which each builds on the previous one. Sometimes each station is longer and within 35 minutes the student may be expected to read the materials provided, then carry out the assessment and the designated activities, and complete the necessary paperwork (Rentschler et al., 2007). The marking is usually carried out at the time of the OSCE by the examiner for each station.

Stuart (2007) reports considerable variation in reported validity and reliability in using OSCEs, including citing several authors who report high validity and reliability of this mode of assessment. However, Phillips et al. reported in 2000 *'that as a form of assessment it is seriously flawed, having neither inter- nor intra-assessor reliability'* and this stance was supported by Hodges in 2003 (both cited by Stuart, 2007: 119). Two major issues have been identified (McWilliam and Botwinski, 2010) which can be enhanced to improve the reliability of OSCEs in formative or summative assessment, but the effort and cost will be considerable:

- the development of case scenarios and updates: these should give detailed information about the patient, and should be updated regularly;
- the role and training of the standardised patient: those playing the patient role require precise training to maintain accuracy and consistency in what they say and do. It is estimated that they require 10 hours training per scenario.

Stuart has summarised a number of approaches to increase reliability (see Box 13.3) and validity (see Box 13.4).

Box 13.3 Increasing Reliability in OSCEs (Stuart, 2007)

- Assessors are carefully trained
- Assessors are experienced
- There is more than one assessor
- Scoring is standardised, e.g. by checklists (although may become trivialised), within structures framework; global ratings by experienced assessors may be as or more reliable
- Large number of stations enables wide sampling across problems and learning tasks
- Separate written test is added to performance at stations
- Periodic review of assessment to confirm it remains unbiased

Box 13.4 Increasing Validity in OSCEs (Stuart, 2007)

- Problems to be used generated by expert groups or formal observation and analysis of what learners will have to undertake
- Tasks within problems or conditions in which students are expected to be competent are defined
- Blueprint constructed to sample items for inclusion, e.g. matrix of one axis showing generic competencies (history taking, communication, management, etc.) with others showing problems or conditions within which competencies will be demonstrated
- Wide sampling across competencies

COMPETENCE ASSESSMENT

As already considered in Chapter 10, competence is '*the combination of skills, knowledge and attitudes, values and technical abilities that underpin safe and effective nursing practice and interventions*' (NMC, 2010a: 11). Thus while different aspects such as skills or knowledge can be assessed individually, assessment of competence has to encompass all of the attributes mentioned within the context of providing '*safe and effective nursing practice*'.

The NMC (2010a) has identified four domains within which competencies are specified and formatively assessed towards the end of each practice learning placement. Successful performance within each domain at each summative assessment stage will include both individual skills and application of knowledge in skilled performance of competencies. The totality of judgement of clinical competence needs to use a combination of different assessment methods.

The overall assessment of competence therefore needs to be multifaceted. Each HEI can determine its own approach to such assessment, as long as it meets the quality assurance mechanisms of the NMC. In most HEIs, assessments associated with practice learning placements consist of two key elements:

- The Clinical Assessment Schedule is completed which incorporates a judgement on the student's achievement of a pass or graded level on the domains and competencies specified by the NMC.
- This is used with written work demonstrating application of knowledge and intellectual skills to practice (see below). This may also contribute to judgements associated with the clinical assessment and this written work also provides a grade or mark that the university may use in calculation for the final award.

Clinical Assessment Schedule

Most HEIs will have developed a clinical assessment schedule, or schedules for different stages, in collaboration with their partner clinical service providers, which is then used by all mentors in formative and summative assessment. This assessment schedule needs to take account of information gathered in several ways, including:

- observation of performance by mentor and other qualified nurses;
- specific checklists or questionnaires depending on particular placement and focus of learning, for example a spiritual care competence scale (van Leeuwen et al., 2009) to help to identify areas where further preparation in providing spiritual care is needed;
- written documentation associated with person-centred patient care, for example admission documents and care plans, observation charts, patient assessment forms;
- other written work which demonstrates evidence-based practice and intellectual input to competence, for example, reflections on practice and student portfolios.

It may also include reports on the meetings between student and mentor throughout the experience, learning contracts and action plans developed and results achieved from these plans.

Assessment of Intellectual Input to Competence

Portfolios

Portfolios are often used to enable students to demonstrate their achievement of competencies by a collection of materials which address the different learning outcomes/competencies. A number of different types of work can be used to demonstrate the application of intellectual skills in the practice context including case studies, care studies, reflections, patient reviews, all of which may be incorporated into or be separate from portfolios of evidence from their clinical experience.

McMullan et al. (2003) discuss the value of portfolios in the holistic assessment of competence, and identify the principles of adult learning as central to their value in promoting student development. Reflection associated with Kolb's experiential cycle (Knowles et al., 2011) enables students to demonstrate the application of knowledge to the clinical care they are providing. There are two broad approaches to using portfolios to demonstrate applied knowledge as part of competence:

- a global approach in which students provide evidence related to the overall outcomes for the programme;
- a more focused submission in which the aspects of practice to be evidenced vary with the context in which practice is set. For example, the highly technical competencies in ICU will demand different outcomes from those in a community context and the portfolio guidelines differ to reflect this.

Some students will have difficulty in converting learning outcomes to practice activities that can be observed and assessed, and supported by evidence in their portfolio. Learning the technique of portfolio writing takes time and effort and is often supported by mentors (who may also need guidance). The difficulty is that this may detract from learning from practice through causing students to focus on learning to prepare the portfolio. It is suggested that the portfolio requirements should move from simple at the beginning of the programme to complex as the students develop their abilities in reflection and analysis throughout the programme (Scholes et al., 2004).

Marking portfolios can take a considerable amount of time, so providing guidelines which will result in students focusing their writing and making the marking more manageable is useful. Formative feedback on students' portfolios can be particularly valuable for development of understanding of situations in practice and for developing skill in reflecting on practice. A suggested marking schedule for portfolios is shown in Table 13.3 With further development, this could help enhance reliability.

Case/Care Studies

These can be used in different ways for teaching and assessment. The case and the care study can be differentiated, although when focused on an individual they may be indistinguishable:

TABLE 13.3 *Possible Marking Grid for Practice Learning Portfolio*

Aspect	Criteria	Marks (out of 100)
Introduction	Learning outcomes and how contents of portfolio demonstrate achievement of different outcomes	10
Clinical expertise	*Evidence of achievement of:* Assessment, planning and evaluation of care demonstrates patient-centred approach Record of performance of skills safely, with attention to patient welfare and comfort Evidence that care provided is evidence-based practice Demonstrates creativity in practice	20
Communications	*Evidence of achievement of:* Demonstrates good communication skills Verbal communication with patients and families that is appropriate and supportive in difficult situations Communicates appropriately with professional colleagues Written communication clear and concise	15
Health promotion	*Evidence of achievement of:* Demonstrates understanding of importance of patient teaching Plans and delivers teaching packages relevant to the patient condition and family needs for providing care Demonstrates health promotion role with patients and families	15
Professional role	*Evidence of achievement of:* Professional behaviour including reliability, accountability Interprofessional teamwork and good relationships with colleagues Takes responsibility for own learning	15
Management	*Evidence of achievement of:* Effective management of resources Delegation and supervision of care for individuals and groups of patients Clear, concise oral and written reporting of patient progress Identifies need for and plans innovation to enhance care	15
Presentation	Correct use of English, i.e. accurate spelling and punctuation, good sentence and paragraph construction Satisfactory structure of document, divided as appropriate	10

- The focus in the care study is on the nursing assessment, care planning, intervention and evaluation of care.
- The case study usually takes a broader perspective (Stuart (2007) identifies components of a case study, see Box 13.5).

In the context of assessment they are more usually presented as a paper submission, but can also be an assessed oral presentation to peers. A case/care study does not permit assessment of clinical skills but does enable some aspects of competence to be assessed, such as:

- knowledge base surrounding the case/care study;
- an understanding of that knowledge;
- application of theory to practice;
- ability to assess, implement appropriate interventions, evaluate effect of intervention;
- it may be possible to assess attitudes and interpersonal skills. (Stuart, 2007: 123).

Box 13.5 Elements of a Case Study

- Orientation to the subject (which can be an individual patient, family or community)
- Socioeconomic background of the subject and the influence of this on the development of the illness, disease condition or health problem and access to health and other services
- Draws on and integrates theory from a range of subjects to explain the nature and cause of the illness, disease condition or health problem(s)
- Problems/difficulties encountered by the subject and the care, support, health promotion or other interventions required
- The rationale for the approach to management and treatment
- Contributions made by other members of the multidisciplinary team and their importance
- Evaluating the effectiveness of the interventions

Reflections

Nursing students are often expected to write reflections on their experience in practice, and reflection is a key element in experiential learning. Assessment of reflection, however, is controversial with some academics considering that reflection is personal to the student and should not have to be submitted for assessment, although students may be encouraged to share parts of it with their mentor or personal tutor. Others consider that reflection on practice is a key skill which students need to develop for continuing professional development, and assessment is the motivating factor for this. Dyment and O'Connell (2011) reviewed eleven research papers examining the level of reflection in HE student journals (portfolios) using eight different models of reflection. Four of these studies involved nursing students and based their assessments on three frameworks. Of the eleven papers, only two, neither of them about nursing students, reported the majority of students reflecting at higher levels (see Chapter 8); five were weakly critical, with the remaining four reporting a moderate level of reflection.

It is important that staff involved with a particular programme have a consistent approach to marking reflections and a number of approaches to this have been described. Dalley (in Bulpitt and Deane, 2009) drew on concepts from other writers in developing guidelines for students (identified as Elements of Reflection), which staff used when marking reflections (see Box 13.6). While students' marks improved significantly due to the clarity of the instructions when this was introduced, the one negative result was a fall in creative approaches in their work. Encouragement of creativity throughout the programme may overcome this. Drawing on his earlier publication (Kember, 2001), Kember et al. (2008) have also developed a scheme for marking reflective writing, shown in Box 13.7, which identifies four levels of reflection and simplifies marking.

Box 13.6 Elements of Reflection (Bulpitt and Deane, 2009)

- Description
  - What happened?
  - This might include details such as Where? Who? When?
- Exploration
  - How did you feel or react?
  - What did the experience mean to you?
  - Why did things happen as they did?
- Insights
  - Did you come to any conclusions?
  - Have you come to any conclusions since?
  - Do you see things differently now?
  - Is there anything you understand better?
- Further development
  - What ideas or plans do you have for improving things?
  - What have you learned?
  - How have you changed:

(Continued)

(Continued)

- Your approach
- Your attitude
- Your ideas
- Or your actions?

- Theory and practice
  - You might use literature to explore your experience, to gain insights or to plan for next time
  - What insights have you gained from the literature?
  - Where does your experience link with the literature?

Box 13.7 Summary of Four Categories of Reflection (Kember et al., 2008)

Non-reflection

- The answer shows no evidence of the student attempting to reach an understanding of the concept or theory which underpins the topic.
- Material has been placed into an essay without the student thinking seriously about it, trying to interpret the material, or forming a view.
- Largely reproduction, with or without adaption, of the work of others.

Understanding

- Evidence of understanding of a concept or topic.
- Material is confined to theory.
- Reliance upon what was in the textbook or the lecture notes.
- Theory is not related to personal experiences, real-life applications or practical situations.

Reflection

- Theory is applied to practical situations.
- Situations encountered in practice will be considered and successfully discussed in relation to what has been taught. There will be personal insights which go beyond book theory.

Critical reflection

- Evidence of a change in perspective over a fundamental belief of the understanding of a key concept or phenomenon.
- Critical reflection is unlikely to occur frequently.

(N.B. Intermediate categories are permitted)

STUDENTS FAILING IN PRACTICE

One of the issues which is of concern to all involved in assessment of competence in practice is that of students who are not achieving the level of performance expected. Duffy (2003) drew on earlier publications in her qualitative study of 'Failing to Fail' in which she explored factors contributing to the impression '*that some student nurses are being allowed to pass clinical assessments without having demonstrated sufficient competence*' (Watson and Harris, cited in Duffy, 2003: 6). As identified earlier, a number of different individuals are involved in assessment but, according to the NMC, the mentor (qualified nurse with additional preparation for the role) is responsible for confirming that the student has achieved the specified competencies. Duffy's work identified a number of reasons why mentors find it difficult to fail students, as shown in Box 13.8.

Box 13.8 Difficulties in Failing Students

- Students receive pass grade even though not performing adequately
  - Concerns raised verbally with lecturers are not acted upon, mentors unwilling to 'put pen to paper'
  - Tensions between HEI and appeals procedure, and professional values of nursing lecturers and mentors
- Lack of validity and reliability of current clinical assessment tools may contribute to the issue of 'failure to fail'
  - Difficulty in defining borderline performance
  - Mentors give benefit of doubt
  - Difficulty in failing on grounds of attitude or inappropriate professional behaviour
- Procedures in failing student
  - HEI needs to be informed early of potential for failure but mentor needs week or two to identify problem and work with student to remedy it
  - Mentors not always identifying and documenting problems early enough
  - Not following procedures resulting in lecturer's inability to support decision which will not be supported at appeal
- Mentor issues
  - Mentors not taught about difficulties in failing students
  - Constraints on mentorship role due to shortage of staff, workload etc.
  - Mentors consider that students will improve so do not fail early in programme
  - Mentors reluctant to fail third year students as is so late in programme
  - Limited experience as mentor results in lack of confidence to fail
  - Lack of acceptance of accountability
  - Lack of support from lecturers

Preparation of mentors is considered elsewhere, but the other key recommendations in relation to failing students in nurse education programmes are:

- tripartite arrangements to support mentors in clinical assessment with some method of recording mentor concerns;
- lecturers should have a role in clinical assessment particularly in relation to the application of theory in practice and academic level;
- professional behaviour and attitudes emphasised in assessment;
- communication mechanisms to support and keep mentor informed of subsequent decisions;
- recognition by managers of additional work for mentor of supporting a failing student (Duffy, 2003).

In addition, an ongoing record of achievement, now required by the NMC (2010a), enables comments on student performance to be passed to succeeding mentors and progress to be monitored. However, several papers and posters at the RCN (2011a) education conference were still identifying some of the difficulties identified by Duffy (2003) and an ongoing concern about some individuals who are admitted to the Professional Register.

The first aspect of working with students who may fail is identification of the failing student. Most HEIs now expect at least three interviews to be held between student and mentor during each placement and recorded formally: the initial, mid-placement and final assessment interviews. In addition, mentors will be working with their students, giving regular feedback on their performance and recording their development. Clinical assessment is carried out as a continuous process of formative assessment throughout the clinical experience, with summative assessment towards the end of the experience. Frequently mentors will identify those students who cause concern early in their experience and are potential failures through identifying the various indicators shown in Box 13.9.

Box 13.9 Indicators of Possible Failure (Duffy and Hardicre, 2007a)

- Inconsistent clinical performance; limited practical, interpersonal and communication skills; unsafe practice and/or does not meet required level of competence for stage of training;
- Lack of interest or motivation, unreliability and persistent lateness/absence; preoccupation with personal issues;
- Does not respond appropriately to feedback; may be lack of insight leading to inability to change following constructive feedback;

- Inappropriate recognition of professional boundaries and/or poor professional behaviour;
- Continual poor health, feeling depressed, uncommitted, withdrawn, sad, tired or listless;
- Lack of theoretical knowledge.

By the mid-placement interview the mentor is able to clearly identify issues of concern in the student's performance in formative assessment. This opportunity can be used to give detailed feedback on performance and develop an action plan to help the student remedy clinical performance and achieve the set outcomes. If a student is giving considerable cause for concern, involving the link lecturer or the student's personal tutor may be helpful to ensure that the necessary HEI procedures are carried out, and intention to fail is not thwarted by incorrect formalities.

The final placement interview incorporates the formal summative assessment and the results should not be a surprise for the student, but frequently students respond in a way that indicates they have not really understood the significance of the feedback they have previously received. Duffy and Hardicre (2007a) identify a number of different ways that students may respond (see Table 13.4) and which will guide the assessor in future interaction.

TABLE 13.4 *Student Responses to a Failed Assessment*

Shock and disbelief	Possible inaccurate self-assessment of their own abilities and competence. Previous experience of being given the benefit of the doubt and passed even with critical feedback
Betrayed and hurt	Some students '*interpret the nurturing, supportive mentorship role as a close friendship*'. Developing a professional supportive role as a mentor requires thought and practice
Crying	Students need time to cry before further discussion of assessment result and implications
Anger/aggression and/or denial	Students may react badly to a failure and not accept the result. Bias, victimisation, personality clashes may all be blamed and legal action may be threatened. If expected, the presence of a personal tutor or other person may be helpful
Blaming others	Students may blame 'previous mentors', 'lack of appropriate placements', and *'their university course'* for their deficits
Relieved and willing	Students may accept a failed assessment and '*often recognise their clinical weaknesses, are concerned by their shortcomings and consequently are relieved when mentors highlight areas that need improvement*'

While this chapter is essentially about assessment, it makes sense to include some consideration of the management of the failing student here.

The key elements of early identification and provision of feedback have been discussed above as ways of helping these students to recognise their own deficits and improve their performance. Duffy and Hardicre (2007b) discuss other important issues for mentors:

- Providing clearly documented evidence of failure: to ensure that the decision to fail a student is not overturned on appeal due to lack of clear evidence of inadequate performance after:
  - development of action plans to remedy deficiencies,
  - repeated opportunities to practise under supervision, and
  - feedback designed to aid improvement.
- Seeking support: failing a student is difficult for the mentor who is concerned about whether they are doing the right thing and whether they are completing all the documentation correctly. The link lecturer, personal tutor or practice education facilitator can support the mentor, ensure that the student is being judged fairly, and provide guidance in completing documentation.

CHAPTER SUMMARY

This chapter has examined some of the issues relating to assessment of skills and competence. This chapter links with the previous one, as knowledge applied in the practice setting is an essential aspect of competence. Attitudes and professional behaviour are two key elements of the judgement to be made, and are issues about which the general public are concerned. This aspect of the assessment of a nursing student is probably the most difficult part of making the range of necessary judgements leading to a student becoming a registered nurse. Some of the different types of work submitted for assessment of application of knowledge in the practice context have been discussed. One of the most difficult issues in clinical assessment is that of failing a student. Approaches which can be used to reduce failure and to deal with the student's response have been considered.

14 STUDENT RECRUITMENT AND SELECTION

INTRODUCTION

Recruitment of suitable people to become nurses is one of the most important aspects of the role of those responsible for nursing education. It is suggested that a nursing degree programme is one of the toughest in the UK with students undertaking longer academic years than most others, completing 2300 hours of clinical practice covering the full 24 hours and seven days a week, and balancing course demands with family responsibilities. It is also, for many students, the most satisfying thing they have ever done with the prospect of an interesting and challenging career.

In previous chapters aspects of the curriculum related to development of knowledge, skills and values essential for a nurse to provide high quality care have been discussed and the criteria to be met are specified by the NMC (2010a and 2010d). In order to achieve the necessary standards, students have to have innate ability and qualities on which to build, as well as the motivation to succeed. Selection of individuals to become nurses, or to undertake more advanced programmes in nursing, needs to take account of these different types of attributes.

NMC STANDARDS AND SELECTION

In the selection of students to start a nursing education programme, the HEI has to work within the Standards specified by the NMC (2010a), as summarised in Table 14.1, and needs to take account of several types of attributes.

TABLE 14.1 *Expected Requirements for Entry to Nursing Education (Most of this content is taken from* Standards for Pre-Registration Nursing Education *(NMC, 2010a: 54–59))*

NMC Standard: indicated by	**Comment**
Good written and spoken English, including reading and comprehension: • Evidence of literacy • Communicates clearly and effectively in writing including using a computer	In Wales, good Welsh may replace English Usually English at GCSE level or other qualification When international students (outside EU) offer IELTS, they must achieve 7 overall and in each of four sections
Evidence of capacity for numeracy to achieve competencies: • Accurate use of numbers for volume, weight and length • Addition, subtraction, division, multiplication, decimals, fractions, percentages • Use of calculator	Usually mathematics at GCSE level or other qualification May be through an appropriate access course
Appropriate academic and professional requirements • Evidence of 10 years of general education	Specified in EHEA document on recognition of professional qualifications Access course acceptable for entry to HE
NMC requirements for good health and good character • Capable of safe and independent practice without supervision • Cautions, convictions or charges pending must be declared before entering and throughout the programme • Checked before admission, at progression points and on completion • International students must also meet UK Government requirements	Self-declaration of good health and character at progression points Other details provided in NMC (2010a): 56–7 Additional information in NMC (2010b) which includes consideration of *'reasonable adjustment'* for those with disabilities.
Accreditation of Prior Learning (APL) as appropriate	As specified in NMC (2010a) pages 57–9
Face-to-face engagement between applicants and selectors	Selectors trained in principles of selection, anti-discrimination and equal opportunities
Selection involves representatives from practice learning providers	Suggested by NMC: include as appropriate nurses in practice, service users, carers, nursing students and people with disabilities

Nursing is an activity which requires a high level of knowledge and decision-making with pre-registration programmes being at (or moving towards) degree level. Thus academic ability (including numeracy and literacy) is an important aspect of selection, usually assessed by formal school-leaving qualifications although it is equally important to consider the various routes which enable people with non-standard qualifications to enter the profession. Equally important are the personal attributes of empathy and caring, which are more difficult to assess but must be addressed, and sensitivity and precision in carrying out psychomotor skills.

There are a number of issues which arise in the process of implementing the NMC specified standards. In particular there is a balance to be struck between two legal requirements:

- firstly, the statutory rationale for the NMC, which is safeguarding the public;
- secondly, the legal requirements of the Equality Act (2010) in England and disability discrimination legislation in other countries.

Academic Qualifications

The move to degree level entry to the nursing profession has increased the level of academic qualification to that normally required in HE. However, nursing has traditionally taken students from a wide section of the population and, to continue to maintain an adequate nursing workforce, needs to maintain a wide entry gate.

HEIs in most of the UK have until recently used Advanced ('A') Levels taken at about 18 years as the main selection criteria and these are still important although there are a range of other acceptable qualifications. A system of Tariff Points is now in use by many universities which simplifies the use of different qualifications (UCAS, 2011). Table 14.2 shows some of these. This is particularly relevant in nursing which has a high proportion of mature applicants and those with experience as healthcare assistants applying. Many of these take access courses at Colleges of Further Education to gain acceptable entry qualifications, with some being seconded by their employing authority.

Accreditation of Prior Learning (APL) for entry to nursing is permitted (NMC, 2011b). While the majority of entrants enter nursing through taking 'A' levels or access courses, there are other routes which widen access. For example, some routes *(for example foundation degrees and vocational programmes) … meet programme entry requirements, but also aim to meet some of the pre-registration programme learning outcomes in theory, practice or both* (NMC, 2011b: 14). NHS Cadet Schemes or Apprenticeship Schemes (NHS Careers, 2011) both combine the necessary theoretical study to enter nurse education with practical work. Cadet Schemes offer a route into nursing education for those lacking adequate academic qualifications and also increase the number of those from black and ethnic minority groups entering nursing (Watson et al., 2005). It appears that as Cadet Schemes become more experienced in selection, their attrition rates drop, resulting in one scheme achieving 100% of cadets progressing into nursing education (Norman et al., 2008).

TABLE 14.2 *Examples of Educational Entry Qualifications for Nursing (University of Ulster, 2011b)*

Qualification	**Entry Level**	**Notes**
A level	A minimum of 280 UCAS Tariff Points to include grades B, B	A non-compulsory academic qualification, generally taken after completion of GCSEs (normally about 18 years), and commonly used to gain access to higher education.
Irish Leaving Certificate	A minimum of 280 UCAS Tariff Points to include grades B2, B2, B2, C2, C2 at Higher Level	Provides students with a range of subjects. Candidates for university entrance normally take seven. All subjects may be studied at Higher and Ordinary Level.
Business and Technician Education Council (BTEC) National Diploma	280 UCAS Tariff Points - Pass overall BTEC ND with DMM (distinction and 2 merits).	BTEC qualifications at different levels, awarded by Edexcel, are a vocational route into higher education. They are on the National Qualifications Framework at various levels but are based primarily on practical work or coursework.
Access Course	Pass Access course with an overall average of 65%.	Aimed at adults (minimum age 19 years) seeking access to higher education, but lacking the necessary educational qualifications.
Acceptable level of Numeracy	Demonstrated through one of a range of qualifications such as: GCSE, appropriate key or essential skills, appropriate element in Access Course, appropriate module in BTEC qualification.	
Acceptable level of Literacy	Students whose first language is not English must pass IELTS test of competence in English with a score of 7 overall and 7 in each of 4 sections: listening, reading, writing and speaking (but see later discussion on EU candidates)	
Acceptable understanding of Science		

Whether the qualifications required for entry enable selectors to identify the problem solving ability that is needed in nursing is debatable.

Literacy and Numeracy

An acceptable level of literacy and numeracy is essential for nursing practice and it is the responsibility of the HEI to ensure that prospective students have achieved this. However, numeracy in particular is often a difficulty with even some of those who have passed GCSE mathematics lacking the necessary ability to calculate drug dosages. A number of institutions now incorporate a mathematics test into their selection process (for example, Cardiff University, 2011).

The directive on the recognition of professional qualifications (EU, 2005) requires the qualifications of the professionals included in the legislation (which includes nurses) who are from countries which are signatories of the directive to be recognised by the relevant statutory bodies. In addition Article 53 states that:

> Persons benefiting from the recognition of professional qualifications shall have a knowledge of languages necessary for practising the profession in the host Member State. (EU, 2005: 50)

Up to the time of publication of this book, the relevant Statuory Bodies (i.e. the NMC for nursing) have been unable to require such professionals to undertake an English test before commencing professional practice. Potential employers or educators have carried the responsibility for ensuring that English competence is adequate for the role or education to be undertaken. In the context of nursing and other health professionals, this is clearly a risk factor for unsatisfactory patient care. However, during 2012, the regulations for professional recognition across Europe are being reconsidered with the likelihood that member states will be able to request evidence of adequate language competence for specific professions.

Applicants from outside the European Economic Area (the EU plus Norway and Switzerland) have to meet the same standards as those from the UK and may demonstrate their fluency in English through taking IELTS (International English Language Testing System) developed and offered by the British Council (Table 14.2).

Good Health and Good Character

The NMC (2010a) requires HEIs to ensure that entrants to nursing programmes meet the requirements of good health and good character and confirm that these are rechecked at progression points, entry to the Register and on transferring from other institutions. These aim to ensure that every nurse, and every nursing student, *'is capable of safe and effective practice as a nurse'* (NMC, 2010d: 6).

As nursing students will be involved with children and/or vulnerable adults, and must be trustworthy, it is a requirement to obtain an Enhanced Disclosure from the Criminal Records Bureau in England, or equivalent in other UK countries, before commencing placement. Students must take responsibility for self-declaration of any convictions, cautions or pending charges against them during their programme, or later as a qualified nurse.

Good health implies that the individual can undertake nursing safely and independently. A chronic illness or disability that does not prevent adequate performance is completely acceptable.

Disability

The disability legislation makes it unlawful to discriminate against people with a disability and requires *'reasonable adjustment'* to be made to enable people with a disability to undertake any activity. The issue is recognition of what is *'reasonable adjustment'* and how this is managed in nursing and in selection of students for nursing education programmes. Someone with a disability acquired after qualifying as a nurse and needing to use a wheelchair may be able to continue to work with *'reasonable adjustment'* by the employer. However, an adult nursing student in the same position might not be able to carry out all the activities required to complete the programme.

It is essential to be creative and access available services to assess whether or not it will be possible for the potential student to undertake the education programme. The point at which a student cannot undertake the programme is when *'reasonable adjustment'* will not make it possible to undertake nursing safely for the patients. Table 14.3 shows some examples of how *'reasonable adjustment'* may, or may not, be achieved.

Normally potential students will submit a medical report which is checked by the Occupational Health Service for fitness to undertake the programme and, when necessary, individuals are seen by the Occupational Health nurse or doctor. However, the Course Director or someone with a clear understanding of the demands on the student must be able to contribute to the decision-making about suitability for the programme.

Personality

Crucial in the selection of nursing students is personality; is this someone you would want to nurse you or your mother? There is a little evidence about personality characteristics and success in nursing, for example higher scores on psychoticism were found to be more common in those who left nurse education programmes early (McLaughlin et al., 2008). The same authors suggest that further investigation on psychological profiling in selection of nursing students is needed. At present it is difficult to assess someone's suitability for nursing although a personal statement, reference and interviews are used to endeavour to achieve this end.

References and Personal Statement

The UCAS application includes a personal statement by the candidate and a reference. In the personal statement, a particularly useful item to note is whether or not the applicant has undertaken any voluntary work or has gained experience in a caring role, either within the family or in a paid capacity. This statement can provide valuable insight into their values, contribution to the community and interaction with others and can indicate a caring approach which is desired in nursing. Unfortunately help

TABLE 14.3 *Reasonable Adjustments for Students with Disabilities*

Dyslexia	Initial screening, then assessed by educational psychologist. Student support identifies and provides necessary help: additional time to complete examinations; coursework scheduled and 2 weeks extra allowed; coaching and proof reading for grammar; computer provided. Placement: advised to tell mentor, yellow filter to help reading, handover sheets photocopied. If a student has such severe dyslexia that examination papers are read aloud and they need a scribe, it is unlikely that they will be able to read and write patient notes adequately to provide safe care.
Unstable, brittle type 1 diabetes mellitus	Numerous reasonable adjustments made to placement (recommended by student health): adjusting shift times (starting time and shift length and patterns); minimum night duty; fixed break times to ensure stable eating patterns; placements closer to home so that she does not have to stay away from home. Regular reviews with HEI Occupational Health.
Stable epilepsy	Occupational health reviews, wears medic-alert, friends know, mentor informed, otherwise course unchanged.
Partial hearing	Used hearing aid and provided with digital stethoscope. Measuring blood pressure only problem. Managed issues herself - for example, sitting at front of lectures.
Profound stammer	Stammer overwhelming. Rejected on first interview but advised to work with people (nursing home) and practise speaking. Accepted at second interview, improvement noticeable but still caused concern. Student Support carried out assessment and contributed to finance to undertake McGuire programme, with exceedingly good results.
Bipolar disorder	Applicant with bipolar affective disorder accepted. During programme became very unwell on two occasions requiring short periods of hospitalisation. However, with support from academic staff, student services, occupational health and student colleagues she completed her programme. Her current employers are equally supportive and she has talked to students about being a user of mental health services.
Severe anorexia	Anorexia identified on health declaration but occupational health physician stated she was fit to do nursing. Lecturer concerned about potential health and safety issues did not permit participation in moving and handling practical classes. Referred back to occupational health physician who asked consultant for review; bone scan performed and student declared unfit for nursing due to osteoporosis. Discontinued from programme.
Latex allergy	Diagnosed with latex allergy towards end of year 1. Thereafter, clinical placements are arranged before other allocations in consultation with service colleagues. Risk assessment of each area carried out. Clinical areas informed (with student's permission), had latex-free gloves, stethoscope etc. Carried epi-pen for immediate use if needed. Completing programme.
Cystic fibrosis and blind in one eye	Adjustments only needed in relation to practice learning settings. Wards with many respiratory patients were avoided. Otherwise student managed unaided.

provided in preparing the personal statement cannot always be ruled out, and plagiarism from statements on the web has become a concern (*The Times*, 2007). Clearly this diminishes the value of the statement. UCAS now use a plagiarism search engine with all university applications and, if plagiarism is identified, informs the HEIs to which the individual has applied.

For school leavers, references often focus on academic ability rather than suitability for nursing and tend to be of limited value. However, for mature applicants the individual they select as referee may provide valuable information about their background and caring experience.

Face-to-face Engagement

The NMC states that:

> AEIs must ensure that the selection process provides an opportunity for face-to-face engagement between applicants and selectors (NMC, 2010a : 59).

This will usually be by some form of interview. However, a number of authors have raised concerns about the traditional individual interviews describing them as: '*difficult to standardize, time consuming and* (with) *high administrative costs*' (cited by Ehrenfeld and Tabak, 2000: 102), although others have found them to be of some value. Overall, their usefulness is doubtful.

The use of multiple mini-interviews (MMI) has been described by Harris and Owen (2007) for the selection of medical students. A Q-sort methodology was used to rank the key factors needed for medicine (very similar to those needed for nursing). These were used to develop ten stations, eight for individual interviews rated by single interviewers and two interviewers in the context of a group activity. Box 14.1 shows the eight interview stations, each of 5.5 minutes with 30 seconds for changeover. The final two stations involved a PBL group session, conducted by an experienced PBL lecturer, during which two trained observers graded qualitative or quantitative observations. Each station has a specific rating scale for the different characteristics with some identified as essential, and each candidate is given an overall rating on a seven-point scale. Those with unsatisfactory ratings on key characteristics were discussed by the interviewer team and a decision made. This approach was used to exclude unsuitable candidates rather than select suitable ones and those rejected had significantly different scores from those who were accepted. Rosenfeld et al. (2008) '*have found that the MMI is more reliable and has better predictive power than our traditional panel interviews*' (43) and report that it is more efficient than traditional interviews. Although time is necessary for developing the scenarios and for staff training, less time is required for the interviews.

Box 14.1 Eight Interview Stations for Selection of Medical Students

1. *Giving instructions*. (Rationale: displaying confidence, technical communication and appropriate social skills, dealing with frustration, maintaining a sense of proportion in the face of the task)
2. *Taking instructions*. (Rationale: displaying confidence, technical communication and appropriate social skills, dealing with frustration, maintaining a sense of proportion in the face of the task and having a realistic outlook)
3. *Emotional communication*. (Rationale: demonstrating mature social skills and a realistic perspective)
4. *Problem-solving*. (Rationale: demonstrating the ability to take a comprehensive approach to a problem while maintaining a sense of proportion)
5. *Resilience and maturity*. (Rationale: demonstrating life experience and a realistic outlook in dealing with problems)
6. *Enthusiasm for medicine*. (Rationale: exploring curiosity and enthusiasm about medicine and lifelong learning)
7. *Ethics*. (Rationale: demonstrating a grounded perspective and an awareness of ethics as an issue)
8. *Awareness of common issues in medicine*. (Using rural medicine as a focus to demonstrate some familiarity with healthcare systems)

While this has been developed for medicine, a similar approach has been used by the University of British Columbia in selection of nursing school applicants (McBurney and Carty, 2009). Students spent eight minutes at each station discussing a specific scenario which addressed several of the desirable attributes. Both academic staff and applicants found this a valuable approach to selection and other Schools may wish to follow this example.

Accreditation of Prior Learning (APL)

The NMC states that *'programme providers must ensure that programmes include opportunities for accreditation of prior learning'* (2010a: 57) in relation to theory and/or practice. This is permitted for up to 50% of the programme and must ensure that students fully meet all specified requirements. In reality, in pre-registration education the proportion of the programme for which APL is allowed is likely to be considerably smaller than this. Nurses transferring into another field of practice may be given unlimited APL and midwives up to 50% APL provided in all cases that all requirements are met in full.

The processes for APL must be:

- robust, valid and reliable, and sufficient to ensure that professional requirements and academic standards are met;
- equally challenging as other methods of assessing learning in higher education;
- rigorous in accrediting practice based learning;
- explicit, unambiguous and fair, and applied in a consistent, transparent and rigorous way;
- well defined, setting out clear roles, responsibilities and accountabilities of staff, applicants and external examiners;
- able to ensure that staff are competent, prepared and developed for their roles;
- clear, explicit and accessible to potential applicants;
- monitored through an institution's quality assurance framework. (NMC, 2011b: 17)

In theory, those who have worked as healthcare assistants can be given credit for prior learning in relation to their learning in practice. However, Scott (2007) found no difference in reported learning between students completing their first year with least one year's prior experience and those with none. Had APL been justified, those with such experience would be expected to perceive less learning in their first year. It appears reasonable that, while some of the psychomotor and other skills will be unchanged, the context of their application as a healthcare assistant and as a student aiming to become a professional nurse is very different and cannot be equated. Thus, the use of APL in this situation is inappropriate.

The most straightforward use for APL is for certificated learning in subjects which are included in the nursing curriculum with some mechanism for ensuring their application within nursing. In addition, someone who has had significant experience with a particular patient group, either through employment or informal caring by, for example, looking after a family member with dementia, could have their practice learning experience modified to offer a different practice learning context.

RECRUITMENT

Different countries of the UK have different circumstances in relation to application for nursing programmes but women, who are still the majority of those entering nursing, now have a much wider range of career options. Thus, recruitment campaigns are important to attract potential healthcare students into nursing and maintain student numbers, particularly in relation to mental health and learning disability fields of nursing.

Understanding factors influencing the choice of nursing is important if recruitment is to be successful. A study of entrants to a range of pre-qualifying professional programmes in healthcare (see Box 14.2) in one university and of qualifying students from the same institution identified major motivations for their selection of career (Miers et al., 2007). These were similar for the different groups with altruism high for all professions, although nursing (children's, learning disability and mental health) and midwifery entrants showed a strong commitment to the client group. However, altruism was associated with longer careers in nursing (Duffield et al. cited by Miers et al., 2007). Older applicants identified prior experience as particularly relevant to their move into healthcare.

Box 14.2 Professional Groups Studied and Motivation for Entering Healthcare Professions

Professional Groups

Adult nursing, Children's nursing, Mental health nursing, Learning disability nursing, Midwifery, Physiotherapy, Occupational therapy, Radiotherapy, Diagnostic imaging (radiography)

Motivation

1 Altruism/being of service (Help others, Hands on, Making a Difference, Teamwork)
2 Personal interest/Abilities (Personal Interest, Own qualities, Setting/milieu)
3 Professional values/rewards (Professional values, Professional rewards, Flexibility of qualification)
4 Prior experience (Extension of current role, Personal experience)
5 Commitment to client group
6 Longstanding motivation
7 Other

Perceptions of Nursing

A career choice of nursing will be influenced by the unrealistic perceptions of nursing held by the general public, many of whom still see nursing as a fairly menial occupation whose members carry out the tasks required by doctors. Brodie et al. found that:

> many students were surprised ... by the high academic standards required of them and came to recognize and value the tremendous knowledge, skills set and responsibilities of nurses. However, their experiences reinforced both society's and their own image of an underpaid, overworked profession that lacks respect and has low morale (Brodie et al., 2004: 721).

To enhance recruitment of suitable applicants, there needs to be greater focus on the reality of the academic demands on the professional nurse and on the scope of clinical practice and career opportunities. Equally important is to improve the student experience and reduce the potential for student disillusionment due to the challenges with which they must cope:

> Many of these were related to the pressures of an under-funded health system whilst others were related to unwelcoming or disorganized clinical placement. (Brodie et al.. 2004: 731).

One of the other key issues to be taken into account is the gender-laden perceptions of nursing. Muldoon and Reilly (2003) carried out a study of gender role orientation (i.e. psychologically feminine or masculine) and the way that different specialisms were perceived with a new intake of nursing students. The perception still exists that nursing is primarily an occupation for women, although in this study different specialisms were considered to be highly female sex-typed, female sex-typed or gender neutral (see Table 14.4).

TABLE 14.4 *Perceived Gender Appropriateness and Popularity of Nurse Specialisms (Muldoon and Reilly, 2003: 95)*

	Gender appropriateness		**Popularity**	
	Mean	**Rank**	**Mean**	**Rank**
Specialisms rated as highly female sex-typed (HF)				
Midwifery	5.98	1	0.77	4
School nurse	5.05	2	0.52	12
District nurse	4.97	3	0.79	3
Health visitor	4.94	4	0.72	6
Paediatrics	4.76	5	0.70	9
Practice nurse	4.50	6	0.79	2
Specialisms rated as female sex-typed (F)				
Palliative care	4.29	7	0.52	15
Oncology	4.24	8	0.56	13
Critical care	4.23	9	0.66	11
Nurse teacher	4.21	10	0.48	16
Elder care	4.20	11	0.46	17
General medical	4.11	12	0.91	1
Specialisms rated as gender neutral (GN)				
Nurse manager	4.06	13	0.71	7
General surgical	4.03	14	0.69	10
Nurse consultant	4.02	15	0.71	7
Theatre	4.02	16	0.54	14
Learning disability	4.02	17	0.38	18
Accident and emergency	3.95	18	0.76	5
Mental health	3.71	19	0.34	19

In endeavouring to recruit applicants to nursing education, it is necessary to provide accurate information to try to change perceptions about nursing to attract bright, creative, articulate, caring individuals. The scope of nursing is great and it is therefore a potential career for a wide variety of people. Recruitment needs to be focused on those coming through schools and the entry courses discussed above (Table 14.2), but also on groups of mature individuals who want to start a career after having children, or have a career change. Those who are older on entry are more likely to finish their programme than younger students (Pryjmachuk et al., 2009). In the next section, characteristics associated with high attrition or with retention are discussed, but rather than being useful in determining who to select or reject, this information is important for identifying those who need additional support in order to be successful.

Structural Issues in Recruitment

Experience with mature students (including some single mothers) has included a significant number with family responsibilities, including care of children or of vulnerable adults. Many of these mature individuals with their caring experience are highly motivated and likely to become excellent nurses who remain in practice. However, it has been clear that, in some cases, the stress of balancing the pressures of the programme with their caring responsibilities has been a major contributing factor in leaving the programme. The aspect of the course causing most difficulty is placement, including a 35-hour week, shift working and night duty.

In many parts of the country, pre-registration nursing programmes are only available full-time and are not manageable for some of these students. To widen access, consideration of part-time pre-registration nursing is necessary. The Open University currently offers a part-time Diploma in Higher Education in adult or mental health nursing for those in healthcare employment. However, other universities could also offer part-time programmes, in which students could complete the theoretical parts of the programme full-time, but undertake the practice learning with a shorter working week, spread out over a longer period of time.

The NMC requirements for the three stages of the new programmes being introduced, will limit the flexibility to deal with small numbers of students through this route. A group large enough to be economical in providing the programme for these students alone will be needed. An additional issue is that while the NMC is willing to approve part-time programmes, in some parts of the UK the commissioning bodies will not approve student funding.

ATTRITION AND RETENTION

Attrition rates from nursing pre-registration programmes, cited by Urwin et al. (2010), are around 25% in 2006, varying from 3 to 65% in different institutions (from RCN), with figures for 2006 for the UK countries (cited by Pryjmachuk et al., 2009) as: England 16%; Scotland 24%; Wales 9%; Northern Ireland 6%. Unfortunately the methods for calculating attrition vary and thus figures are not readily compared and are of questionable validity. However, the financial and personal investment in becoming a nurse is considerable and thus it is important to minimise the attrition rate during both pre- and post-registration education programmes.

Understanding attrition is important in order to identify those students at particular risk of leaving their programme and provide appropriate support. Attrition has been defined in several ways including: *'the difference between the number of students beginning each cohort and the number who completed that cohort'* (Glossop, 2002: 377) which is a straightforward definition allowing comparisons. However, using this definition, attrition includes students who change cohort, or HEI, during their programme and still qualify as nurses, so that the attrition figures obtained produce an inflated figure in relation to those who start and eventually qualify as nurses. Attrition has also been defined as: *'failure to complete a programme of nursing leading to admission to the professional register, for any reason'* (Cameron et al., 2010: 1088), which provides a more positive view of those completing their education.

Some level of attrition is expected and reflects the reality that some of those who commence nurse education will discover that they are not suited to nursing. However, it is important to know why individuals decide to leave nursing and to provide support to enable those who are suited to nursing and who really wish to complete their education to enter the profession.

Causes of Attrition

Cameron et al. (2010, 2011) have reviewed the literature since 1995 on causes of leaving and of staying in nurse education programmes (see Table 14.5). Many factors are involved but it is clear that personality characteristics are particularly important and relate to the ability to cope with stress and burnout. Deary et al. also identified that:

> those with a more open personality, those who were more original, daring and liberal were more likely to be emotionally exhausted, suggesting that those who

were less open (conventional, unadventurous and conservative) suffered less from EE. (Deary et al., 2003: 78)

Thus, the individuals whom we want to see in nursing are those who will suffer the most from the very nature of the role and preparation for the role. Support throughout their programme is essential.

TABLE 14.5 *Why They Leave and Why They Stay (papers cited by Cameron et al., 2010, 2011; Pryjmachuk et al., 2009; Mulholland et al., 2008)*

(– increases attrition: + reduces attrition: ? effect unclear from research)

Theme	Issue	Comment	Effect
Society/ Profession	Career choice	Stereotyping of nursing as hands-on, following instructions. Reality of contrast with 'knowledgeable doer' in programme	–
		Lack of personal experience of nursing care (as patient or healthcare assistant)	–
	Knowledge of career	Knowledge of role and experience of being nursed	+
		Professional autonomy	+
Prediction	Personality	Less agreeable and conscientious, apathetic and impulsive, higher psychoticism scores	–
		Introverted tend to get higher scores on assessment	?
		High self-efficacy	+
	Age	Younger students (24 years or less)	–
		Mature students	+
	Entry qualifications	Lower or non-conventional qualifications	–
		Already holding a degree	–
	Ethnicity	Black and ethnic minority students - academic or disciplinary reasons	–
		From overseas English speaking countries	+
	Gender	Male	–
		Female	+
Programme	Academic expectations	Unexpected academic demands	–
		Lack of preparation for academic study at degree level	–
		Failing to get academic support	–
	Emotional factors	Stress and burnout not strongly associated with attrition	?
	Placements	Organisation of care, support by mentor, poor quality placements	?
	Support	Personal tutor support	+
		Peer support	+
Personal	Family	Managing family commitments	–
		Practical support with chores and children	+
		Parents not university educated	–
		Lower socio-economic status	–
		Family members who were nurses	+
	Finances	Difficulty in taking part-time work to support lifestyle	–
		Bursary inadequate for those with family responsibilities	–

Rarely is there a single cause for attrition and different factors will interact to create difficulties for individual students. One of the major changes since nursing education moved into HE is an increase in the number of mature people, predominantly women, who undertake nursing education and often have family responsibilities and need adequate support (financial, family or social care) to manage these.

Attrition varies between the different branches of nursing, with one of the factors increasing attrition being the recruitment of students under the age of 21 years. Those below 21 can still be identified as adolescents (Shepherd, 2008) and are still going through the transition to adulthood and setting their own self-identity, while adapting to university life and the different expectations for study of an andragogical approach. The numbers in this age group undertaking the different branches vary considerably (see Table 14.6) with a particularly high proportion of those doing children's training being in this category and having particularly high attrition rates (Department of Health, cited by Shepherd, 2008). Those entering mental health and learning disability nursing tend to be older than those entering other branches, although those becoming learning disability nurses tend to be in small student cohorts so are difficult to compare with other groups. In a robust study, Pryjmachuk et al. found that '*Those completing tended to be (3 years) older at entry than those not completing, and those with only the minimum entry qualifications were less likely to complete*' (2009: 157).

TABLE 14.6 *Example of BSc Students Between 18 and 24 at University of Greenwich 2005–6 (Shepherd, 2008)*

Child Branch	Adult Branch	Mental Health	Midwifery
69%	32%	22%	26%

A small study by Owen and Standen found high attrition rates in learning disability nursing. While many who commenced their professional education had previous experience, either within their family or through working as healthcare assistants, others had very little idea about what it entails. The paper recommends that all candidates have some experience before starting their education programme (Owen and Standen, 2007).

Retention

The work on attrition is useful in that it highlights characteristics of students who, for some reason, have not completed their programme. An interesting question is why students who have thought of leaving do not leave before completing their programme, but there appears to be little research on this. A small qualitative study (Bowden, 2008) interviewed eight of ten students (22%) in one cohort who had replied positively to '*I seriously considered leaving on one or more occasion(s)*'. The results are summarised in Table 14.7, and are similar to those already discussed in relation to those who do leave. In this study seven of the eight participants had non-traditional entry qualifications. This study, although non-generalisable due to the small sample size, reinforces several points which lecturers would intuitively identify as important in providing support for students. Interestingly, few students accessed the university support services.

TABLE 14.7 *Reasons Why Students Nearly Left Nursing and Why They Did Not (Bowden, 2008)*

Reasons why students seriously considered leaving – combination of issues			N = 8
1	Academic issues	Stress of examinations Writing assignments – difficulties in acquiring the skill of writing academic work, particularly for mature students and those with non-traditional qualifications	N = 6
2	Placement issues	Constantly being 'the new student', not being part of the team (2) Dealing with sick and dying patients (2) Not knowing what to expect from clinical practice (1)	N = 5
3	Financial issues	Unable to support themselves on bursary, working left little time for study (2) Male student – felt he had lost provider role in relationship (1)	N = 4
4	Personal issues	Serious personal issues potentially long-term pre-dated course (1), death or ill-health of parent (3) Combination of personal problem with other stresses of student life	N = 4
Factors which enabled them to stay – support			
1	University staff	Personal tutors – providing personal and instrumental support (6) Link lecturer – placement issues, trusting they will be treated fairly (3) University support mechanisms (3)	
2	Peers	Emotional and practical support Similar characteristics important to mature students` Group affiliation	N = 5
3	Family and friends	Parents, partners and friends supportive (3) Mothers – significant support to 3 youngest students (3) Partners (including 2 nurses) provided support (3)	

CHAPTER SUMMARY

This chapter has considered the NMC Standards for entry to nursing education and some of the difficulties in applying these in selecting suitable entrants. Approaches to recruitment are discussed. Causes of attrition and how this knowledge can assist us in managing the student experience to enhance retention are examined. The potential value of part-time programmes in recruitment of highly motivated, mature students with family responsibilities is indicated. In this chapter a number of factors are identified which course planning teams should be taking into consideration in developing programmes to meet the needs of potential students.

15 STUDENT SUPPORT

INTRODUCTION

For some students the academic and personal demands of the pre-registration nursing programme are considerable and they need support to overcome these challenges. In addition, nursing is an occupation in which students are exposed to the traumatic situations which their patients face and have to learn to provide support for their patients and families. They also have to learn to cope with the resulting emotions in themselves. There are a number of circumstances which many, if not most, nursing students find traumatic, such as caring for a dying patient and their family, facing the death of a child, or caring for someone who has just received bad news. They need sympathetic support to learn how to manage the care professionally and deal with their own emotions.

The aim of the support provided is to help the students successfully complete their programme and obtain their nursing qualification, while still maintaining standards which safeguard the public (NMC, 2010a). In the previous chapter factors associated with attrition were identified and help to identify areas where support is needed.

UNIVERSITY-BASED SUPPORT

Personal Tutor/Studies Adviser

At the beginning of their course, each student is allocated to a member of academic staff who has a responsibility for supporting their students, with the aim of helping them to achieve successful completion of their programme or to make a decision which is right for them to change course or leave university. The terminology for this role varies but personal tutor or studies adviser are the most common. The primary aim of this role has been described by Wheeler and Birtle as:

- to facilitate personal development of tutees;
- to monitor progress of tutees;
- to provide a link between students and university authorities;
- to be a responsible person within the organisation in whom the student can confide;
- to intervene with the university authorities on behalf of their tutees. (Cited by Wisker et al. 2008: 44)

Figure 15.1 summarises role requirements and aspects of the role of the personal tutor.

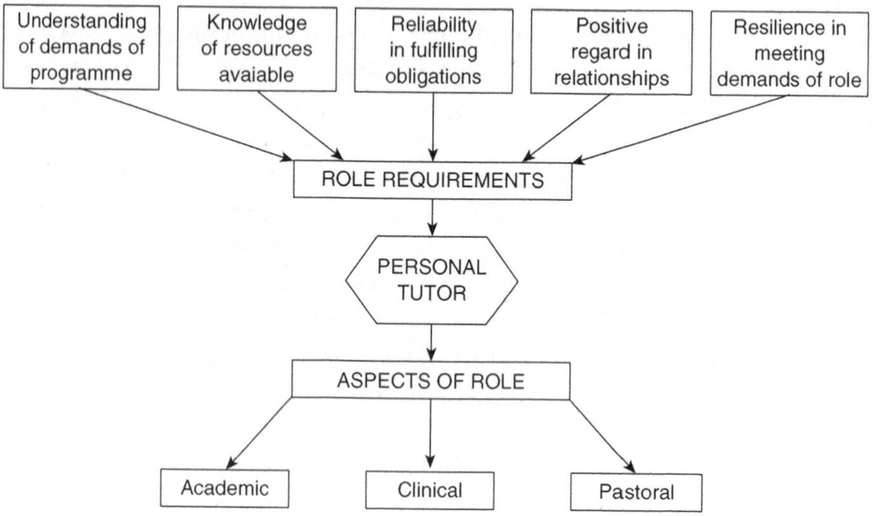

FIGURE 15.1 *The Personal Tutor*

Modes of Personal Tutoring

Neville (2007) has proposed a personal tutoring model comprising the three 'R's of care, regard, reliability and resilience interacting to create care and achieve an effective personal tutor. While this is presented as applicable to the lecturer acting as a personal tutor, the attributes are also relevant in students. Reliability is a characteristic expected in nurses, and by demonstrating this in keeping appointments and expecting students to cancel a meeting if they are unable to attend, students will begin to understand the importance of developing this attribute. Students treated with positive regard using the approach described by Rogers (Rogers and Freiberg, 1994) are likely to develop the same attribute. To cope with the challenges of nursing, students need to be resilient, so support during their programme needs to help them develop the ability to cope with the circumstances they will meet in practice.

In the context of being a personal tutor in nursing, three main components to the role have been described (Gidman, 2001): clinical, pastoral and academic. Although Gidman identifies the clinical component of the personal tutor role, the difficulties in providing clinical support over the range of clinical environments militates against this. The NMC (2010a) states that HEIs *'should ensure that nurse teachers are able to spend part of their normal teaching hours supporting student learning in practice'* (89). In many HEIs a link lecturer who has clinical expertise in the area is allocated to specific clinical areas and works with mentors and students in that context (see p.269).

Being available to listen and provide support for students with personal, family or financial difficulties is a critical part of the pastoral role of the personal tutor and necessitates the development of an appropriate personal relationship with the student. It is essential that the personal tutor knows about the various services available to help students and how to refer and encourage them to use such services as necessary (see below).

Moving into higher education can leave some students finding difficulty with the academic skills needed for studying at HE level and becoming a self-directed learner. The personal tutor may need to provide some individual tuition to help students understand and develop the necessary intellectual skills. At the beginning of most programmes time is spent on developing study skills, but some students will need additional help. Students also need to be clear on the expected workload in the programme. As already discussed, one credit point is considered equivalent to 10 hours of study, so that a student should put in 100 hours for a 10-credit module. However, Snelling et al. (2010) found that students were in general spending significantly fewer hours studying than expected for each module and, therefore, that the 4600 hours specified by the NMC (2010a) is unlikely to be achieved. This time specification corresponds with the EU requirements for general nursing preparation and there are implications for recognition across Europe if these hours cannot be guaranteed. Personal tutors should emphasise the expectations and students need guidance on how to use the study hours expected.

Various approaches to managing the role of personal tutor exist. In some universities personal tutors arrange to meet their students in induction week, or very soon after, to explain their role and how to arrange contact with them, but in general leave it to the student to make such arrangements.

Other HEIs may have a more structured organisation and variations exist in between. Watts (2011) describes structured personal tutoring with the characteristics shown in Box 15.1.

Box 15.1 Characteristics of Structured Personal Tutoring (Watts, 2011)

Students allocated to tutorial group for whole programme

Entitled to:	minimum of 6 individual and 3 group tutorials per year
First week:	written information about tutorial system, students' and personal tutors' responsibilities, University's student support services initial group meeting with tutor in first week followed by individual meeting
1st semester:	individual tutorial midway, before first placement
Thereafter:	individual meeting before and after placement group tutorial after placement

Watts' reflection on this approach reports that *'effective personal tutoring can positively enhance the student's learning experience and act as a catalyst for transferring professional values'* (Watts, 2011: 217). However, this approach will have a significant impact on the workload of academics and a balance between efficacy and cost has to be achieved.

Skills of Personal Tutoring

At some point in their programme many students will have some concerns that they wish to discuss. These tend to fall into the following groups:

- inadequate academic skills which have not previously been developed, such as revising for and sitting examinations, or writing essays;
- difficulties in managing time to undertake enough study combined with other aspects of living;
- continuing difficulty with specific learning skills, possibly needing referral for dyslexia or other specific learning difficulty;
- difficulties in understanding specific subject area or modules;
- interpersonal difficulties with other students or staff members;
- particularly after the first placement, concern about whether they have selected the right career.

Sometimes the student will be able to clarify the issues clearly and discuss them calmly, but on other occasions the student may be very upset and need calming before any real discussion can take place. While the personal tutor will sometimes be able to deal with the issues raised, it is also a part of the role to explain the range of other resources available to help and to refer students to these as appropriate.

The most important thing to recognise is the importance of the personal tutor role in enabling students, especially those at greater risk of attrition, to successfully achieve registration as nurses. The skills identified (Wisker et al., 2008) as needed by a good personal tutor are comparable to skills held by many nurses:

- engagement one-to-one with the student's needs and development;
- being able to provide a range of responses;
- observation;
- active listening skills;
- empathy;
- non-judgemental behaviour;
- organisation and planning;
- an ability to keep a professional distance;
- ability to give feedback;
- exhibiting the caring qualities that support students.

Student Support Services

Most HEIs provide a range of support services for students (University of Ulster, 2011c) covering a range of areas which personal tutors need to know about (see Figure 15.2). Many students have personal and family issues which they need to deal with during the period of their study and the aim of these services is to provide support to help students successfully complete their programme. In Bowden's (2008) study only three out of eight students seriously considering leaving their course consulted the HEIs support services so the personal tutor's guidance is crucial in facilitating and encouraging students' access to such services.

Of particular importance is the wide range of services provided in relation to mental health and counselling. These aim to help:

> students to gain the greatest advantage from their education through enabling the individual to face difficult and challenging situations in such a way as to encourage the development of self-awareness, interpersonal skills and personal resourcefulness. … outcome studies give evidence of the fact that access to counselling can be a key factor in enabling a student to complete a course of study. (University of Ulster, 2011c).

Leaflets are available to provide information and guidance for students who can then arrange to see a counsellor if needed; an example of guidance for dealing with examination stress is shown in Box 15.2.

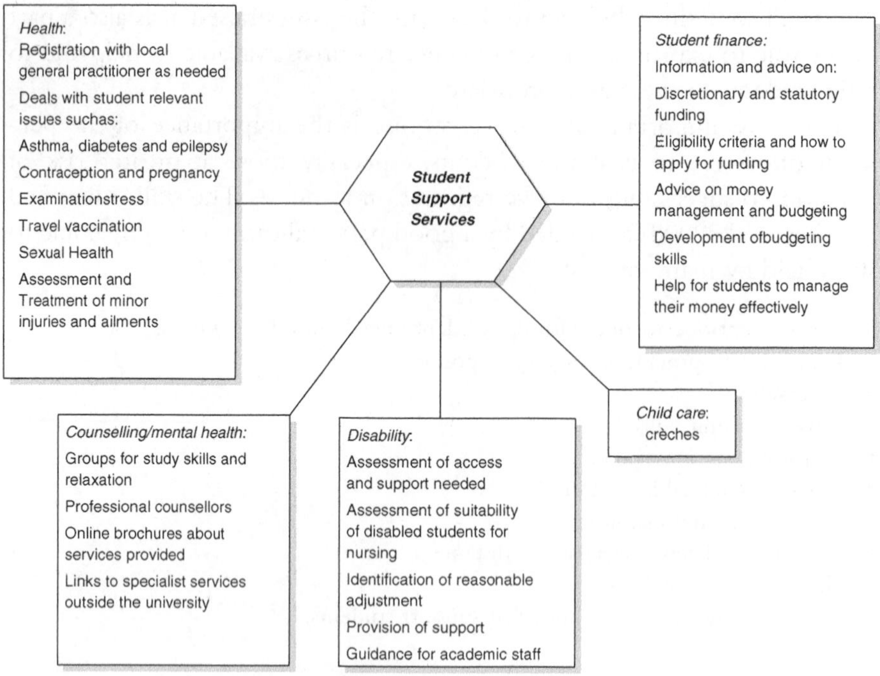

FIGURE 15.2 *Student Support Services*

Box 15.2 Strategies for Handling Exam Stress (University of Ulster, 2011c)

Introduction

Dealing with a degree of anxiety whilst preparing for and doing examinations is a normal behavioural pattern. Some anxiety indicates heightened motivation and is likely to improve performance (getting psyched up for the test after the year's preparation). The psyched up feeling or being in a state of readiness is like butterflies in the stomach but is one of being in control, and purposeful, and in this state you will do your best possible.

For some students the feelings of anxiety can become so exaggerated that coping with them becomes their intellectual focus and less attention is paid to preparation and taking examinations. As a human being can tolerate an enormous amount of stress this does not necessarily mean failure in exams, but the experience can make life hell and performance will not reflect your abilities.

The feelings and thoughts associated with overstress/overanxious state are many and no two people will have quite the same experiences. Examples of what people do experience are:

- poor concentration
- sleep disturbance
- strange lonely feelings
- feelings and thoughts of running away
- nausea
- headaches
- dread and loss of self-esteem
- depression

You can of course have all these symptoms and others and still pass your examination. You may, however, want to reduce or be in control of anxiety and if so there are many strategies open to you. The Counselling Service is available on campus to help you in such circumstances.

Strategies to Consider

- Peer Group Support: Your university peer group can be a helpful emotional and listening source and can also be used for group-study arrangements. Be mindful that fellow students have exams also and may not have the time to listen and encourage you as much as you would like.
- Reassuring tutor/academic: Seek out a friendly lecturer, tutor or studies adviser, and bend his/her ear – they do want you to pass your exams and can help with academic problems and exam techniques.
- Actively seek support: Help can be got at the last minute, but plan ahead if you are anticipating anxiety problems; see the university nurse, the university counsellors or psychologist, the university doctors, studies advisers. As well as having specific skills, they will all have done examinations in the past.
- Read about exam preparation: Look at the many short books which are available in the library.
- Living arrangements: If you are living away from home and it helps to move back home or vice versa should it help (see the accommodation officer and explain).
- Take time out: Keep a social life going.
- Exercise: Regular exercise can provide an outlet for tension and enables you to focus your attention.
- Maintain routine: Unless this has been successful for you in the past, don't change dramatically your eating or sleeping habits. Strive to keep a balance between study and other pastimes.
- Counselling and Guidance Service: Visit the University Counselling and Guidance Service early or late in the year. It could be helpful to talk over your feelings, gain understanding of your responses and plan to deal with them. The service also runs study skills and relaxation groups each semester on all sites.
- Relaxation: Audio-tapes to aid relaxation (both pre-recorded and specially made to suit your requirements) are available from the University Counselling and Guidance Service.
- No list of strategies can be exhaustive. It is important to consider your individual needs. Do you have some personal problem and the anxiety attached to it is being brought into focus by your examinations?

Pre-registration nursing courses have a large number of mature students who may not have been involved in academic study for some time and need help with study skills and reassurance about their abilities; mature students (over 26) tend to get higher marks than younger students (McCarey et al., 2007).

The knowledge and skills of the disability services staff are particularly valuable in working with academic staff to identify methods to enable *reasonable adjustment* for students in relation to their academic study but also for practice learning. The nursing academic professional input in consultation with health service colleagues is essential in deciding what is reasonable and what is not in undertaking nurse education programmes.

The student health services play an important role in providing information, advice, support and referral as necessary to deal with students' health issues, as well as dealing with minor injuries and ailments. This is particularly important for international students and those away from home, who must register with a local general practitioner. Occupational Health Services necessary for assessment of nursing students' suitability for nursing may be provided by the University Student Services or by the clinical services partner in education.

The Student Funding Advisors provide professional and impartial information and advice to students on a range of issues aiming to help students manage their finances in order to enhance their university experience. In many HEIs they are also responsible for the administration of the government Support Funds and University Hardship Funds.

In addition, the University Careers Service may collaborate with the School in helping students prepare themselves for applying for and successfully obtaining employment after qualifying.

Students' Union

The Students' Union is an important resource for supporting and advising students facing challenges during their course of study. Because the officers are still or have just finished being students themselves, current students may find them more approachable than university staff. They will provide representation for students in negotiation with lecturers aiming to act as 'middlemen' between students and the university. They play an important and responsible role in helping the university to identify and meet student needs.

CLINICAL PLACEMENT SETTINGS

Fifty per cent of the pre-registration nursing programme occurs in practice settings and support is at least as important in this context. A number of different people are available to provide this support but mentors are the most important, as they are the people most in contact with students.

Mentor

The role of mentor has been described as *'giving support, assistance and guidance in learning new skills, adopting new behaviours and acquiring new attitudes'* (Jordon, cited in Huybrecht et al., 2011: 274). The mentor's role in teaching and assessment, and ensuring appropriate experience to meet outcomes, has already been discussed and is the principal focus of their relationship. Successfully enabling students to achieve the skills and competence for registration is satisfying for the mentor and a foundation for developing a good relationship with the student. In addition, the mentor's guidance and support in completing practice-related written work such as portfolios helps the student develop confidence in their choice of materials.

However, the mentor is also usually the most important person who provides emotional support for students in practice learning. The supportive relationship is important in helping students adapt to the new and strange environment and experiences. Mentors are present when students are faced with traumatic situations and challenges in practice and are available to enable students to talk through their feelings. Students experience a range of challenges during practice learning and the mentor's presence, listening and support enables students to continue to develop as professionals.

The relationship which develops between mentor and mentee is important in facilitating student learning and giving appropriate feedback. However, they are also the assessors of student competence and, although they may find it difficult, they cannot allow friendship to distort their professional judgement.

Link Lecturer

The link lecturer's role has been described as: *'to support students and clinical staff and undertake innovations, assessments and audits'* (Smith and Gray, 2001: 233) with visits reported as about every two weeks. However, the way in which this role (or some equivalent) is organised and carrieed out varies between universities (see Chapter 16). The link lecturer plays an important role in relation to placement and helping students to apply theory to practice, and ensuring that each student is gaining suitable experience. They provide support for the mentor as well as the student, working with the mentor to monitor the student's progress and ensure that the mentor gives adequate feedback early enough to be useful. They can provide an independent view of the student's performance, particularly in relation to the intellectual aspects of competence.

The expertise in teaching and assessment held by the lecturer who holds, or is working towards, a qualification as a teacher recorded by the

NMC (2008a), the fourth and highest level of achievement for supporting learning and assessment in practice (Table 16.1 in the following chapter), is useful in supporting the mentor. While the mentor is responsible for clinical assessment (NMC, 2008a), it is recommended that the link lecturer is also involved in clinical assessments (papers cited by Rutkowski, 2007). In particular, when having to fail students, many mentors want university support from the link lecturer.

Service Resources

Some practice learning settings have appointed Practice Education Facilitators, or staff with other titles, to play a role in managing the practice learning environment. They provide support to mentors and monitor and record their regular updating. They are also available for students to consult when necessary. If students are ill or injured while in the placement setting, they can access the occupational health service.

OTHER SUPPORT

Peer Support

Making friends and generating a social support network was the main factor identified as important in the first year at university (Wilcox et al., 2005) and lack of this was a major consideration in students who decided to leave. Sharing accommodation with incompatible companions made it much more difficult to become part of a social group and feel at home. The organisation of accommodation was relevant in facilitating or not the development of social groups. Small flats shared by a few students were particularly difficult if any individual was incompatible.

In the same study, personal tutors were generally found to be helpful although less important than peers. Working in small (about 12 students) tutorial or group activities provided another source of potential friends and were appreciated, while some students formed small independent study groups.

While on placement, peer support is particularly important. It is helpful to try to ensure that students in a particular clinical area know each other and are aware of the importance of peer support and their responsibility to each other. While each student has a mentor, their peer group are going through similar experiences as themselves and they often find it easier to discuss their activities, what they are learning, feelings about their work and their relationships in the practice setting, while maintaining patient confidentiality.

Nursing Professional Organisation

Nursing students are eligible for student membership of the Royal College of Nursing, and of other health unions. The RCN as a professional organisation as well as a trade union provides a range of benefits (shown in Table 15.1) for students (RCN, 2011b) including amongst other things:

- access to the largest nursing library in the UK and to learning opportunities on the Learning Zone;
- advice and support through student information officers and workplace representatives;
- telephone and online information, advice and support service;
- a publication to help students make the most of their practice learning opportunities (RCN, 2002).

TABLE 15.1 *Benefits of RCN Membership*

Protection	Indemnity protection of up to £3 million against claims of clinical negligence at work or on a placement. Advice and representation by experienced lawyers on a matter of employment law that occurs in the course of employment or placement.
Learning and development	Access to one of the largest specialist nursing libraries in Europe with over 64,000 books, key nursing databases, 700 ejournals and 600 ebooks. The elibrary can save money through accessing materials through the RCN elibrary free and online. The Learning Zone permits creation of an online evidence-based portfolio and access to bite-sized chunks of learning. It includes tools and exercises for individual use.
Advice and support	RCN student information officers in every university are a point of contact for university-related problems, as well as providing information and guidance. Workplace representatives can ensure health and safety requirements are met and terms and conditions are satisfactory on placement. RCN Direct is the information, advice and support service open 8.30am to 8.30pm by phone and online 24 hours/365 days a year. The RCN Careers Service provides advice on writing CVs and application forms, interview techniques and careers. RCN Immigration Services are authorised by the Office of the Immigration Services Commissioner and offer free consultations to members. The welfare service offers practical financial advice.
Networking opportunities	RCN's specialist forums provide opportunities to start networking with other healthcare professionals within the specialism who can provide advice and guidance on all areas of nursing and possible nursing careers. Every fortnight RCN Bulletin magazine is sent out which is packed with news and nursing jobs.
Campaigning voice	Campaigning and lobbying to gain improvements in the lives of nurses and healthcare assistants - improving studying, working conditions, and training opportunities. The RCN works alongside other unions when negotiating with decision-makers to ensure that pay and conditions are the best they can possibly be.
Discounts	Available on insurance, utilities, high street stores, supermarkets, dining out, leisure attractions, DVDs, holidays and more.

Online Resources

Online resources and communication strategies can be of considerable value in enabling students to access support while on placement. The use of discussion fora within the VLE (Chapter 11) while on placement can enable students to maintain contact with peers, personal tutors and link lecturers. NIPEC's Development Framework has already been discussed.

CHAPTER SUMMARY

Understanding the factors which increase the risk of attrition will help academic and clinical staff to provide the support, or refer students to relevant sources of assistance, to help them to successfully complete their programme and become registered nurses. The complexity of issues which arise in a programme of theory and practice means that academic staff, particularly personal tutors, need to be aware of the full social context in which students learn. They also need to know about the range of resources available to help students including those provided by the HEI, the clinical facilities, the students' union, professional organisation and peers.

16 RESOURCES AND THEIR MANAGEMENT

INTRODUCTION

This chapter considers the resources needed for nursing education which fall into three main categories: people, material resources for learning, and placements for practice learning. In addition, most universities provide residential and recreational resources for students which are not discussed here.

In earlier parts of this book the roles of academic and clinical staff have been considered in relation to teaching, assessment and support of students. What has not been considered is the preparation and continued updating of these staff to ensure that they are able to undertake their roles. It is important to have some knowledge of these aspects in order to be able to function effectively as part of the team involved in delivering nursing education. Also important are the range of support and administrative staff in HEIs who contribute to different aspects of the academic responsibilities. For someone moving into HE it is helpful to have some idea of how the institution functions.

Resources for learning also need to be considered, including the academic learning resources, simulation facilities and skills laboratories. Finally the clinical facilities where students undertake practice learning are discussed.

STAFF WHO TEACH

Nursing staff in both HEIs and service providers are involved in the teaching of nursing students, including:

- all registered nurses in practice;
- mentors (registered nurses who have completed the required mentor training);
- practice teachers;
- positions primarily within practice settings under a range of job titles and responsibilities, including practice education facilitators or academics in practice;
- lecturer-practitioners;
- teachers/lecturers (university academics).

In addition, members of the multidisciplinary team play an important role in preparation of students for professional practice which involves working within a multi-professional team. The preparation, roles and responsibilities of the mentor, practice teacher and teacher in supporting learning and assessment in practice are specified by the NMC (2008a). The principles underpinning these roles are summarised in Box 16.1 and must be met by all involved in these roles. The teaching aspects of the other nursing roles identified above are not regulated.

Box 16.1 Principles of Roles in Teaching and Learning

Nurses and midwives involved in making judgements on proficiency of students in practice must:

- be on the same part or sub-part of the register as that which the student is intending to enter;
- have developed their own knowledge, skills and competency beyond that of registration through CPD – either formal or experiential learning – as appropriate to their support role;
- hold professional (as opposed to academic) qualifications equal to, or at a higher level than, the students they are supporting and assessing;
- have been prepared for their role to support and assess learning and met NMC defined outcomes ... in practice and (where relevant) academic settings, ... including abilities to support interprofessional learning.

Nurses and midwives who have completed an NMC approved teacher preparation programme may record their qualification on the NMC register. Other teaching qualifications may be assessed ... through the NMC accreditation route.

The NMC (2008a) *Standards to Support Learning and Assessment in Practice* includes a developmental framework showing the expectations at the four levels of preparation in eight aspects of supporting learning and assessment in practice. The outline is indicated in Table 16.1 but the details on the

TABLE 16.1 *Outline Of Developmental Framework to Support Teaching and Assessment in Practice*

Domain	Stage 1: Nurses and Midwives	Stage 2: Mentor	Stage 3: Practice Teacher	Stage 4: Teacher
	The particular attributes for every domain and each of the four stages are specified by NMC (2008: 50–8)			
Establishing effective working relationships	Demonstrate effective relationship building skills sufficient to support learning, as part of a wider interprofessional team, for a range of students in both practice and academic learning environments.			
Facilitation of learning	Facilitate learning for a range of students, within a particular area of practice where appropriate, encouraging self-management of learning opportunities and providing support to maximise individual potential.			
Assessment and accountability	Assess learning in order to make judgements related to the NMC standards of proficiency for entry to the register or for recording a qualification at a level above initial registration.			
Evaluation of learning	Determine strategies for evaluating learning in practice and academic settings to ensure that the NMC standards of proficiency for registration or recording a qualification at a level above initial registration have been met.			
Create an environment for learning	Create an environment for learning, where practice is valued and developed, that provides appropriate professional and interprofessional learning opportunities and support for learning to maximise achievement for individuals.			
Context of practice	Support learning within a context of practice that reflects health care and educational policies, managing change to ensure that particular professional needs are met within a learning environment that also supports practice development.			
Evidence-based practice	Apply evidence-based practice to their own work and contribute to the further development of such a knowledge and practice evidence base.			
Leadership	Demonstrate leadership skills for education within practice and academic settings.			

TABLE 16.2 *Outline of Preparation of Mentors, Practice Teachers and Teachers*

Aspect	**Mentor**	**Practice Teachers**	**Teachers**
Prerequisites	1 year post-registration practice	At least 2 years post-registration practice. Additional qualifications to support specialist students	At least 3 years post-registration practice. Extended their knowledge to at least first degree level
Academic level	HE Intermediate level (i.e. level 5)	Honours degree level, (i.e. level 6)	Postgraduate level (i.e. level 7)
Length of education	10 days (5 days protected time)	30 days protected learning time	1 academic year
Context of preparation	Academic and practice settings	Academic and practice settings	Academic and practice settings
Period of programme	Normally completed within 3 months	Normally completed within 6 months	1 academic year
Work-based learning	Includes mentoring student under supervision with reflection	Includes critical reflection on e.g. acting as practice teacher to specialist nursing student under supervision	Include a minimum of 12 weeks teaching practice
Focus of role	Student's practice learning	Student's practice learning	Student's academic and practice learning
Content	To achieve outcomes in 8 attributes in Table 16.1 at stage 2. Preparation for teaching, supervision and assessment mainly in clinical context, skills training in simulated setting. Disability awareness training	To achieve outcomes in 8 attributes in Table 16.1 at stage 3 Similar to mentor Includes criteria for sign-off mentor	To achieve outcomes in 8 attributes in Table 16.1 at stage 4 Theory and practice of education in academic and clinical contexts
APEL	Up to 100% permitted	Up to 100% permitted	Recognition of other teaching qualifications with required nurse teaching practice
Maintenance of qualification	Meeting mentor requirements Annual updating Reviewed 3-yearly, mentored at least 2 students	Meeting practice teacher requirements Annual updating Reviewed 3-yearly, supervised at least 1 student	Maintain and develop knowledge, skills and competence as teacher by regular updating Must ensure that knowledge of practice is contemporaneous and, where appropriate, skills fit for safe and effective practice
Qualification	Maintained on local register	Maintained on local register	Recorded on NMC Register

NMC website demonstrate the increasing knowledge and breadth of the role at each stage.

Those involved contribute in different ways to student learning in the clinical and academic contexts. While the roles of mentors and practice educators focus on practice learning in the clinical environment, the teacher's role is more comprehensive covering both academic and practice learning. Table 16.2 outlines the NMC requirements for preparation and continuing recognition for the three different roles identified.

Mentors and Sign-off Mentors

Mentors play the major role in enabling students to achieve and assess the necessary competencies in practice by being responsible and accountable for the activities shown in Box 16.2, covering all aspects of managing the student's experience. Mentors have to balance these activities with their responsibilities for patient care, which usually will have to take priority. The ward manager needs to be kept aware of any issues arising with the student requiring additional time from the mentor.

Box 16.2 Responsibilities of Mentors

- Organising and co-ordinating student learning activities in practice.
- Supervising students in learning situations and providing them with constructive feedback on their achievements.
- Setting and monitoring achievement of realistic learning objectives.
- Assessing total performance – including skills, attitudes and behaviours.
- Providing evidence as required by programme providers of student achievement or lack of achievement.
- Liaising with others (e.g. mentors, sign-off mentors, practice facilitators, practice teachers, personal tutors, programme leaders) to provide feedback, identify any concerns about the student's performance and agree action as appropriate.
- Providing evidence for, or acting as, sign-off mentors with regard to making decisions about achievement of proficiency at the end of a programme.

Each student is required to work under direct or indirect supervision for at least 40% of their time in practice learning, with the mentor determining the type of supervision required. In addition, during the final placement, the student will spend the equivalent of an hour a week with the sign-off mentor to receive feedback on performance.

Sign-off Status

The sign-off mentor is a mentor who meets additional criteria specified by the NMC (2010e) to undertake the role of confirming that the student has met the required outcomes for entry on the Professional Register at the end of the programme for nursing pre-registration students and at the end of each placement for midwifery students. Amongst other criteria, they must have completed three sign-off assessments under the supervision of an existing sign off mentor, although the first two of these may be in simulated conditions. Lecturers may only sign off practice if they have a practice-based role and have met the necessary criteria for a sign-off mentor. All midwifery mentors must meet the criteria for sign-off mentors (NMC, 2010e).

Practice Teachers

These are required for supervision and clinical assessment of specialist public health nurses. However, some are also involved in supervision and assessment of other specialist nurses and may play a role in supervision of student nurse clinical education.

Positions in Practice Settings

These are held by experienced nurses with an interest in education working primarily in practice contexts and may be employed by the HEI or service under a range of different job titles. For example, in Northern Ireland, practice education facilitators are employed by the health service and they undertake an important role in liaising with the HE institution. They are responsible for managing the allocation and monitoring of mentors, undertaking the triennial review necessary to remain a mentor, maintaining the mentor/practice teacher local register, and undertaking audits for approval of clinical settings for student experience in collaboration with the link lecturer.

Lecturer/Practitioner

There are now a substantial number of lecturer/practitioners who hold posts jointly between higher education and clinical service. The focus of the role within the health service can vary enormously covering such activities as research, practice development and expert clinical practice, while covering the usual range of activities of academic staff in HE. A lecturer/practitioner who has undertaken mentor training can carry responsibility for clinical assessments of students.

Teacher

Aspects of the role of teachers in the HE context have already been discussed in earlier chapters focusing primarily on teaching, but university lecturers may specialise in or combine activities in education, research, knowledge transfer and/or practice development. They may also become involved in university committees and developments, and local, national and international activities. In relation to education, the NMC (2008a) specifies their role as shown in Box 16.3. Their role is set out in much less detail than for the mentor, recognising the difficulty of prescribing the breadth of their educational and other responsibilities. In comparison with the mentor, the teacher is expected to be able to function in both academic and practice environments and they '*are expected to spend a proportion of their time supporting student learning in practice*' (NMC, 2008a: 40).

Box 16.3 Responsibilities of Teachers

- Organising and co-ordinating learning activities in both academic and practice environments.
- Supervising students in learning situations and providing them with constructive feedback on their achievements.
- Setting and monitoring achievement of realistic learning objectives in theory and practice.
- Assessing performance and providing evidence as required of student achievement.
- Their teaching role will be supported by appropriate professional and academic qualifications and ongoing research, education and/or practice development activity to provide an evidence base for their teaching. Only teachers who work in both practice and academic settings e.g. lecturer practitioners may assess practice.

New Lecturers

Many newly appointed nurse lecturers are moving from clinical positions where they had recognised expertise and respect into a situation where they perceive tension between their previous and their new role. In comparison with working in the health service, a new lecturer in HE finds the '*jobs, culture and organizations ... very different, and possibly more different than they had expected*' (McArthur-Rouse, 2008: 405). In comparison with clinical practice, there is a perceived lack of structure in the organisation of the work involved and multiple roles to encompass. New staff may have difficulty in identifying what they are expected to achieve and how to achieve it. In addition, they do not understand the structure of the institution and how it functions. Initially, their recognition as clinical experts by students is important in bolstering their self-esteem, while they draw on mentorship within the academic department to develop a critical approach to their new roles in scholarship and research (Boyd and Lawley, 2009).

Allocation to a colleague as mentor is an important approach to aiding their adaptation. Some new lecturers have found that a very experienced lecturer has more difficulty in identifying the details of their activities than a more recently appointed lecturer who still has learning about their role at the forefront of their minds. A mentor who identifies aspects of the work of the School to observe or attend, and tasks to learn to do, was found helpful for recently appointed staff in coming to terms with their new role and developing into 'nurse lecturers' (McArthur-Rouse, 2008).

Personal Tutor

One of the aspects of their role that they often come across first is that of personal tutor (see Chapter 15) and it may well be a role for which they have had no preparation. Some of the issues which students raise can cause distress for the personal tutor, who may not have the skills needed to help the student and who finds that they also need support (Neville, 2007).

In some HEIs, student services provide courses to help personal tutors develop the knowledge and skills they need for the role, and staff can always contact expert staff in student services for advice about specific issues. Students with mental health problems may need referral but be reluctant to accept it, causing additional difficulties for staff involved who should obtain advice from student services. It is important to differentiate the role of personal tutor from that of therapist – there may be a particular temptation for specialist mental health nurses to move into the role of therapist and this should be avoided.

Link Lecturers (see also Chapter 15)

Some institutions identify link lecturers who take responsibility for liaising with specified wards, departments or units within the health service, monitoring the performance of students and supporting mentors based in the specified clinical areas. Other HEIs function on the personal tutor model where the lecturer follows 'their' students through all their placements. Each system has advantages and disadvantages. The link lecturer approach enables lecturers to work in clinical areas in which they have the relevant expertise and can develop relationships with the practitioners, but they do not necessarily know the students before their allocation to that setting. With this approach, it is essential that a system is implemented to ensure good communication between lecturers who have worked with individual students. The personal tutor system ensures that the lecturer knows their students and their strengths and weaknesses, but is unlikely to be clinically credible in the area of practice and will have limited opportunity to develop good working relationships with clinical staff (Humphreys et al., 2000). Gillespie and McFetridge (2006) emphasise the importance of the lecturer's relationship with mentors to ensure they understand the curriculum and are kept up-to-date with changes. This helps to bridge the theory–practice gap and develop the application of decision-making skills in clinical practice. It is important to arrange placement support to enable this relationship to continue and develop.

Whichever system is used, there is considerable variation in the way in which individuals undertake this role. One of the key elements is to support the application of theoretical knowledge in the practice setting. Some academics, particularly those recently moved into HE from practice, use their expertise in clinical practice by focusing on skills and clinical competence (Boyd and Lawley, 2009) while others focus more specifically on applying theory to practice by using some of the other approaches shown in Table 16.3.

TABLE 16.3 *Approaches to Lecturer's Teaching in Clinical Context*

Patient care focus	Providing patient care with their students drawing on theoretical knowledge to support students in clinical decision-making
Mind/concept-mapping	Students develop a concept map demonstrating all aspects of knowledge, skills and values relevant to care of individual patient, followed by discussion with lecturer
Clinical rounds	Students introduce link lecturer and give report on patient's treatment and care. The theoretical background to care is then elaborated in discussion
Care/case studies	Allows an in-depth examination of the evidence-based care of an individual patient
Clinical presentations	One or two students give short presentation on a clinical issue to a small group of students, and possibly clinical staff, which acts as the focus for discussion

In using any of the approaches shown in Table 16.3, it is an essential professional requirement to maintain patient confidentiality. Many of these approaches can be carried out without the lecturer knowing the patient or details that would allow identification. The patient must give permission before becoming involved in situations with lecturers and students in which confidentiality is breached

While nurse lecturers mainly relinquish hands-on care with increasing time in HE (Carr, 2007), to be able to support practice-based learning the teacher must maintain their clinical relevance and the NMC identifies a range of methods to achieve this (see Box 16.4). However, individual teachers need to identify a method(s) which suits their own expertise and personality, and negotiate this with the clinical setting and their Head of School. Some academic staff arrange their work to spend a few weeks each year in clinical practice, often returning to their previous place of work with an honorary contract.

Box 16.4 Maintaining Clinical Relevance (NMC, 2008a: 40–41)

- Acting as a clinical teacher or a link lecturer.
- Preparing, supporting and updating mentors and practice teachers.
- Taking part in practice-based action learning groups.
- Contributing to practice development.
- Undertaking practice-based research activity.
- Other strategies that would enable teachers to maintain practice knowledge and awareness, and where appropriate, practice skills, ... for example, nurse teachers in specialist areas may maintain a limited caseload.

An issue that receives a lot of attention is the 'theory–practice gap' and the lecturer seeing students in practice is aiming to minimise this gap through helping students to apply theory to practice (Landers, 2000). However, it can be argued that, as university staff are expected to develop new knowledge through research and to teach this knowledge, it will be reasonable to find that sometimes the knowledge taught in the university has not yet reached practice. Link lecturers may have a role in facilitating this transfer.

Interprofessional Team

Nursing practice takes place within the context of an interprofessional team (see Chapter 6). Thus, students need to learn about interprofessional team working both in the university and in practice. Academics from the range of healthcare professions collaborate in planning interprofessional learning opportunities and endeavour to facilitate some interprofessional activities in the clinical setting. Clinicians from healthcare professions will often agree to provide opportunities for observation and experience in their field and demonstrate collaborative working on different clinical issues.

Continuing Professional Development (CPD)

All nurses are required to complete at least 450 hours of practice and 35 hours of CPD in the previous three years in order to maintain their registration, although the mechanism for monitoring this is currently being reviewed. In addition there are specific requirements related to the roles in teaching, learning and assessment. Mentors are expected to '*maintain and develop their knowledge, skills and competence as a mentor through regular updating*' (NMC, 2008a: 30), including annual updating to ensure that they are aware of issues related to nursing education that are relevant to mentoring and assessment of competence and fitness for practice. Similar requirements must be met by practice teachers. Evidence of this updating is confirmed at the triennial review in relation to accurate recording of the qualifications on the local Register of Mentors and Practice Teachers. Similarly, the NMC (2008a: 40) '*also requires that teachers focus on the practice aspects of their roles and ensure their knowledge of practice is contemporaneous and that, where appropriate, their skills are fit for safe and effective practice*', as well as meeting any requirements of the HEI. Most HEIs now require new lecturers to undertake a course of preparation for their role as a teacher in HE within their first few years of employment. This equally applies to those nurse lecturers who have not yet obtained a recorded qualification as a nurse teacher.

One of the major ways of continuing to learn has already been discussed in relation to nursing students and is equally relevant to academic staff. Reflection can be used by the educators in exactly the same way as by the students to learn from experience, to generalise from that learning and to experiment in using that general understanding in different aspects of teaching. Cowan (2006) emphasises the importance of reflection in becoming an innovative university teacher.

However, there are other ways of undertaking CPD. Most of those involved in teaching healthcare professionals are experienced in teaching their own discipline, but few have been prepared for working in the different context of interprofessional education (IPE) and this an important area on which to focus. A two-day masters level course in IPE for those involved in teaching from a range of professions and with a range of preparation for education (from none to master's qualifications) aimed to achieve the competencies prepared under the auspices of the Centre for the Advancement of Interprofessional Education (CAIPE) shown in Box 16.5. The programme was highly effective in achieving a significant difference between pre-and post-course knowledge questionnaires in relation to: drivers and benefits of IPE; generic, underpinning concepts; teaching approaches with theoretical underpinnings; relevant perspectives for teaching and learning with the relevant professions; quality standards; diversity issues; leading and developing IPE within the relevant sphere of practice. (Anderson et al., 2009)

Box 16.5 CAIPE Competencies for Interprofessional Teaching (Freeth et al., cited by Anderson et al., 2009: 83)

- A commitment to interprofessional education and practice
- Credibility in relation to the particular focus of the IPE to which the educator contributes
- Positive role modelling
- An in-depth understanding of interactive learning methods and confidence in application
- A knowledge of group dynamics
- Valuing diversity and unique contributions
- Balancing the needs of individuals and groups
- Inner conviction and good humour in the face of difficulties

STAFF WHO PROVIDE SUPPORT

Universities are large institutions with a range of staff who in different ways support the education of nursing students. Organisationally some of these are defined as academic-related staff, often with comparable qualifications to academic staff, who are intimately involved in educational activities such as learning resources and computer services. Secretaries and technicians are important in the everyday running of the institution and its activities. Others play a crucial role in maintaining the functioning of the university through security, housekeeping, catering services and others. The contribution of all these staff is essential for the smooth running of the university and progress of educational activities, particularly when an event, such as a professional awards ceremony, is being held. Development opportunities are normally available for all grades of staff and some universities recognise exceptional contributions to the work of the institution.

It is important for academic staff to understand the roles and responsibilities of these different staff in order to know who to contact about various issues and to use their expertise most effectively. Good working relationships with all groups and grades of staff enhance effective functioning and increase the pleasure of work.

School-Based Staff

Secretarial and technical staff are an integral part of the staff of the School and collaboration between academic and support staff is essential for the smooth running of the School. They arrange to accept submitted coursework, arrange meetings, produce necessary documentation for academic and clinical work, and ensure that all the necessary equipment and resources are available and in working order. They get to know both staff and students and, because they are often in contact with students, they may be the first people to identify students with personal problems.

Faculty Administrative Staff

In some universities the Faculty administrative staff play an important role in managing the selection and admissions process, implementing the standards agreed with the School for proceeding to interview, arranging interviews and dealing with all the communications etc. In addition they play an important role in managing Faculty-level activities in relation to research, research students, education and a range of other issues.

University-Level Staff

The key elements of the university mission are managed in most HEIs by pro-vice-chancellors and some specialist senior officers (e.g. finance, human resources) under the overall direction of the vice-chancellor and senate, with the university council providing oversight. Many of the activities involving academic staff are determined at university level by senior academics with a major involvement in setting policy and senior administrative staff with support implementing that policy. The senior administrative and support staff are essential in smooth running of many activities including those shown in Table 16.4, and good relationships with these different staff can make operationalising the curriculum considerably simpler and more pleasant.

UNIVERSITY FACILITIES

The HEI has a number of resources which will help students and staff in promoting learning. The organisation and range of materials now available has changed radically in the past 15 years.

TABLE 16.4 *Activities Dependent on Senior Administrative and Support Staff*

Teaching and learning	Examinations, international students, English language support, technology-facilitated learning, university regulations, academic planning, marketing, quality management
Research	Ethics committee, research repository, knowledge transfer, research funding, research students
Students	Equality and diversity services, student support, career development
Staff issues	Access and educational partnerships, purchasing, salaries and wages, health and safety, staff development, information services
Security, domestic, catering	Arranging special events e.g. Professional Awards Ceremonies

Learning Resources

Libraries

These used to consist of books and journals with, in the older universities, back-runs of journals from centuries past which will still be residing in the archives. Resources such as *Index Medicus* in book form were essential for reviewing the literature, and books or journals not held in the HEI library were requested via inter-library loan from the British Library or other resource. Inter-library loan is still a valuable resource for academic and postgraduate students, although many HEIs will restrict its use by undergraduates.

The world has changed. Libraries still contain books and journals, with back-runs, but much of the space is now taken up by computers and study rooms which can be booked by small groups of students. Academic staff are regularly asked to review books on the shelves to determine whether any are now out-of-date and can be disposed of or archived; they are also responsible for ensuring that adequate new books are requested for purchase for the courses offered.

HEI libraries have a number of online databases, suitable for the areas of study within the institution, and many online journals. However, no library can afford to have all the journals they would like and again academic staff play an important role in working with the librarians to select the most important journals for their discipline. Often, due to financial constraints, a new journal can only be acquired by dropping another considered of less importance. Most HEI libraries will focus on the peer-reviewed academic journals which are of significance in assessment of research output in the Research Excellence Framework (REF). Professional journals are perceived as of less value although they play an important role in disseminating knowledge of professional developments. The RCN Library is valuable in enabling members to access a range of professional, as well as academic, nursing journals.

The expertise of librarians is invaluable in providing induction to the library and its resources for new students, but also for students at later stages in their course. Courses on different aspects of library use are provided but librarians can always be approached for help. Students about to start work on their dissertation are usually grateful for a revision session on literature searching.

Computer Facilities

Some HEIs now provide all their students with laptops. However, all HEIs have computers available for student use, and some HEIs will have selected computer laboratories accessible 24 hours a day, seven days a week. Most entrants to nursing education now are able to use computers, and indeed the NMC (2010a) now require this, although some may need additional help in developing their skills. HEIs will almost always have short courses available to help these students. Of particular value is the Computer Services Helpdesk.

Online Learning Materials

Courses vary in their use of online learning materials. While nursing cannot wholly be learnt using online materials, they can play an important role in the context of blended learning. As well as materials prepared by the staff of the School of Nursing, a number of publishers and other organisations have prepared online materials. Most HEIs will have departments containing academics with specialist expertise in online learning materials who work with the subject experts in developing appropriately structured materials in the discipline.

Clinical Skills Laboratories

Facilities in which students can practice their clinical skills play an important role in preparation for practice. These frequently take the form of a mock-up ward environment with the range of equipment necessary, kept in good order by technical support. The technician is responsible for maintaining the electronic and IT based equipment but also managing the equipment and supplies needed for students to develop their clinical skills. The skills required cover a range not usually found in university technicians, although an experienced, highly motivated, healthcare assistant can learn the additional skills required to undertake this role effectively. Development and oversight of these facilities needs to be provided by a lecturer with an interest in the area of skills teaching. It is important that students learn to use the equipment in use in the clinical areas, and often it is possible to arrange to borrow up-to-date equipment from the service partners.

CLINICAL FACILITIES

A pre-registration nursing programme is offered in partnership between an HEI and the service organisations in which practice learning takes place. Programme providers are required to ensure that *'Practice learning opportunities must be safe, effective, integral to the programme and appropriate to the learning outcomes'* (NMC, 2010a: 76). The HEI has to work in partnership with NHS, private and voluntary care providers to ensure that sufficient suitable practice learning places are available for the students undertaking the programme, and has to confirm to the NMC that this is so. The HEI in collaboration with its service partners have a number of responsibilities in relation to practice learning indicated in Box 16.6.

Box 16.6 Responsibilities for Practice Learning (NMC, 2010a: 76–78; NMC, 2008a)

- Mentors and practice teachers meet NMC requirements.
- Local register of mentors and practice teachers maintianed, including details of sign off status, updates, triennial review.
- Objective criteria and processes used for approving practice learning settings which are audited two-yearly.
- Range of suitable practice learning opportunities to enable programme outcomes to be achieved.

Quality of Practice Settings

Crucially, the quality of care in placement settings must be acceptable and this is primarily the responsibility of the health service. However, both parts of the partnership involved in providing nursing education are responsible for ensuring that the quality of care in placement settings is of an acceptable standard and that the staff providing supervision are able to undertake their mentoring role effectively. There are a number of indicators of potential problems of quality (Chapter 17) but link lecturers must raise any issues giving rise to concern with the relevant clinical managers and senior managers in service and the placement coordinator in the HEI. Very occasionally a clinical unit may need remedial measures to achieve a suitable standard for practice learning.

The NMC requires programme providers to '*use objective criteria and processes for approving new practice learning environments, and audit them at least every two years. … [to] show how the nature, scope and quality of the learning experience supports programme outcomes*' (2010a: 76–7). The key element in promoting learning is the quality of the learning environment and, if the area is to continue to be used for student learning, this must be audited at least two-yearly or if use of the clinical environment is changed (see Chapter 17).

Clinical Learning Environment

Some of the earliest UK research publications examining the ward as a learning environment were by Fretwell (1982) and Orton (1981) and, although at that time student nurses were employees and an important part of the ward team, many of the findings of these studies are still valid. The ward sister still plays the key role in determining the quality of patient care and of the clinical learning environment through her own values and expectations of staff and students. Although the mentor is responsible for teaching, supervision and assessment of students, the ward sister still creates the emotional environment through *'teamwork, negotiation and good communication'*; students learn more in wards *'in which sisters make a conscious effort to make teaching a reality'* (Fretwell, 1982: 111) through ensuring mentors have time available to work with students. Similarly clinical areas still exist where students do not feel welcome (low-student-orientated wards) or do feel that all staff aim to help them learn (high-student-orientated wards) as described by Orton (1981).

Nursing students will gain experience in both institutional and community settings. In either case a number of groups of factors contribute to the quality of the clinical learning environment: people, learning opportunities and experiences, staff commitment to teaching and learning, and material resources. These are elaborated on in Table 16.5. A welcoming social climate, and enthusiasm for caring and teaching among all staff are infectious and will help to motivate student learning. The mentor aims to ensure that the clinical setting is a learning environment and helps students to make the most of the experiences available, including opportunities for interprofessional learning (Gopee, 2008).

Practice Learning Opportunities

During the overall programme students must be able to experience all the necessary practice learning opportunities to meet the NMC and university programme outcomes, including:

- direct contact with healthy and ill people and communities;
- to organise, deliver and evaluate nursing care on the basis of the knowledge and skills they have acquired;

- across a range of community, hospital and other settings;
- experience of 24-hour, 7-days a week care;
- meeting EU requirements for general care (adult nursing students). (NMC, 2010a: 77–8)

In addition, before students under 18 can enter the placement setting, the HEI must carry out a risk assessment.

TABLE 16.5 *The Clinical Learning Environment* (Stuart, 2007)

The people	
Leader of team	Wide diversity of roles to fulfil, with limited direct contact with students. However, indirect influence on positive learning climate is important.
Members of team	Team committed to delivering high quality patient care and to promoting learning activities helps create positive learning environment. Students need opportunities to fit into the nursing and multi-professional team.
Students	Students come with varying levels of knowledge and skills. Support and encouragement appropriate to their level of education is needed.
Mentors and assessors	Mentor is 'friend, role model, able advisor, and the person who supports in many different ways' (218) plus assessor, major contributor to learning environment.
Learning opportunities and experiences provided by:	
Patient/client care	Provision of care is major learning opportunity and is planned with mentor to provide a wide range of experience to meet learning outcomes.
Other clinical activities	Interprofessional learning experiences particularly important, including multi-professional team meetings. Management experience in later stages of programme. Learning about record-keeping and using equipment. Teaching/learning sessions.
Staff commitment to teaching and learning	
Support and supervision of learners	Welcome to ward. Information pack to help student adapt to ward. Help students to cope with stress and anxiety. Provide ongoing support and supervision, answer questions and discuss progress and learning needs with students.
Continuing professional development	An environment where lifelong learning is embraced by qualified staff who are regularly involved in learning activities themselves, students are likely to be motivated to take advantage of learning opportunities.
Material resources	Philosophy of care for area, policy/procedure manuals, learning resources relevant to area, resource room/space, IT access for evidence for care, health promotion materials, someone to develop and maintain resources.

Planning allocations for practice learning experience must be carried out in collaboration between HEI and service colleagues. Patient admissions to healthcare settings may have to be altered unexpectedly at different seasons of the year or due to outbreaks of infection. It is essential that the HEI is immediately informed so that contingency arrangements can be agreed.

CHAPTER SUMMARY

This chapter has considered the resources necessary to provide a programme of nursing education. The staff are the most important aspect of this as the quality of the work they undertake will determine the quality of the students' learning in academic and clinical environments. In pre-registration education, the mentors are essential in the practice learning context. It is important that those performing this role have undertaken the necessary preparation and, most importantly, that they understand the importance of the role and want to carry it out.

Academic staff have to adapt from expert clinical nurse to novice nurse-academic, a transformation which requires the learning of a new set of knowledge and skills and developing an understanding of the scope of the role. Effective support and guidance is needed early on in this new stage of their career as they progress towards becoming an expert nurse-academic. The wide scope of their role involves interaction with a range of other staff in both the academic and clinical settings, and the management of resources to provide the high quality education needed for nursing graduates to provide high quality care for patients in hospital and community settings.

17 QUALITY MANAGEMENT

INTRODUCTION

The planners of nursing education programmes aim to prepare nurses able to provide high quality care and, to achieve this aim, they must provide high quality programmes. Ensuring the ongoing quality and appropriateness of nursing education programmes is a major concern. The provision of high quality education should be the goal of every person involved in course planning, delivery and educational support, and is one of the major aims of the partners providing nursing education.

While originally developed in the context of health care, Donabedian's (1980) work is still relevant to managing quality in nursing education. It provides a framework for managing quality through examining:

- *Structure:* for example, the human, physical, financial resources, and the organisational structure in which they function, which will influence the
- *Process:* how education is planned and provided, in both academic and clinical settings, which will influence the
- *Outcome:* such as academic results, suitability for professional practice, student satisfaction, high quality patient care.

In essence, quality is managed by setting standards for structure, process and outcome for all aspects of the activity, endeavouring to implement those standards, monitoring whether those standards are met, and taking necessary action to remedy any deficiencies (see Figure 17.1). In reality they combine to form an integrated system, although initially they will be considered separately. However, HEIs tend to develop systems which

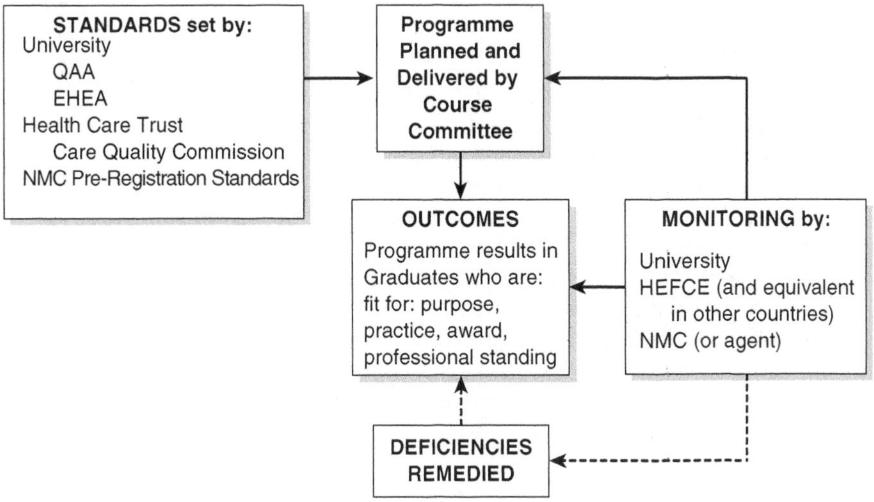

FIGURE 17.1 *Achievement of Quality in Nursing Programmes*

integrate standards and quality management and meet QAA's Code of Practice (2004–10). An example is shown in Box 17.1.

Box 17.1 Principles of Standards Assurance and Quality Management (University of Ulster, 2010a)

In relation to standards the system seeks to ensure that:

- the academic standards of the programmes of study offered by the university are appropriate to their related awards;
- the university's programme structures accord with the requirements of the national Framework for Higher Education Qualifications (FHEQ) and all awards conform to the approved structure;
- the standards of awards are kept under review to ensure the continued validity of the award and that student achievement is commensurate with these;
- standards are externally benchmarked and validated through, inter alia, the input of external examiners and professional, statutory and regulatory bodies and by reference to relevant national subject benchmarks;
- the learning resources provided are sufficient to support students in achieving the award for which they are registered.

In relation to quality the system seeks to ensure that:

- the processes in place for programme approval, monitoring and review are working effectively;

(Continued)

(Continued)

- the views of students, staff, academic subject peers, employers and professional and statutory bodies are fully integrated into the process of programme planning, development and change;
- appropriate quality management arrangements are in place to ensure that all aspects of learning resources are working effectively in support of student learning;
- timely and appropriate action is taken where change is necessary or where matters of concern have been identified;
- excellence in teaching is recognised and rewarded;
- excellence in research and the support of research study is promoted;
- good practice and innovation are recognised and promulgated.

As nursing programmes are complex, with different institutions involved in delivery of formal teaching and promoting learning in a range of clinical environments, the arrangements for assuring quality are also complicated, involving the different organisations and approaches. For those involved in nursing education it is useful to understand the overall structure for quality assurance of nursing and higher education as well as the detail of each part of the process. Because universities are self-governing institutions, each can arrange its own procedures as it wishes and these will vary in different institutions. In this chapter most of the examples given that are related to HE are from the home university of the authors but underpinned by QAA principles.

It is worth noting that healthcare is one of the areas devolved to the authority of the four countries of the UK and the organisations involved in quality management vary. In this chapter, the references to quality within the health service are based primarily on English structures and practices. In the other UK countries the detail may be different but the principles are similar. At present within the NHS in England, Health **Trusts** are responsible for provision of hospital and community services although reorganisation of the NHS is currently under consideration. However, the principles of quality management should not alter.

STANDARDS

The two main partners in providing nursing education are the HEI and the healthcare provider, and each organises the management of quality through standard setting quite separately. HEIs following QAA guidance set standards related to structure, process and outcomes for education (see Chapter 4) while Trust Boards are responsible for the quality of care provided within their organisation where students undertake practice learning. It is important that, in the context of quality of nursing education, they try to speak a common language for quality assurance. In addition, the Statutory Body (NMC in the UK) sets the standards for the specific educational programme for preparing nurses.

Higher Education

The QAA sets standards for higher education, which are compatible with the Bologna Process structures (discussed in Chapter 4), within the Academic Infrastructure, shown in Figure 17.2 and defined as:

> a set of UK-wide nationally agreed reference points that give all higher education providers a shared starting point for setting, describing and assuring the quality of the learning experience and standards of higher education awards or programmes. (QAA, 2011a)

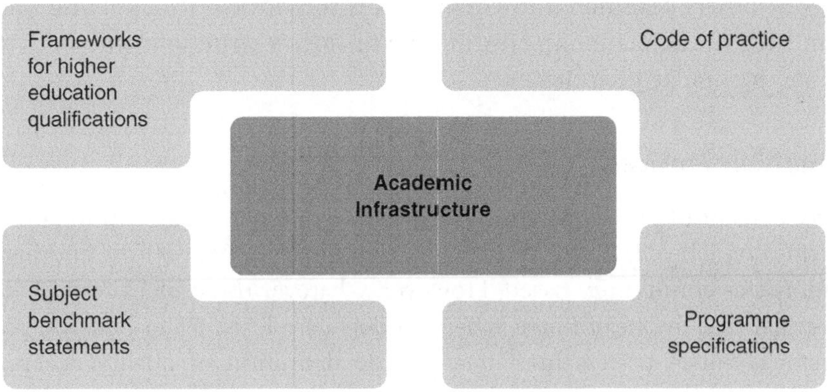

FIGURE 17.2 *Academic Infrastructure*

It is currently being restructured as a new UK Quality Code for Higher Education containing much of the current content but updated and modified to meet current requirements. The new version should replace the current documentation for the academic year 2012–13 and will be presented in three sections:

Part A: Setting and maintaining threshold academic standards;

Part B: Assuring and enhancing academic quality;

Part C: Providing information about higher education. (QAA, 2011b)

Universities in the UK are self-governing organisations and can determine how they meet the QAA standards (discussed in Chapter 4) and achieve benchmark statements for healthcare and nursing (QAA, 2001) (see Chapter 2). Funding for most HEIs is dependent on demonstrating suitable quality of provision, as assessed by QAA.

University

Within the guidelines of QAA, each university will state its requirements for each programme including the structures, processes and outcomes to ensure quality. Normally a university will have a senior officer (probably a Pro-Vice-Chancellor) with overall responsibility for quality of teaching and learning, with different areas of work within this area managed by senior administrative staff. Documents to provide guidance for academic staff on different aspects of educational provision are developed, such as *Programme Approval, Management and Review Handbook* (University of Ulster, 2010a), or *Assessment Handbook* (University of Ulster, 2010b), to ensure that standards required are clear. The course planning team, consisting of both academic and health service staff, as well as others considered in Chapter 3, is responsible for applying these standards to the planning, creating the necessary structures, and delivery of the particular programme.

Healthcare Provider

Fifty percent of pre-registration nursing programmes occur within clinical settings which may be NHS, private or voluntary organisations, and institutional or community based. However, whatever the type of setting, it is essential that the health care where students are learning to become professional nurses is of a high quality. The definition of quality accepted within the NHS was specified in 2008 as follows:

> Care provided by the NHS will be of a high quality if it is:
>
> - Safe;
> - Effective
> - with positive Patient Experience. (Darzi, cited by National Quality Board, 2011: 2)

Within the context of clinical governance in the NHS, Health Trusts are held responsible for quality of care provision. Clinical governance has been defined as:

> a system through which NHS organisations are accountable for continuously improving the quality of their services and safeguarding high standards of care by creating an environment in which excellence in clinical care will flourish. (Scally and Donaldson 1998: 62)

This requires the integration of several approaches to achieve quality of care, as shown in Figure 17.3 which identifies details in the management of the six approaches: infrastructure, culture, coherence, risk avoidance, dealing with poor performance and quality methods.

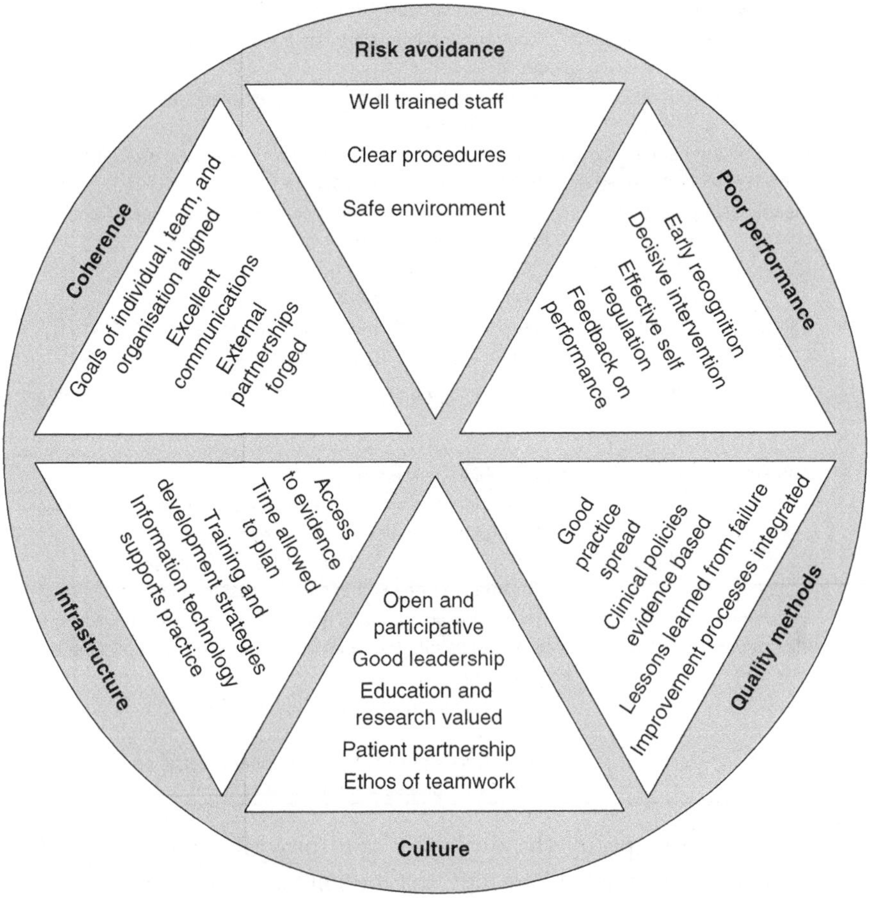

FIGURE 17.3 *Integrating Approaches of Clinical Governance (Scally and Donaldson, 1998)*

All health and social care service providers in England are expected to meet the 28 Government Standards, 16 of which are directly related to the quality of care and safety, shown in Table 17.1 with the expected outcomes (CQC (Care Quality Commission), 2011a), and which incorporate structures, processes and outcomes. These apply to hospitals, care homes and community care.

TABLE 17.1 *Government Standards for Health and Social Care*

	Outcomes	Expected Behaviour
1	Respecting and involving people who use services	People should be treated with respect, involved in discussions about their care and treatment and able to influence how the service is run.
2	Consent to care and treatment	Before people are given any examination, care, treatment or support, they should be asked if they agree to it.
4	Care and welfare of people who use services	People should get safe and appropriate care that meets their needs and supports their rights.
5	Meeting nutritional needs	Food and drink should meet people's individual dietary needs.
6	Cooperating with other providers	People should get safe and coordinated care when they move between different services.
7	Safeguarding people who use services from abuse	People should be protected from abuse and staff should respect their human rights.
8	Cleanliness and infection control	People should be cared for in a clean environment and protected from the risk of infection.
9	Management of medicines	People should be given the medicines they need when they need them, and in a safe way.
10	Safety and suitability of premises	People should be cared for in safe and accessible surroundings that support their health and welfare.
11	Safety, availability and suitability of equipment	People should be safe from harm from unsafe or unsuitable equipment.
12	Requirements relating to workers	People should be cared for by staff who are properly qualified and able to do their job.
13	Staffing	There should be enough members of staff to keep people safe and meet their health and welfare needs.
14	Supporting workers	Staff should be properly trained and supervised, and have the chance to develop and improve their skills.
16	Assessing and monitoring the quality of service provision	The service should have quality checking systems to manage risks and assure the health, welfare and safety of people who receive care.
17	Complaints	People should have their complaints listened to and acted on properly.
21	Records	People's personal records, including medical records, should be accurate and kept safe and confidential.

These standards specify the quality of care provision which should be demonstrated in settings where nursing students are undertaking practice learning. While the health and social service organisations are responsible for the quality of care, all programme providers must be sure that students will gain satisfactory experience to achieve their practice learning outcomes. Thus the educational audit (discussed later in this chapter) should demonstrate that the necessary standards for care and for practice education are met and in essence is a contract between the two partners in nursing education. Academic staff noting, or hearing from students, any deficiencies in care should first take it up through the appropriate management structure within the Trust and expect action to be taken to remedy the situation. It may be necessary to remove students from the placement area. However, it must also be recognised that nursing lectures have a professional responsibility for protection of the public and under exceptional circumstances may need to take further action by reporting concerns to the Care Quality Comission and/or the Nursing and Midwifery Council.The NMC (2010f) guidance on raising and escalating concerns provides relevant information and organisations which can be of assistance.

Statutory Body

The Standards set by the NMC (2010a) specify details of required structures, the processes for delivery of the programme and the anticipated outcomes, and have already been discussed.These have been developed in consultation with the profession and other interested stakeholders and should ensure the quality of the programme and, thus, high quality care provided for patients by the students and future registered nurses.

PROGRAMME PLANNING AND DELIVERY

Programme planning and delivery are joint activities between HEI and the health services and both are responsible for the quality of the programme. Indeed every individual involved with students or education is responsible for quality. In ward settings, the quality of the patient care provided is mainly determined by the ward sister and, similarly, in a university the Head of School largely determines the social climate and enthusiasm of the staff for high quality education.A positive atmosphere within the institution provides an environment in which the ward or School leaders are motivated and enjoy their work and which motivates their staff.

The people at the sharp end of delivering nursing education are lecturers and mentors and the quality of their delivery depends on a range of factors indicated in Figures 17.4 and 17.5. Both need enthusiasm for their work, a supportive environment in which to work, and willingness to continue to develop using feedback and a range of CPD activities. The differences lie in the scope and context of their work, preparation for the role, and possible acquisition of research expertise in lecturers.

Higher Education Institution

The organisation of universities varies, but in all cases the management of quality is important and may be implemented through a top-down or a bottom-up approach. A top-down approach involves carrying through the

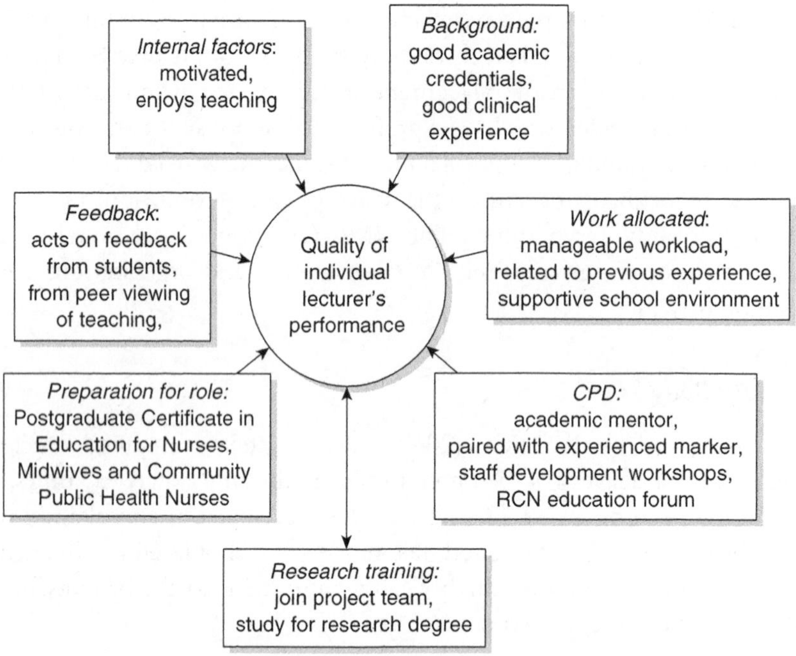

FIGURE 17.4 *Quality of Individual Lecturer*

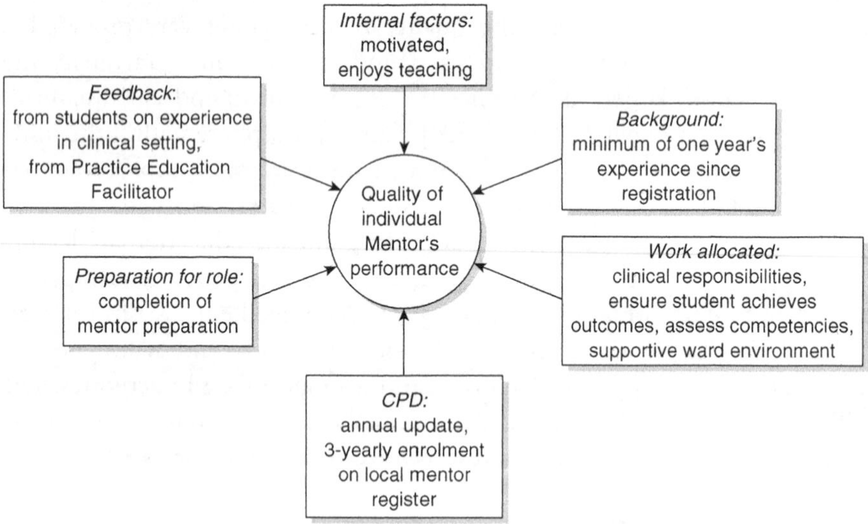

FIGURE 17.5 *Quality of Mentor Input to Education*

instructions issued by senior management. However, the bottom-up approach is becoming more generally accepted. It places responsibility firmly with the Course Committee, with Faculty, and university-level monitoring and initiation of action if deficiencies are noted. The university carries the responsibility for ensuring that the necessary structures, both physical and organisational, are provided. The standards and guidelines developed at university level are implemented at school level.

The School

The programme is developed by a planning team which may be organised in different ways. In some Schools this activity is carried out mainly by senior academics while other Schools endeavour to involve all staff who will be contributing to delivery of the education. Senior staff guide the planning process and ensure that the various standards discussed previously are incorporated in the programme. However, many junior academic staff join HE with a strong clinical background and/or research expertise and can make a valuable contribution to programme planning.

Whatever the university and School structures and support mechanisms, the quality of delivery of education is determined at individual lecturer level within the course team. The programme is managed by the Course Committee, guided by the Course Director, and including all academic staff who contribute to the teaching, representatives from the health service, student representatives and service user representatives. The Course Committee is responsible for ensuring the quality of all aspects of the education provided. The university may produce a detailed checklist of issues as a guide for the Course Committee through the year, covering all activities necessary to deliver the course effectively, provide a good student experience, and continue to enhance quality (University of Ulster, 2011d). The main areas are identified in Box 17.2.

Health Service Organisations

The major responsibility for the quality of placement for practice learning is held by the organisations providing health care. Many of the NHS organisations have appointed staff members (for example, Practice Education Facilitators) with specific responsibilities associated with ensuring the quality of practice settings (Chapter 16). However, private healthcare facilities are less likely to have such appointments and the university staff have to ensure the quality of the placement.

Box 17.2 Outline of Areas of Responsibility of Course Committee (derived from University of Ulster, 2011d)

The areas of responsibility of the course committee include:

- recruitment and selection of students, and managing student issues;
- ensuring that the programme is delivered as planned in both university and practice learning environments;
- managing assessment as planned and liaising with External Examiner;
- student progression and award;
- receiving and acting on feedback from a range of sources;
- responding to communications from other committees;
- liaising with the Statutory Body and other relevant organisations;
- providing required information for the university and statutory body;
- considering issues raised from the Staff-Student Consultative Committee;
- programme and subject development.

MONITORING

A number of different organisations are involved in monitoring the quality of the programme using a wide range of indicators of structure, process and outcomes. In addition, there are numerous stakeholders with an interest in the results including the funding bodies, the education commissioning bodies, professional and statutory bodies, students, potential students, patients, potential employers and others.

Monitoring by HE

Each HEI is responsible for ensuring that all their courses achieve an acceptable standard and all students receive a good education. However, the HE system monitors achievement of institutions and their programmes through the activities of QAA, which has:

> responsibility to safeguard the public interest in sound standards of higher education qualifications, and to encourage continuous improvement in the management of the quality of higher education ... by reviewing standards and quality, and providing reference points that help to define clear and explicit standards. (QAA, 2009)

Through institutional reviews, QAA determines whether confidence can be placed in an HEI's ability to maintain the quality of their programmes and the standards of their academic awards. The growing acceptance of this approach to quality is indicated by '*the Council of Europe* [which] *proposed that quality assessment mechanisms should be built on trust and give due regard to internal quality development processes*' (Kohler et al. cited by Rosa et al., 2011).

The university plays an oversight role in quality management of its education by reviewing reports from Course Committees and, if necessary, taking appropriate action. In addition, themed audits are carried out across the university of selected aspects of course provision or the student learning experience. These audits provide detailed information about qualitative and quantitative aspects of the university's activities in relation to the usual teaching and learning but also about national and local priority areas.

School Responsibilities and Response

Within the bottom-up approach, each course committee is responsible for monitoring the quality of the programme they run, using guidance from the university in doing so, by reviewing all the data available, identifying any risk factors and determining remedial action. A risk management approach is used in many HEIs in which areas causing concern are identified and monitored in depth. In this context, one of the major aspects of the Course Committee's role is module review to identify 'at-risk' modules and plan appropriate action to remedy deficiencies and ensure quality of the module. This is achieved by two key elements: the student survey and module monitoring.

The student survey asks for student opinions about all aspects of the module. It consists of 11 closed questions about module delivery, assessment, feedback, learning resources, the tutor etc. and two open questions about what is particularly good and what they would like to see improved. Students are asked to complete this online at the end of each semester for each module that they have studied. The quantitative information and a list of the open question comments are available to the module coordinator very shortly after the survey closes to encourage rapid improvement of the module.

Module monitoring is the second approach used and is carried out by the Head of School. One of the aims is to reduce the overall amount of reporting required. Modules are selected for detailed examination at the end of each semester on the basis of statistical information showing either higher than expected or lower than expected student performance. Box 17.3 shows the usual range of approaches used by the Head of School in undertaking this review. Following completion of the review the Head of School and Module Coordinator jointly develop an action plan to improve the quality.

Box 17.3 Detailed Module Review by Head of School

- Discussion with module coordinator.
- Review of Staff/Student Consultative Committee minutes.
- Review of student survey on the quality of teaching outcomes/comments.
- Discussion with a group of students who have completed the module, including successful and unsuccessful students.
- Review of past performance on the module to establish if the unexpected level of performance is a 'one-off' or a recurring theme.
- DEVELOPMENT OF ACTION PLAN TO REMEDY DIFFICULTIES

National Student Survey

In addition to university-organised monitoring, the external National Student Survey is carried out and results are displayed on *Unistats* (2011) to help potential students with their choice of university, and these are also available to institutions. These results reflect the quality of programmes as demonstrated through some of the data from above and student views. From 2012, Key Information Sets (KIS) are expected to be available on university websites for each course and should include material which students have reported as useful, such as

- student satisfaction
- course information
- employment and salary data
- accommodation costs
- financial information, such as fees
- students' union information. (HEFCE, 2011)

Each HEI aims to enhance its reputation by a strong performance in the different indicators, with the hope of attracting increasing numbers of high quality students.

External Examiner

In the UK and Ireland, each university course appoints an experienced examiner (or examiners) within the particular discipline from another institution. Examiners should have no current or recent relationship with the host institution, and their primary role is to be the guardian of academic standards. QAA (2004) described the aims of this system as threefold:

- The external examining function should help institutions to ensure that: the academic standard of each award and its component parts is set and maintained by the awarding institution at the appropriate level, and that the standards of student performance are properly judged against this;
- the assessment process measures student achievement appropriately against the intended outcomes of the programme, and is rigorous, fairly operated and in line with the institution's policies and regulations;
- institutions are able to compare the standards of their awards with those of other higher education institutions. (QAA, 2004: 6)

These still represent a reasonable description of the role although the 2004 document has now been replaced and the expectations of the external examiner are discussed in detail in QAA (2011b). Typical responsibilities are shown in Box 17.4.

Box 17.4 Typical Responsibilities of External Examiners

Plays key role in guarding the academic standards of the programme and contributing to comparability in the discipline across academic institutions through:

- Reviewing assessment strategy: may recommend/agree modifications to assessment regulations
- Reviewing proposed individual examinations and coursework assessment and may suggest modification
- Reviewing clinical assessment procedures, process and results
- Moderating marking of examination and coursework to ensure equity and consistency and appropriate standard of internal marking. Plays particular attention to fail and first class graded work
- Comparing student performance with students from comparable programmes in other institutions
- Discussing issues arising from marking with internal examiners prior to examination board
- Attending examination board meetings, contributing to discussion and (almost always) endorsing recommendations for conferment of academic awards
- Reporting to the institution on the assessment process

Appointment of an external examiner is an important event in managing quality and the UK-wide criteria to be considered are shown in Box 17.5. In addition, the substantial increase in nursing student numbers in HE since nursing education moved into HE in the 1990s, has resulted in an increased need for external examiners. The NMC has integrated their quality approval mechanisms with those of QAA, but incorporating involvement in practice learning:

> AEIs (Approved Education Institutions) must appoint external examiner(s) who can demonstrate currency in education and practice with due regard and engage with assessment of both theory and practice. (NMC, 2010a: 87)

Box 17.5 Criteria for Appointment as External Examiner (QAA ,2011c)

Person specification

(a) Institutions appoint external examiners who can show appropriate evidence of the following:

1. knowledge and understanding of UK sector agreed reference points for the maintenance of academic standards and assurance and enhancement of quality
2. competence and experience in the fields covered by the programme of study, or parts thereof
3. relevant academic and/or professional qualifications to at least the level of the qualification being externally examined, and/or extensive practitioner experience where appropriate
4. competence and experience relating to designing and operating a variety of assessment tasks appropriate to the subject and operating assessment procedures
5. sufficient standing, credibility and breadth of experience within the discipline to be able to command the respect of academic peers and, where appropriate, professional peers
6. familiarity with the standard to be expected of students to achieve the award that is to be assessed
7. fluency in English, and where programmes are delivered and assessed in languages other than English, fluency in the relevant language(s) (unless other secure arrangements are in place to ensure that external examiners are provided with the information to make their judgements)
8. meeting applicable criteria set by professional, statutory or regulatory bodies
9. awareness of current developments in the design and delivery of relevant curricula
10. competence and experience relating to the enhancement of the student learning experience.

Conflicts of interest

(b) Institutions do not appoint as external examiners anyone in the following categories or circumstances:

1 a member of a governing body or committee of the appointing institution or one of its collaborative partners, or a current employee of the appointing institution or one of its collaborative partners
2 anyone with a close professional, contractual or personal relationship with a member of staff or student involved with the programme of study
3 anyone required to assess colleagues who are recruited as students to the programme of study
4 anyone who is, or knows they will be, in a position to influence significantly the future of students on the programme of study
5 anyone significantly involved in recent or current substantive collaborative research activities with a member of staff closely involved in the delivery, management or assessment of the programme(s) or modules in question
6 former staff or students of the institution unless a period of five years has elapsed and all students taught by or with the external examiner have completed their programme(s)
7 a reciprocal arrangement involving cognate programmes at another institution
8 the succession of an external examiner by a colleague from the examiner's home department and institution
9 the appointment of more than one external examiner from the same department of the same institution.

Care Environments

Most health service organisations maintain data about incidents, complaints, and a range of issues related to the essential standards previously discussed. These, with information from other organisations, are used by CQC in monitoring compliance with the standards.

Care Quality Commission (CQC)

The standards for care published by CQC have already been discussed. CQC is also responsible for monitoring that these standards of quality and safety are met in all contexts where care is provided, and for ensuring that vulnerable people's interests are protected. While these inspections are not focused on education, they are focusing on the quality of the care provided in settings where students are undertaking practice learning and are thus highly relevant. When carrying out the unannounced inspections the inspectors:

- ask people about their experiences of receiving care;
- talk to care staff;
- check that the right systems and processes are in place;
- look for evidence that care isn't meeting government standards. (CQC, 2011b)

These are similar to some of the areas that are considered when carrying out educational audits.

Educational Audits

The NMC expects those involved in supporting students in practice to:

> Create an environment for learning, where practice is valued and developed, that provides appropriate professional and interprofessional learning opportunities and support for learning to maximise achievement for individuals. (NMC, 2008a: 55)

Gopee (2008) discusses approaches to ensuring that a suitable environment for learning is provided and the educational audits monitor that the specified standards are being achieved. The partners providing nursing education are required by the NMC to undertake audits of the educational environment at least two-yearly, and many carry them out annually, to ensure that they are suitable for practice learning and will enable students to achieve the expected outcomes.

In general each university, with its health service partners, devises its own educational audit documentation. In Northern Ireland, the three Universities (the Open University, Queen's University Belfast, University of Ulster) with the five Health and Social Care Trusts and representatives from the independent sector devised documentation to cover all the programmes offered in Northern Ireland. The audit is carried out by a HEI educationalist with a Trust/independent sector representative and the results are shared between all the universities. An outline of the content is shown in Table 17.2.

Statutory Body

The NMC is responsible for ensuring the quality of nursing education, although this may be delegated to a suitable external organisation. Some understanding of the process enables those involved in nursing education to make an appropriate contribution. Details of the processes are available in the *Quality Assurance Handbook* (NMC/Mott MacDonald, 2011) and includes:

- approval of new programmes;
- re-approval and modifications of existing programmes;
- annual monitoring of approved education institutions and their practice partner.

At present an agent carries out these activities on behalf of the NMC.

TABLE 17.2 *Outline of Content within Educational Audits for Practice Placement*

Topic	Information about
Placement details	Provider, site, clinical setting; date of audit, review date
Students	Maximum number of students Courses for which suitable, pre- and post-registration, field of practice Exclusions - not suitable for e.g. first placement
Contact details	Ward/team manager, practice education facilitator, link lecturer
Description of placement area	Field of practice, type of unit, number and types of patients, patient turnover
Experience	Will enable skills and/or standards for specified programme to be met
NMC Standards to support learning and assessment in practice	Number and availability of (full-time equivalent) mentors and sign-off mentors, regular updating and triennial review, local register of mentors, support of mentors, mentorship preparation programme
Mentor information	Students' programme, outcomes for placements, practice assessment, students' ongoing record of achievement
Student support	Mentors allocated before students arrive, student orientation pack. Placement can facilitate 40% time for mentors to work with students, sign-off mentors 1 hour/week
Guidelines	Specified documents are available in relation to: relevant trust and university policies, patient health and safety, professional behaviour, quality of care Policies and guidelines are implemented, any identified complaints or incidents noted
Additional experience	Voluntary organisations, members of multidisciplinary team
Learning resources	Evidence for practice can be accessed, study area, protocols for care
Organisation of care	Framework/model of care used, shift system in use
Quality assurance	Quality audits of patient/client care, patient satisfaction surveys
Staff development	CPD, staff appraisal, clinical supervision, mandatory training etc.
Staffing	Full-time/part-time, part of register, field of practice, post-registration qualifications, CPD currently in progress
Results of audit	Suitable (or not) for practice learning allocation, suitability for specified programmes and clinical modules. Action agreed for next 12-24 months and those responsible

Approval and Re-approval of Nursing Education Programmes

The academic and professional aspects of a nursing education programme are integrally linked and conjoint approval events of the whole are carried out jointly by the HEI and the NMC. The membership of the Validation Panel is agreed by the University and the NMC (or their agent) and includes both University and NMC representatives and possibly patient/carer and student representatives. Although a University senior officer chairs the event, the position of the NMC is preeminent in that they hold the legal responsibility for '*setting and maintaining standards of education, training and conduct*' (NMC, 2010a: 4) in relation to nursing.

The Panel meets with the senior academic staff responsible for the programme and then with the course planning team to discuss the programme and any issues identified for attention. Box 17.6 shows the key concerns of the approval process. Members of the panel also meet with representatives from service, mentors, practice education facilitators and clinical managers.

Box 17.6 Joint Approval Process (NMC/ Mott MacDonald, 2011)

The approval process is designed to ensure that:

1 The rules and standards of the NMC are explicit in the intended programme.
2 Arrangements for the proper supervision, teaching and assessment of students are in place.
3 Practice learning placements have been quality assured.
4 External examining arrangements are applied as rigorously for assessment of practice as for academic assessments.
5 The programme addresses contemporary knowledge and practice.
6 The general rules of the programme provider are compatible with the NMC rules and requirements.

The result of the validation is graded as:

Outstanding:	Exceptionally and consistently high performance with examples of effective practice which is innovative and worthy of dissemination and emulation by other programme providers.
Good:	The element/programme enables students to achieve stated learning outcomes without need for specific improvements.
Satisfactory:	The element/programme enables students to achieve stated learning outcomes but improvement is needed to overcome specific weaknesses.
Unsatisfactory:	Exceptionally low performance. The element/programme makes less than adequate contribution to the achievement of stated learning outcomes. Significant and urgent improvement is required to become acceptable. (NMC/Mott MacDonald, 2011: 18).

The outcome can be:

- approval, normally for a five year period;
- approval subject to specified conditions which must be met if the programme is to continue;
- withhold approval.

Annual Risk-Based Monitoring

Annual monitoring takes place in two stages.

Firstly, programme providers are required to submit an annual report to the NMC to demonstrate that they are meeting all the necessary standards and requirements. This self-evaluation must provide information about all aspects of the programme, as detailed in the *Quality Assurance Handbook* (NMC/Mott MacDonald, 2011); no specific format is required, enabling re-use of reports generated for other purposes (e.g. for HEI use). A risk-based review plan is used as a guide for this annual report which identifies the key risks (as shown in Table 17.3) and provides the detail of how the risks are identified and can be controlled (NMC/Mott MacDonald, 2011).

TABLE 17.3 *Key Risks for NMC Monitoring (NMC, 2011c)*

Theme	Key Risks
Resources	Programme providers have inadequate resources to deliver approved programmes to the standards required by the NMC Inadequate resources available in practice settings to enable students to achieve learning outcomes
Admissions and Progression	Inadequate safeguards are in place to prevent unsuitable students from progressing to qualification
Practice learning	Inadequate governance of practice learning Programme providers fail to provide learning opportunities of suitable quality for students Confirmation of achievement unreliable or invalid
Fitness for practice	Approved programmes fail to address all required learning outcomes
Quality assurance	Programme providers' internal QA systems fail to provide assurance against NMC Standards

A visit prior to the monitoring event is used to identify issues for consideration, materials required and the programme for the event, including identification of placement visits. The managing reviewer prepares a Pre-Review Commentary (PRC) based on the self-evaluation and the preliminary visit. At the monitoring event itself the reviewers are responsible for identifying the status of risks or good practice identified through review of documentation, placement visits, and meetings with '*programme leaders, students, service managers, mentors and practice teachers, patients and carers'* (NMC/Mott MacDonald, 2011: 29). In the context of the review of the whole programme each key risk is assessed and graded using similar judgements as for the whole programme but with the descriptors shown below:

> Outstanding: Exceptional and consistently high performance. Strong risk controls are in place across the provision and in addition, reviewers **must** identify specific features within the risk control systems that are worthy of dissemination and emulation by other programme providers.
>
> Good: The element/programme enables students to achieve stated learning outcomes. Appropriate risk control systems are in place without need for specific improvements.
>
> Satisfactory: The element/programme enables students to achieve stated learning outcomes. But improvements are required to address specific weaknesses in risk control processes.
>
> Unsatisfactory: The element/programme makes less than adequate contribution to the achievement of stated learning outcomes. Risk control systems and processes are weak and significant and urgent improvements are required to become satisfactory. (NMC/Mott MacDonald, 2011: 34)

FITNESS FOR PROFESSIONAL PRACTICE

The graduate nurses are the major outcomes of a nursing programme and the quality must be satisfactory. An HEI offering programmes of nursing (and other comparable professional) education needs a mechanism for ensuring that those being recommended for entry to the professional register at the end of their programme are suitable to be nurses. This is usually achieved through

> the Fitness for Professional Practice procedure which exists to protect:
>
> (a) the public interest, by safeguarding client/patient wellbeing:
>
> (b) the student's interests by ensuring that students do not proceed into a career for which they may well not be suited or for which a regulatory body may not register them. (University of Ulster, 2011e: 75)

The circumstances which may lead to a student being dealt with under these procedures are shown in Box 17.7. Anyone who has concerns about a student in relation to any of these circumstances can initiate the Fitness for Professional Practice procedure which investigates the complaint and determines appropriate action, with possible options shown in Box 17.8. Care is taken to ensure that the proceedings are fair to the student and the public by the composition of the Fitness for Professional Practice Panel which, as well as members of the School, includes an academic from another professional area, and a registered nurse from practice.

Box 17.7 Grounds for Consideration under Fitness for Professional Practice (University of Ulster, 2011e: 75)

Students may be considered unfit for practice on the grounds of:

(a) physical or mental health reasons;
(b) criminal or other serious misconduct:
(c) unprofessional conduct or action:
(d) academic unsuitability for the demands of the professional training.

Box 17.8 Possible Actions by Fitness for Professional Practice Panel (University of Ulster, 2010e: 77)

(a) no action may be required
(b) the student may be referred to Occupational Health, which may result in a period of leave of absence;
(c) recommend to the Faculty Board that the student discontinue studies on the course with or without possibility of transfer to another course;
(d) if the student is at an appropriate stage in his/her programme, he/she may be offered an alternative award which does not lead to a professional qualification;
(e) the student may be referred to the University Disciplinary Committee;
(f) other action as deemed appropriate to the situation.

Where concerns are related to physical or mental health every effort will be made to resolve the issue through medical or counselling services, and the full procedure is only applied if this is unsuccessful. Care is taken to safeguard the student and provide support throughout the period of suspension and investigation, and appeal if applicable.

It is hoped that student indexing will eventually be reintroduced by the NMC to enable HEIs to check whether applicants have previously been enrolled on a pre-registration nursing programme. This would enhance protection of the public through enabling identification of those who have previously been discontinued from a programme as unfit for practice.

CHAPTER SUMMARY

Quality management of nursing education programmes is complex involving HEIs, health service providers and the Statutory Body. The previous chapter considered the necessary resources for nursing education, and this one has examined structure, process and outcome in terms of standards set, implementing these through programme planning and delivery, and monitoring their implementation. It aims to help all those involved to understand how their role fits into the totality of quality management. This whole book endeavours to help all those involved in nursing education to provide a high quality programme to prepare nurses able to provide high quality care.

The overall aim of nursing and nursing education is '*to safeguard the public by ensuring that nurses and midwives consistently deliver high quality healthcare*' (NMC/Mott MacDonald, 2011, 3). In the UK, nursing education is moving towards requiring a degree level qualification in nursing for entry to the profession. The evidence by Aiken et al. (2003) indicates that having a higher proportion of nurses with bachelor's degrees resulted in better patient outcomes, including lower mortality rates in patients receiving surgical interventions. Thus the importance of achieving a high quality bachelor's level education is emphasised and it is hoped that this book will help to achieve this.

GLOSSARY

Academic Staff	The term used in the UK for faculty.
Honours Degrees	In most UK universities Bachelor's degrees are awarded as 1st, upper 2nd, lower 2nd, or 3rd class honours degrees or unclassified degrees. An honours degree requires a higher standard of academic achievement.
Lecturer	A specific grade of academic staff, but also used generically to refer to all university teachers.
Link Lecturer	Term used by most HEIs to refer to a lecturer with responsibility for working with students and mentors in clinical practice.
Mentor/ Preceptor and Sign-off Mentor	The term mentor is usually applied in the context of a long-term relationship in which a more senior colleague provides counselling and facilitates career development. In the UK, they are responsible for supporting and assessing pre-registration nursing students. A preceptor has been described as someone who provides transitional role support and learning experiences within a collegial relationship for a specific time while continuing to perform some or all of the other responsibilities of their position.www.hspcanada.net/glossary.asp. In the UK they provide support for newly qualified nurses. A sign-off mentor is a mentor who has undertaken additional preparation in order to undertake the responsibility of confirming that a nursing student has achieved a level of competence to permit registration on the NMC Register of Nurses.

Module	A unit of learning within a programme, sometimes known as a course.
NHS Trust	Organisation which provides health care within UK National Health Service.
Nursing Statutory Body	An organisation set up by law which is responsible for maintaining the register of nurses within that country and for setting the standards to permit registration.
Personal Tutor	Lecturer with responsibility for monitoring progress and supporting students throughout their programme. Sometimes known as studies adviser.
Professor	In the UK, Professor is the title used only for those of the most senior academic rank.
Programme	The complete curriculum experience leading to a formal qualification. Sometimes known as a course (but see Module above).
School	The term used in this book to mean the grouping of staff responsible for offering the programme. It may be a school or department within a university or multi-professional college, or a hospital-based school or college of nursing.
Service	This refers to the range of statutory, private and voluntary organisations which provide health care.

REFERENCES

Adair, J. (2007) *Decision Making and Problem Solving Strategies.* London: Kogan Page.

Aiken, L. H., Clarke, S. P., Cheung, R. B., Sloane, D. M. and Silber, J. H. (2003) Educational levels of hospital nurses and surgical patient mortality. *Journal of the American Medical Association,* 290 (12). 1617–23. http://jama.ama-assn.org (accessed 21/4/2012).

Alligood, M.R. and Tomey, A.M. (2010) *Nursing Theorists and Their Work* (7th edn). Maryland Heights, MO: Mosby Elsevier.

An Bord Altranais (2005) *Requirements and Standards for Nurse Registration Education Programmes* (3rd edn). Dublin: An Bord Altranais.

Anderson, E.E. and Kiger, A.M. (2008) 'I felt like a real nurse' – Student nurses out on their own. *Nurse Education Today*, 28, 3–9.

Anderson, E.S., Cox, D. and Thorpe, L.N. (2009) Preparation of educators involved in interprofessional education. *Journal of Interprofessional Care*, 23(1): 81–94.

Anderson, L.W. and Krathwohl, D.R. (eds) (2001) *A Taxonomy for Learning, Teaching, And Assessing: A Revision of Bloom's Taxonomy of Educational Objectives.* New York: Longman.

Applin, H., Williams, B., Day, R. and Buro, K. (2011) A comparison of competencies between problem-based learning and non-problem-based graduate nurses. *Nurse Education Today* 31: 129–34.

Aston, L. and Molassiotis, A. (2003) Supervising and supporting student nurses in clinical placements: the peer support initiative. *Nurse Education Today,* 23(3): 202–10.

Atherton, J.S. (2011) *Learning and Teaching; Bloom's Taxonomy* [Online: UK] http://www.learningandteaching.info/learning/bloomtax.htm (accessed 22/2/2011).

Ausubel, D.P., Novak, J.D. and Hanesian, H. (1978) *Educational Psychology: A Cognitive View* (2nd edn). New York: Holt, Rinehart and Winston.

Bandura, A. (1986) *Social Foundations of Thought and Action: A Social Cognitive Theory.* Englewood Cliffs, NJ: Prentice-Hall.

Barnett, R. and Coate, K. (2005) *Engaging the Curriculum in Higher Education* (The Society for Research into Higher Education). Maidenhead: Open University Press.

Barr, H., Helme, M. and D'Avray, L. (2011) *Developing Interprofessional Education in Health and Social Care Courses in the United Kingdom: A Progress Report.* (Occasional Paper 12, Health Sciences and Practice Subject Centre). London: Higher Education Academy.

Barrett, D. (2007) The clinical role of nurse lecturers: past, present, and future. *Nurse Education Today*, 27: 367–74.

Barrett, T. and Moore, S. (2011) *New Approaches to Problem-Based Learning: Revitalising your Practice in Higher Education.* Abingdon: Routledge.

Beckett, A., Gilbertson, S. and Greenwood, S. (2007). Doing the right thing: nursing students, relational practice, and moral agency. *Journal of Nursing Education*, 46: 28–32.

Belbin, R.M. (2010) *Team Roles at Work* (2nd edn).T Oxford: Butterworth-Heinemann.

Benner, P.E. (1984) *From Novice to Expert: Excellence and Power in Clinical Nursing Practice*. Menlo Park, CA: Addison-Wesley.

Bennett, P.N., Gum, L., Lindeman, I., Lawn, S., McAllister, S., Richards, J. Kelton, M. and Ward, H. (2011) Faculty perceptions of interprofessional education. *Nurse Education Today*, 31: 571–6.

Bevis, E.O. and Watson, J. (2000) *Toward a Caring Curriculum*. Sudbury, MA: Jones and Bartlett.

Biggs, J. and Tang, C. (2007) *Teaching for Quality Learning at University: What the Student Does* (3rd edn) (The Society for Research into Higher Education). Maidenhead: Open University Press (McGraw-Hill).

Biley, F.C. and Smith, K.L. (1998) 'The buck stops here': accepting responsibility for learning and actions after graduation from a problem-based learning nursing education curriculum. *Journal of Advanced Nursing*, 27: 1021–9.

Billings, D.M. and Halstead, J.A. (2009) *Teaching in Nursing: A Guide for Faculty* (3rd edn). St Louis, MO: Saunders (Elsevier).

Bligh, D. (1998) *What's the Use of Lectures?* (5th edn). Exeter: Intellect.

Bloom, B.S. (ed.) (1956) *Taxonomy of Educational Objectives, Handbook I: The Cognitive Domain*. New York: David McKay Co Inc (Longman).

Blumenstyk, G. (2010) Beyond the Credit hour: old standards don't fit new models. *The Chronicle of Higher Education,* January 3. http://chronicle.com/article/News-Analysis-Thinking-Beyond/63349/

BNF (2012) *British National Formulary*. London: BMJ Publishing and RPS Publishing. http://bnf.org/bnf

Bologna Process (2005a) *The European Higher Education Area – Achieving the Goals: Communiqué of the Conference of European Ministers Responsible for Higher Education*, Bergen, 19–20 May 2005. www.bologna-bergen2005.no/Docs/00-Main_doc/050520_Bergen_Communique.pdf

Bologna Process (2005b) *The Framework for Qualifications of the European Higher Education Area (FQ-EHEA)*. Copenhagen: Ministry of Science, Technology and Innovation. www.bologna-bergen2005.no/Docs/00-Main_doc/050218_QF_EHEA.pdf

Boore, J. and Porter, S. (2011) Education for entrepreneurship in nursing. *Nurse Education Today*, 31(2): 184–91.

Boud, D. and Associates (2010) *Assessment 2020: Seven propositions for assessment reform in higher education*. Sydney: Australian Learning and Teaching Council.

Boud, D. and Falchikov, N. (eds) (2007) *Rethinking Assessment in Higher Education: Learning for the Longer Term*. Oxford: Routledge.

Boud, D. and Feletti, G. (eds) (1997) *The Challenge of Problem-Based Learning* (2nd edn). London: Kogan Page.

Bowden, J. (2008) Why do nursing students who consider leaving stay on their courses? *Nurse Researcher*, 15(3): 45–58.

Bowles, A. and Bowles, N.B. (2000) A comparative study of transformational leadership in nursing development units and conventional clinical settings. *Journal of Nursing Management,* 8(2): 69–76.

Boyd, P. and Lawley, L. (2009) Becoming a lecturer in nurse education: the work-place learning of clinical experts as newcomers. *Learning in Health and Social Care*, 8(4): 292–300.

Brimble, M. (2008) Skills assessment using video analysis in a simulated environment: An evaluation. *Paediatric Nursing*, 20(7): 26–31.

Broadfoot, P. (2007) *An Introduction to Assessment*. London: Continuum International Publishing.

Brodie, D.A., Andrews, G.J., Andrews, J.P., Gail, B., Thomas, G.B., Wong, J. and Rixon, L. (2004) Perceptions of nursing: confirmation, change and the student experience. *International Journal of Nursing Studies*, 41: 721–33.

Brown, G., Bull, J. and Pendlebury, M. (1997) *Assessing Student Learning in Higher Education*. London: Routledge.

Bryan, C. and Clegg, K. (eds) (2006) *Innovative Assessment in Higher Education*. Abingdon: Routledge.

Bryar, R. and Sinclair, M. (eds) (2010) *Theory for Midwifery Practice*. London: Palgrave Macmillan.

Buckwell, K. (2010) *Pilot for introducing service user/carer feedback in pre-registration nursing*. Abstract 4.2.6 in Education: Partners in Practice, RCN Education Forum Conference, Blackpool, February 2010.

Bulpitt, H. and Deane, M. (2009) *Connecting Reflective Learning, Teaching and Assessment*. (Occasional Paper 10. Health Sciences and Practice Centre). London: Higher Education Academy.

Burnard, P. (2002) *Learning Human Skills: An Experiential and Reflective Guide for Nurses and Health Care Professionals* (4th edn). Oxford: Butterworth-Heinemann.

Burns, D., Haggart, M., Pryjimachuk, S., Keeley, P. and Wood, P. (2011) *Students as Partners: An Evaluation of the Role of Peer Educator within a School of Nursing*. Abstract 1.3.2, RCN Joint Education Forums' 3rd International Conference, 15 – 17 June, Belfast, NI.

Callanan, C. (2009) Academic Ambitions. *Nursing Standard*, 24(8): 62–3.

Cameron, J., Roxburgh, M., Taylor, J. and Lauder, W. (2010) Why students leave in the UK: an integrative review of the international research literature. *Journal of Clinical Nursing*, 20: 1086–96.

Cameron, J., Roxburgh, M., Taylor, J. and Lauder, W. (2011) An integrative literature review of student retention in programmes of nursing and midwifery education: Why do students stay? *Journal of Clinical Nursing*, 20: 1372–82.

Cant, R.P. and Cooper, S.J. (2010) Simulation-based learning in nurse education: Systematic review. *Journal of Advanced Nursing*, 66(1): 3–15.

Cardiff University (2011) www.cardiff.ac.uk/sonms/degreeprogrammes/undergraduate/applications/selectionpolicy/index.html (accessed, 17/8/2011).

Carlisle, S. and Scott, A. (2011) *Developing Clinical Nursing Skills in Year 1 Undergraduate Curricula*. Abstract, RCN Joint Education Forums' 3rd International Conference, 15–17 June, Belfast, NI.

Carr, G. (2007) Changes in nurse education: Being a nurse teacher. *Nurse Education Today*, 27, 893–9.

Carr, S., Unwin, N. and Pless-Mulloli, T. (2007) *An Introduction to Public Health and Epidemiology* (2nd edn). Maidenhead: Open University Press/McGraw-Hill.

Casey, A. (1995) Partnership nursing: influences on involvement of informal carers. *Journal of Advanced Nursing*, 22(6): 1058–62.

Christiansen, B. (2009) Cultivating authentic concern: Exploring how Norwegian students learn this key nursing skill. *The Journal of Nursing Education*, 48(8): 429–33.

Clarke, A. (2000) Using biography to enhance the nursing care of older people. *British Journal of Nursing*, 9(7): 429–33.

Clark, R.C. and Mayer, R.E. (2008) *E-Learning and the Science of Instruction: Proven Guidelines for Consumers and Designers of Multimedia Learning* (2nd edn). San Francisco, CA: Pfeiffer (John Wiley).

Cook, N.F. and Robinson, J. (2006) Effectiveness and value of massage skills training during pre-registration nurse education. *Nurse Education Today*, 26: 555–63.

Cooke, M. and Moyle, K. (2002) Students' evaluation of problem-based learning. *Nurse Education Today*, 22: 330–9.

Cooper, S., Kinsman, L., Buykx, P., McConnell-Henry, T., Endacott, R. and Scholes, J. (2010) Managing the deteriorating patient in a simulated environment: Nursing students' knowledge, skill and situation awareness. *Journal of Clinical Nursing*, 19: 2309–18.

Cowan, J. (2006) *On Becoming an Innovative University Teacher: Reflection in Action* (2nd edn). (The Society for Research into Higher Education). Maidenhead: Open University Press.

CQC (2011a) *The Essential Standards*. Care Quality Commission. http://www.cqc.org.uk/organisations-we-regulate/registered-services/essential-standards

CQC (2011b) *About Us*. Care Quality Commission. http://www.cqc.org.uk/public/about-us

Cresswell, M.J. (1986) Examination grades: How many should there be? *British Educational Research Journal*, 12(1): 37–54.

Daniels, R., Grendell, R.N. and Wilkins, F.R. (2010) *Nursing Fundamentals: Caring and Clinical Decision Making* (2nd edn). Clifton Park, NY: Delmar Cengage Learning.

Davies, C.S. and Lunn, K. (2009) The patient's role in the assessment of students' communication skills. *Nurse Education Today*, 29(4): 405–12.

Deary, I.J., Watson, R. and Hogston, R. (2003) A longitudinal cohort study of burnout and attrition in nursing students. *Journal of Advanced Nursing*, 43: 71–81.

De Bono, E. (1990) *Lateral Thinking: A Textbook of Creativity*. Harmondsworth: Penguin.

De Bono, E. (2000) *Six Thinking Hats*. London: Penguin.

DeSanto-Madeya, S. (2007) Using case studies based on a nursing conceptual model to teach medical-surgical nursing. *Nursing Science Quarterly*, 20: 324–9.

Dickoff, J. and James, P. (1968) A theory of theories: a position paper. *Nursing Research*, 17: 197–203.

Dickson, D., Hargie, O. and Morrow, N. (1997) *Communication Skills Training for Health Professionals* (2nd edn). London: Chapman and Hall.

Donabedian, A. (1980) *Explorations in Quality Assessment and Monitoring: Volume 1, the Definition of Quality and Approaches to its Assessment*. Ann Arbor, MI: Health Administration Press.

Dowie, I. and Phillips, C. (2011) Supporting the lecturer to deliver high-fidelity simulation. *Nursing Standard*, 25(49): 35–40.

Drummond, J.S. and Standish, P. (2007) *The Philosophy of Nursing Education*. Basingstoke: Palgrave Macmillan.

Duffy, K. (2003) *Failing students: a qualitative study of factors that influence the decisions regarding assessment of students' competence in practice.* Glasgow: Caledonian Nursing and Midwifery Research Centre, Glasgow Caledonian University. www.nmc-uk.org/Documents/Archived%20Publications/1Research%20papers/Kathleen_Duffy_Failing_Students2003.pdf

Duffy, K. and Hardicre, J. (2007a) Supporting failing students in practice 1: Assessment. *Nursing Times*, 103(47): 28–9.

Duffy, K. and Hardicre, J. (2007b) Supporting failing students in practice 2: Management. *Nursing Times*, 103(48): 28–9.

Dyer, J. (2003) Multidisciplinary, interdisciplinary and transdisciplinary educational models and nursing education. *Nursing Education Perspectives*, 24(4): 186–8.

Dyment, J.E. and O'Connell, T.S. (2011) assessing the quality of reflection in student journals: A review of the research. *Teaching in Higher Education*, 16(1): 81–97.

ebookpedia (2010) *The Carnegie Unit: How to Calculate Student Contact Hours.* http://ebookpedia.net/The-Carnegie-Unit--What-is.html (accessed 27/10/2010).

Edwards, H., Nash, R., Sacre, S., Courtney, M. and Abbey, J. (2008) Development of a virtual learning environment to enhance undergraduate nursing students' effectiveness and interest in working with older people. *Nurse Education Today*, 26(8): 672–9.

Edwards, H., Smith, B. and Webb, G. (2001) *Lecturing: Case Studies, Experience and Practice.* London: Kogan Page.

Ehrenfeld, M. and Tabak, N. (2000) Value of admission interviews in selecting of undergraduate nursing students. *Journal of Nursing Management*, 8: 101–6.

El Ansari, W. and Phillips, C.J. (2004) The costs and benefits to participants in community partnerships: a paradox? *Health Promotion Practice*, 5(1): 35–48.

Emerson, R.J. (2007) *Nursing Education in the Clinical Setting.* St. Louis, MO: Mosby (Elsevier).

Equality Act (2010) *Chapter 15.* London: HMSO.

Eraut, M. (2000) Non-formal learning and tacit knowledge in professional work. *British Journal of Educational Psychology*, 70: 113–36.

EU (2005) Directive 2005/36/EC of the European Parliament and of the Council of 7 September 2005 on the recognition of professional qualifications. *Official Journal of the European Union.* L 255/22, 30.9.2005. http://eur-lex.europa.eu/LexUriServ/LexUriServ.do?uri=OJ:L:2005:255:0022:0142:en:PDF

EURYDICE (2010) *Focus on Higher Education in Europe 2010: The Impact of the Bologna Process.* Brussels: Education, Audiovisual and Culture Executive Agency. http://eacea.ec.europa.eu/education/eurydice/documents/thematic_reports/122EN.pdf

Exley, K. and Dennick, R. (2004a) *Giving a Lecture: From Presenting to Teaching* (Key guides for effective teaching in higher education series). London: Routledge Falmer.

Exley, K. and Dennick, R. (2004b) *Small Group Teaching: Tutorials, Seminars and Beyond* (Key guides for effective teaching in higher education series). London: Routledge Falmer.

Fawcett, J. (2005) *Contemporary Nursing Knowledge: Analysis and Evaluation of Nursing Models and Theories* (2nd edn). Philadelphia, PA: F A Davis.

Fawcett, J. (1989) *Conceptual Models of Nursing* (2nd edn). Philadelphia, PA: FA Davis.

Forbes, H., Duke, M. and Prosser, M. (2001) Students' perceptions of learning outcomes from group-based, problem-based teaching and learning activities. *Advances in Health Sciences Education*, 6: 205–17.

Fowler, J. (2008) Experiential learning and its facilitation. *Nurse Education Today*, 28: 427–33.

Fretwell, J.E. (1982) *Ward Teaching and Learning*. London: Royal College of Nursing.

Fry, H., Ketteridge, S. and Marshall, S. (2009) *A Handbook for Teaching and Learning in Higher Education: Enhancing Academic Practice* (3rd edn). London: Kogan Page.

Gantt, L.T. and Webb-Corbett, R. (2010) Using simulation to teach patient safety behaviors in undergraduate nursing education. *Journal of Nursing Education*, 49(1): 48–51.

Gibson, F., Fletcher, M. and Casey, A. (2003) Classifying general and specialist children's nursing competencies. *Journal of Advanced Nursing*, 44(6): 591–602.

Gidman, J. (2001) The role of the personal tutor: A literature review. *Nurse Education Today*, 21: 359–65.

Gillespie, M. and McFetridge, B. (2006) Nurse education – The role of the nurse teacher. *Journal of Clinical Nursing*, 15: 639–44.

Glen, S. and Wilkie, K. (2000) *Problem-Based Learning in Nursing*. Palgrave: Basingstoke.

Glossop, C. (2002) Student nurse attrition: Use of an exit-interview procedure to determine students' leaving reasons. *Nurse Education Today*, 22: 375–86.

Gopee, N. (2010) *Practice Teaching in Healthcare*. London: Sage.

Gopee, N. (2008) *Mentoring and Supervision in Healthcare*. London: Sage.

Grayling, A.C. (1995) *Philosophy: A Guide through the Subject*. Oxford: Oxford University Press.

Grindle, N. (2000) *The Role of the Arts in Teaching Caring: An Evaluation*. Unpublished PhD Thesis. Coleraine: University of Ulster.

Gutteridge, R. and Dobbins, K. (2010) Service user and carer involvement in learning and teaching: A faculty of health staff perspective. *Nurse Education Today*, 30: 509–14.

Habeshaw, D., Gibbs, G. and Habeshaw, T. (1998) *53 Interesting Ways to Assess Your Students* (Interesting Ways to Teach). Bristol: Technical and Educational Services.

Haigh, C. (2010) Legality, the web and nurse educators. *Nurse Education Today*, 30(6): 553–6.

Haigh, J. (2004) Information Technology in health professional education: Why IT matters. *Nurse Education Today*, 24(7): 547–52.

Hammick, M. and Reid, C. (eds) (2010) *Contemporary Issues in Assessment in Health Sciences and Practice Education* (Occasional Paper 11, Health Sciences and Practice Subject Centre). London: Higher Education Academy.

Harden, R.M. and Stamper, N. (1999) What is a spiral curriculum? *Medical Teacher*, 21(2): 141–3.

Harris, S. and Owen, C. (2007) Discerning quality: Using the multiple mini-interview in student selection for the Australian National University Medical School. *Medical Education*, 41: 234–41.

HEFCE (2011) *Key Information Sets*. www.hefce.ac.uk/learning/infohe/kis.htm

HEIDI (2011) *Higher Education Information Database for Institutions*. Higher Education Statistics Agency (HESA). www.hesa.ac.uk/index.php

Henderson, V. (1966) *The Nature of Nursing: A definition and its implications for practice, research and education*. New York: Macmillan.

Heron, J. (1999) *The Complete Facilitator's Handbook*. London: Kogan Page.

Heywood, J. (2000) *Assessment in Higher Education: Student Learning, Teaching, Programmes and Institutions* (Higher Education Policy Series 56). London: Jessica Kingsley.

Hinchliff, S. (ed.) (2009) *The Practitioner as Teacher* (4th edn). Edinburgh: Churchill Livingstone-Elsevier.

Humphreys, A., Gidman, J. and Andrews, M. (2000) The nature and purpose of the role of the nurse lecturer in practice settings. *Nurse Education Today*, 20: 311–17.

Huybrecht, S., Loeckx, W., Quaeyhaegens, Y., De Tobel, D. and Mistiaen, W. (2011) Mentoring in nursing education: Perceived characteristics of mentors and the consequences of mentorship. *Nurse Education Today,* 31: 274–8.

ICN (2010) *Definition of Nursing*. Geneva: International Council of Nurses. www.icn.ch/about-icn/icn-definition-of-nursing (last updated on 12/4/2010).

Jacobs, B.B. (2001) Respect for human dignity: a central phenomenon to philosophically unite nursing theory and practice through consilience of knowledge. *Advances in Nursing Science*, 24(1): 17–35.

Jarvis, P. (2010) *Adult Education and Lifelong Learning: Theory and Practice* (4th edn). London: Routledge.

Jarvis, P. (ed.) (2002) *The Theory and Practice of Teaching*. London: Routledge Falmer.

Jeffries, P.R. (ed.) (2007) *Simulation in Nursing Education: From Conceptualization to Evaluation*. New York: National League for Nursing,

Jeffries, P.R., Rew, S. and Cramer, J.M. (2002) A comparison of student-centred versus traditional methods of teaching basic nursing skills in a learning laboratory. *Nursing Education Perspectives,* 23(1): 14–19.

Jetté, S., St-Cyr Tribble, D., Gagnon, J. and Mathieu, L (2010) Nursing students' perceptions of their resources toward the development of competencies in nursing informatics. *Nurse Education Today*, 30: 742–6.

Johns, C. (2009) *Becoming a Reflective Practitioner* (3rd edn). Oxford: Wiley-Blackwell.

Jones, M.C. and Johnston, D.W. (2006) Is the introduction of a student-centred, problem-based curriculum associated with improvements in student nurse well-being and performance? An observational study of effect. *International Journal of Nursing Studies,* 43: 941–52.

Kelly, M., Lyng, C., McGrath, M. and Cannon, G. (2009) A multi-method study to determine the effectiveness of, and student attitudes to, online instructional videos for teaching clinical nursing skills. *Nurse Education Today,* 29(3): 292–300.

Kember, D. (ed.) (2001) *Reflective Teaching and Learning in the Health Professions*. Oxford: Blackwell Science.

Kember, D., McKay, J., Sinclair, K. and Wong, F.K.Y. (2008) A four-category scheme for coding and assessing the level of reflection in written work. *Assessment and Evaluation in Higher Education*, 33(4): 369–79.

Ker, J., Mole, L. and Bradley, P. (2003) Early introduction to interprofessional learning: A simulated ward environment. *Medical Education*, 37: 248–55.

Kirk, M., Tonkin, E and Skirton, H. (2011) *Fit for Practice in the Genetics/Genomics Era: a revised competence based framework with learning outcomes and practice indicators. A guide for nurse education and training*. Birmingham: NHS National Genetics Education and Development Centre. www.geneticseducation.nhs.uk/media/45814/ffpgge%20learning%20outcomes%20for%20nurses%20report.pdf

Knowles, M.S., Swanson, R.A. and Holton, E.F. (2011) *The Adult Learner: The Definitive Classic in Adult Education and Human Resource Development* (7th edn). Burlington, MA: Butterworth Heinemann (Elsevier).

Kocaman, G., Dicle, A. and Ugur, A. (2009) A longitudinal analysis of the self-directed learning readiness level of nursing students enrolled in a problem-based curriculum. *Journal of Nursing Education*, 48(5): 286–90.

Krathwohl, D.R., Bloom, B.S. and Masia, B.B. (1964) *Taxonomy of educational objectives: The Classification of Educational Goals. Handbook 2, Affective Domain.* London: Longman.

Landers, M.G. (2000) The theory-practice gap in nursing: the role of the nurse teacher. *Journal of Advanced Nursing*, 32(6): 1550–6.

Laurillard, D. (2002) *Rethinking University Teaching: a conversational framework for the effective use of learning* (2nd edn). London: RoutledgeFalmer (Taylor & Francis Group).

Leininger, M. and McFarland, M.R. (2002) *Transcultural Nursing: Concepts, Theories, Research and Practice* (3rd edn). New York: McGraw-Hill.

Lekalakala-Mokgele, E. (2010) Facilitation in problem-based learning: Experiencing the locus of control. *Nurse Education Today*, 30: 638–42.

Levett-Jones, T.L. (2005) Self-directed learning: Implications and limitations for undergraduate nursing education. *Nurse Education Today*, 25: 363–8.

Macdonald, J. (2008) *Blended Learning and Online Tutoring: Planning Learner Support and Activity Design* (2nd edn). Aldershot: Gower Publishing,

Marquis, B.L. and Huston, C.J. (2012) *Leadership Roles and Management Functions in Nursing: Theory and Application* (6th edn). Philadelphia, PA: Wolters Kluwer/ Lippincott Williams and Wilkins.

Marriner-Tomey, A. (2009) *Guide to Nursing Management and Leadership* (8th edn). St. Louis, MO: Mosby (Elsevier).

Maslow, A.H. (1987) *Motivation and Personality* (3rd edn). New York: Harper Collins.

McArthur-Rouse, F.J. (2008) From expert to novice: An exploration of the experiences of new academic staff to a department of adult nursing studies. *Nurse Education Today*, 28(4): 401–8.

McBurney, S. and Carty, E. (2009) Using multiple mini-interviews to assess nursing school applicants. *The Canadian Nurse*, 105(1): 8–10.

McCarey, M., Barr, T. and Rattray, J. (2007) Predictors of academic performance in a cohort of pre-registration nursing students. *Nurse Education Today*, 27: 357–64.

McCaughey, C.S. and Traynor, M.K. (2010) The role of simulation in nurse education. *Nurse Education Today*, 30: 827–32.

McClune, B. and Franklin, K. (1987) The Mead model for nursing. *Intensive and Critical Care Nursing*, 3(3): 97–105.

McConville, S.A. and Lane, A.M. (2006) Using on-line video clips to enhance self-efficacy toward dealing with difficult situations among nursing students. *Nurse Education Today*, 26(3): 200–8.

McCormack, B. and McCance, T. (2006) Development of a framework for person-centred nursing. *Journal of Advanced Nursing*, 56(5): 472–9.

McCormack, B. and McCance, T. (2010) *Person-centred Nursing: Theory, Models and Methods.* Oxford: Wiley-Blackwell.

McEwen, M. and Wills, E. (2011) *Theoretical Basis for Nursing* (3rd edn). London: Wolters Kluwer Health/Lippincott Williams and Wilkins.

McGavock, H. (2005) *How Drugs Work: Basic Pharmacology For Healthcare Professionals.* (2nd edn). Oxford: Radcliffe.

McGloin, H. (2012) *An Exploration of Telephone Coaching in Type 2 Diabetes.* Unpublished PhD Thesis. Coleraine: University of Ulster.

McLaughlin, K., Moutray, M. and Muldoon, O.T. (2008) The role of personality and self-efficacy in the selection and retention of successful nursing students: A longitudinal study. *Journal of Advanced Nursing*, 61: 211–21.

McMullan, M., Endacott, R., Gray, M., Jasper, M., Miller, C., Scholes, J. and Webb, C. (2003) Portfolios and Assessment of Competence: A Review of the Literature. *Journal of Advanced Nursing*, 41(3): 283–94.

McWilliam, P. and Botwinski, C. (2010) Developing a successful nursing objective structured clinical examination. *Journal of Nursing Education*, 49(1): 36–41.

Meleis, A.I. (2011) *Theoretical Nursing: Development and Progress* (5th edn). Philadelphia, PA: Wolters Kluwer/Lippincott Williams and Wilkins.

Melo, K., Williams, B. and Ross, C. (2010) The impact of nursing curricula on clinical practice anxiety. *Nurse Education Today*, 30: 773–8.

Mencap (2010) www.mencap.org.uk/(accessed 20/09/2011).

Meyer, J.H.F. and Land, R. (eds) (2006) *Overcoming Barriers to Student Understanding: Threshold Concepts and Troublesome Knowledge.* London: Routledge, Taylor Francis Group.

Miers, M.E., Rickaby, C.E. and Pollard, K.C. (2007) Career choices in health care: Is nursing a special case? A content analysis of survey data. *International Journal of Nursing Studies,* 44: 1196–209,

Mikkelsen, J., Reime, M.H. and Harris, A.K. (2008) Nursing students' learning of managing cross-infections – scenario-based simulation training versus study groups. *Nurse Education Today*, 28: 664–71.

MIND (2010) www.mind.org.uk/ (accessed 20/09/2011).

Muldoon, O.T. and Reilly, J. (2003) Career choice in nursing students: Gendered constructs as psychological barriers. *Journal of Advanced Nursing,* 43: 93–100.

Mulholland, J., Anionwu, E.N., Atkins, R., Tappern, M. and Franks, P.J. (2008) Diversity, attrition and transition into nursing. *Journal of Advanced Nursing,* 64: 49–59.

National Quality Board (2011) *Quality Governance in the NHS – A Guide For Provider Boards.* www.dh.gov.uk/prod_consum_dh/groups/dh_digitalassets/documents/digitalasset/dh_125239.pdf

Neuman, B. and Fawcett, J. (2010) *The Neuman's Systems Model* (5th edn). New York: Prentice Hall.

Neville, L. (2007) *The Personal Tutor's Handbook* (Palgrave Study Guides). Basingstoke: Palgrave Macmillan.

Nielsen, A.P., Hansen, J., Skorupinski, B., Ingensiep, H-W., Baranzke, H., Lassen, J. and Sandoe, P. (2006) *Consensus Conference Manual.* The Hague: LEI.

NHS Careers (2011) www.nursing.nhscareers.nhs.uk/index.shtml (accessed 23/8/2011).

NIPEC (2011) *Northern Ireland Practice & Education Council for Nursing and Midwifery, Development Framework.* http://www.nipecdf.org/default.asp

NMC (2008a) *Standards to Support Learning and Assessment in Practice: NMC Standards for Mentors, Practice Teachers and Teachers*. London: Nursing and Midwifery Council.

NMC (2008b) *Good Practice Guidance for Selection of Candidates to pre-registration Nursing and Midwifery Programmes*. Circular 13/2008. London: Nursing and Midwifery Council.

NMC (2008c) *The Code: Standards of Conduct, Performance and Ethics for Nurses and Midwives*. London: Nursing and Midwifery Council. www.nmc-uk.org/Nurses-and-midwives/The-code/

NMC (2010a) *Standards for Pre-Registration Nursing Education*. London: Nursing and Midwifery Council. http://standards.nmc-uk.org/Pages/Downloads.aspx

NMC (2010b) *Guidance on Professional Conduct for Nursing and Midwifery Students*. London: Nursing and Midwifery Council.

NMC (2010c) www.nmc-uk.org/Get-involved/Consultations/Past-consultations/By-year/Pre-registration-nursing-education-Phase-2/Glossary/ (accessed 23/10/2011).

NMC (2010d) *Good Health and Good Character: Guidance for Approved Education Institutions. London: Nursing and Midwifery Council*. www.nmc-uk.org/Documents/Guidance/nmcGoodHealthAndGoodCharacterGuidanceForApprovedEducation-Institutions20101105.PDF

NMC (2010e) *Sign-off Mentor Criteria*. NMC circular 05/2010. London: Nursing and Midwifery Council

NMC (2010f) *Raising And Escalating Concerns: Guidance For Nurses And Midwives*. London: Nursing and Midwifery Council. www.nmc-uk.org/Documents/RaisingandEscalatingConcerns/Raising-and-escalating-concerns-guidance-A5.pdf

NMC (2011a) *Requirements, Guidance And Advice For Learning Outside The Uk For Pre-Registration Nursing And Midwifery Students; Annexe 1*. London: Nursing and Midwifery Council.

NMC (2011b) *Advice and supporting information for implementing NMC standards for pre-registration nursing education*. London: Nursing and Midwifery Council. http://standards.nmc-uk.org/PreRegNursing/non-statutory/Pages/supporting-advice.aspx

NMC/Mott MacDonald (2011) *Quality Assurance Handbook*. Nursing and Midwifery Council/Mott MacDonald. www.nmc.mottmac.com/review/

Norman, I., Normand, C., Watson, R., Draper, J., Jowett, S. and Coster, S. (2008) Calculating the costs of work-based training: The case of NHS Cadet Schemes. *International Journal of Nursing Studies*, 45: 1310–18.

O'Donohue, W. and Ferguson, K.E. (2001) *The Psychology of B. F. Skinner*. Thousand Oaks, CA: Sage.

OED (2006) *Concise Oxford English Dictionary*. Oxford: Oxford University Press.

Orem, D., McLaughlin, K. and Taylor, S. (2003) *Self-care Theory in Nursing*. New York: Springer Publishing Company.

Orton, H.D. (1981) *Ward Learning Climate*. London: Royal College of Nursing.

Owen, S. and Standen, P. (2007) Attracting and retaining learning disability student nurses. *British Journal of Learning Disabilities*, 35: 261–8.

Ozturk, C., Muslu, G.K. and Dicle, A. (2008) A comparison of problem-based and traditional education on nursing students' critical thinking dispositions. *Nurse Education Today*, 28: 627–32.

Parahoo, K. (2006) *Nursing Research: Principles, Process and Issues* (2nd edn). Basingstoke: Palgrave Macmillan.

Patient and Client Council (2012) www.patientclientcouncil.hscni.net (accessed 02/02/2011).

Peelo, M. and Wareham, T. (eds) (2002) *Failing Students in Higher Education* (The Society for Research into Higher Education). Buckingham: Open University Press.

Peplau, H.E. (1993) *Interpersonal Nursing Theory*. Washington, DC: Sage.

Popil, I. (2011) Promotion of critical thinking by using case studies as teaching method. *Nurse Education Today*, 31: 204–7.

Price, B. (2003) *Studying Nursing using Problem-Based and Enquiry-Based Learning*. Basingstoke: Palgrave Macmillan.

Prosser, M. and Trigwell, K. (1999) *Understanding Learning and Teaching: The Experience in Higher Education* (The Society for Research into Higher Education). Buckingham: Open University Press.

Pryjmachuk, S., Easton, K. and Littlewood, A. (2009) Nurse education: Factors associated with attrition. *Journal of Advanced Nursing,* 65: 149–60.

QAA (2011a) *Academic Infrastructure*. Quality Assurance Agency. www.qaa.ac.uk/AssuringStandardsAndQuality/AcademicInfrastructure/Pages/default.aspx (accessed 03/11/2011).

QAA (2011b) *Changes to the Academic Infrastructure: Final Report*. Quality Assurance. Agency. http://www.qaa.ac.uk/Documents/qualitycode.pdf(accessed03/11/2011).

QAA (2011c) *UK Quality Code for Higher Education, Chapter B7: External Examining.* Quality Assurance Agency. www.qaa.ac.uk/Publications/InformationAndGuidance/Documents/Quality_Code_for_Higher_Education_Chp_B7_External_examining.pdf (accessed 03/11/2011).

QAA (2009) *An Introduction to QAA*. Quality Assurance Agency. http://www.qaa.ac.uk/Publications/InformationAndGuidance/Documents/IntroQAA.pdf (accessed 03/11/2011).

QAA (2008a) *The Framework for Higher Education Qualifications in England, Wales and Northern Ireland*. Gloucester: The Quality Assurance Agency for Higher Education.

QAA (2008b) *Higher Education Credit Framework for England: Guidance on Academic Credit Arrangements in Higher Education in England*. Gloucester: The Quality Assurance Agency for Higher Education.

QAA (2004–2010) *Code of Practice for the Assurance of Academic Quality and Standards in Higher Education. Sections 1–10*. Gloucester: The Quality Assurance Agency for Higher Education. www.qaa.ac.uk/AssuringStandardsAndQuality/code-of-practice/Pages/default.aspx

QAA (2004) *Code of Practice for the Assurance of Academic Quality and Standards in Higher Education. Section 4: External Examining*. Gloucester: The Quality Assurance Agency for Higher Education. www.qaa.ac.uk/Publications/InformationAndGuidance/Documents/COP_external.pdf

QAA (2001) *Benchmark statement: Health care programmes, nursing*. www.qaa.ac.uk/Publications/InformationAndGuidance/Documents/nursing.pdf (accessed 15/10/2011).

Quinn, F.M. and Hughes, S.J. (2007) *Quinn's Principles and Practice of Nurse Education* (5th edn). Cheltenham: Nelson Thornes.

Race, P. (2005) *Making Learning Happen: A Guide for Post-Compulsory Education.* London: Sage.

Race, P., Brown, S. and Smith, B. (2005) *500 Tips on Assessment* (2nd edn). Abingdon: RoutledgeFalmer.

RCN (2011a) Joint Education Forums' 3rd International Conference, 15th–17th June, Belfast, NI

RCN (2011b) *Why Should Nursing Students Join the RCN*? London: Royal College of Nursing. www.rcn.org.uk/membership/?a=343080 (accessed 28/8/11).

RCN (2003) *Defining Nursing.* London: Royal College of Nursing.

RCN (2002) *Helping Students Get the Best from their Practice Placements: A Royal College of Nursing Toolkit.* London: Royal College of Nursing.

Registered Nursing Home Association (RNHA) (2011) http://www.rnha.co.uk/MANKWD82154 (accessed 20/09/2011).

Rentschler, D.D., Eaton, J., Cappiello, J., McNally, S.F. and McWilliam, P. (2007) Evaluation of undergraduate students using objective structured clinical evaluation. *Journal of Nursing Education*, 46(3): 135–9.

Rhodes, C.A. and Nyawata, I.D. (2011) Service user and carer involvement in student nurse selection: Key stakeholder perspectives. *Nurse Education Today*, 31: 439–43.

Richardson, E. (2011) *Developing and Teaching Intercultural Competence.* Abstract, RCN Joint Education Forums' 3rd International Conference, 15–17 June, Belfast, NI.

Robshaw, M. and Smith, J. (2004) Keeping afloat: Student nurses' experiences following assignment referral. *Nurse Education Today*, 24: 511–20.

Rodgers, B.L. (2005) *Developing Nursing Knowledge: Philosophical Traditions and Influences.* Philadelphia, PA: Lippincott Williams and Wilkins.

Rogers, C. and Freiberg, H.J. (1994) *Freedom to Learn* (3rd edn). Upper Saddle River, NJ: Prentice-Hall.

Roper, N., Logan, W.W. and Tierney, A.J. (2002) *The Elements of Nursing – A Model for Nursing Based on a Model for Living* (5th edn). Edinburgh: Churchill Livingstone.

Rosa, M.J., Cardoso, S., Dias, D. and Amaral, A. (2011). The EUA Institutional Evaluation Programme: An account of institutional best practices. *Quality in Higher Education*, 17(30): 369–86.

Rosenfeld, J.M., Reiter, H.I., Trinh, K. and Eva, K.W. (2008) A cost efficiency comparison between the multiple mini-interview and traditional admissions interviews. *Advances in Health Sciences Education,* 13: 43–58.

Roy, C. (2008) *The Roy Adaptation Model* (3rd edn). London: Pearson Education.

Rutkowski, K. (2007) Failure to fail: Assessing nursing students' competence during practice placements. *Nursing Standard,* 22(13): 35–40.

Sanford, P.G. (2010) Simulation in nursing education: a review of the research. *The Qualitative Report*, 15(4): 1006-11. www.nova.edu/ssss/QR/QR15-4/sanford.pdf

Savin-Baden, M. and Major, C.H. (2004) *Foundations of Problem-Based Learning* (The Society for Research into Higher Education). Maidenhead: Open University Press.

Scally, G. and Donaldson, L.J. (1998) Clinical governance and the drive for quality improvement in the new NHS in England. *British Medical Journal*, 317(7150): 61–5.

Scholes, J., Webb, C., Gray, M., Endacott, R., Miller, C., Jasper, M. and Mcmullan, M. (2004) Making portfolios work in practice. *Journal of Advanced Nursing*, 46(6): 595–603.

Schön, D. (1987) *Educating the Reflective Practitioner.* San Francisco, CA: Jossey-Bass.

SCIE (2007) *Guide 17. Practice Guide: The Participation of Adult Service Users, Including Older People, in Developing Social Care*. London: Social Care Institute for Excellence. www.scie.org.uk/publications/guides/guide17/files/guide17.pdf

Scott, I. (2007) Accreditation of prior learning in pre-registration nursing programmes: Throwing the baby out with the bath water? *Nurse Education Today*, 27: 348–56.

Sears, K., Goldsworthy, S. and Goodman, W.M. (2010) The relationship between simulation in nursing education and medication safety. *Journal of Nursing Education*, 49(1): 52–5.

Secomb, J. (2008) A systematic review of peer teaching and learning in clinical education. *Journal of Clinical Nursing,* 17: 703–16.

Seren, S. and Ustun, B. (2008) Conflict resolution skills in problem-based compared to conventional curricula. *Nurse Education Today*, 28: 393–400.

Sharples, K. (2009) *Learning to Learn in Nursing Practice. Transforming Nursing Practice Series.* Exeter: Learning Matters.

Shepherd, J. (2008) Adolescent student nurses: Implications for retention. *Paediatric Nursing*, 20(3): 42–5.

Smith, P. and Gray, B. (2001) Reassessing the concept of emotional labour in student nurse education: Role of link lecturers and mentors in a time of change. *Nurse Education Today*, 21: 230–7.

Snelling, P., Lipscomb, M., Lockyer, L., Yates, S. and Young, P. (2010) Time spent studying on a pre-registration nursing programme module: An exploratory study and implications for regulation. *Nurse Education Today*, 30: 713–19.

Staddon, J. (2001) *The New Behaviorism: Mind, Mechanism, and Society*. Philadelphia, PA: Taylor and Francis (Psychology Press).

Standing, M. (ed.) (2010) *Clinical Judgement and Decision-Making in Nursing and Interprofessional Healthcare.* Maidenhead: Open University Press (McGraw-Hill).

Stickley, T., Stacey, G., Pollock, K., Smith, A., Betinis, J. and Fairbank, S. (2010) The practice assessment of student nurses by people who use mental health services. *Nurse Education Today*, 30: 20–5.

Stuart, C.C. (2007) *Assessment, Supervision and Support in Clinical Practice: A Guide for Nurses, Midwives and other Health Professionals* (2nd edn). Edinburgh: Churchill Livingstone (Elsevier).

Taylor, B.J. (2006) *Reflective Practice: A Guide for Nurses and Midwives* (2nd edn). Maidenhead: Open University Press.

The Practice Education Group (2006) *Mentoring: A Resource for Those who Facilitate Placement Learning.* (Version 2). (Making Practice-Based Learning Work Series). Oxford: School of Health and Social Care, Oxford Brookes University.

The Times (2007) The applicants who all had burnt pyjamas. London: *The Times*, 8 March.

Thompson, C. and Dowding, D. (2002) *Clinical Decision Making and Judgement in Nursing*. Edinburgh: Churchill Livingstone.

Trigwell, K., Prosser, M. and Waterhouse, F. (1999) Relations between teachers' approaches to teaching and students' approaches to learning. *Higher Education,* 37: 57–70.

Tufte, E.R. (2003) *The Cognitive Style of PowerPoint*. Cheshire, CT: Graphics Press.

Tuning Project (2004) www.unideusto.org/tuningeu/ (accessed 21/09/2011).

Twomey, A. (2004) Web-based teaching in nursing: lessons from the literature. *Nurse Education Today*, 24: 452–8.

UCAS (2011) http://www.ucas.com/ (accessed 23/8/2011).

UK HE Europe Unit (2006) *Guide to the Diploma Supplement*. London: Universities UK. www.europeunit.ac.uk/sites/europe_unit2/resources/GuideDS.pdf (accessed 21/09/2011).

UK Statutory Instrument (2002) *No. 253. The Nursing and Midwifery Order 2001*. London: HMSO.

Unistats (2011) *National Student Survey*. (accessed 03/11/2011).

Universities UK (2007) *Beyond the Honours Degree Classification: The Burgess Group Final Report*. London: Universities UK. www.universitiesuk.ac.uk/Publications/Documents/Burgess_final.pdf

University of Ulster (2011a) *Blackboard Learn*. https://learning.ulster.ac.uk/webapps/portal/frameset.jsp

University of Ulster (2011b) *University of Ulster Prospectus*. http://prospectus.ulster.ac.uk

University of Ulster (2011c) *Student Support*. http://www.studentsupport.ulster.ac.uk/

University of Ulster (2011d) *Annual Checklist of Items to be Considered by Course Committee*. Coleraine: University of Ulster.

University of Ulster (2011e) *University of Ulster: Charter, Statues and Ordinances 2011–2012*. Coleraine: University of Ulster.

University of Ulster (2010a) *Programme Approval, Management and Review Handbook*. Coleraine: University of Ulster.

University of Ulster (2010b) *Assessment Handbook*. Coleraine: University of Ulster

Urwin, S., Stanley, R., Jones, M., Gallagher, A., Wainwright, P. and Perkins, A. (2010) Understanding student nurse attrition: Learning from the literature. *Nurse Education Today*, 30: 202–7.

USA Education (2010) *Education US*. www.usaeducation.us (accessed 27/10/2010).

Uys, L.R. and Gwele, N.S. (2005) *Curriculum Development in Nursing: Process and Innovation*. Abingdon: Routledge.

Van Leeuwen, R., Tiesinga, L.J., Middel, B., Post, D. and Jochemsen, H. (2009) The validity and reliability of an instrument to assess nursing competencies in spiritual care. *Journal of Clinical Nursing*, 18(20): 2857–69.

Warne, T., Johansson, U-B., Papastavrou, E., Tichelaar, E., Tomietto, M., Van den Bossche, K., Moreno, M.F.V. and Saarikoski, M. (2010). An exploration of the clinical learning experience on nursing students in nine European countries. *Nurse Education Today*, 30: 809–15.

Watkins, R. and Schlosser, C. (2002) Moving past time as the criteria: The application of capabilities-based educational equivalency units in education. *Online Journal of Distance Learning Administration*, 5(3). http://www.westga.edu/~distance/ojdla/fall53/watkins53.html

Watson, R., Norman, I.J., Draper, J., Jowett, S., Wilson-Barnett, J., Normand, C. and Halliday, D. (2005) NHS cadet schemes: Do they widen access to professional healthcare education? *Journal of Advanced Nursing*, 49: 276–82.

Watts, T.E. (2011) Supporting undergraduate nursing students through structured personal tutoring: Some reflections. *Nurse Education Today,* 31: 214–18.

Waugh, A. and Grant, A. (2010) *Ross and Wilson Anatomy and Physiology in Health and Illness* (11th edn). Edinburgh: Churchill Livingstone/Elsevier.

Wellard, S. and Heggen, K. (2010) Are laboratories useful fiction? A comparison of Norwegian and Australian undergraduate nursing skills laboratories. *Nursing and Health Sciences,* 12(1): 39–44.

WHO (2011) *Healthy Cities Project.* www.euro.who.int/en/what-we-do/health-topics/environmental-health/urban-health/activities/healthy-cities. (accessed 20/09/2011).

WHO (2009) *Zagreb Declaration for Healthy Cities: Health and Health Equity in all Local Policies.* Copenhagen, Denmark: WHO Regional Office for Europe.

Wikipedia (2011) Virtual learning environment. *Wikipedia, the free encyclopedia* (accessed 10/28/2011).

Wilcox, P., Winn, S. and Fyvie-Gauld, M. (2005) 'It was nothing to do with the university, it was just the people': The role of social support in the first-year experience of higher education. *Studies in Higher Education,* 30(6): 707–22.

Wilkie, K. and Burns, I. (2003) *Problem-Based Learning: A Handbook for Nurses.* Basingstoke: Palgrave Macmillan.

Wisker, G., Exley, K., Antoniou, M. and Ridley, P. (2008) *Working One-to-One with Students: Supervising, Coaching, Mentoring and Personal Tutoring* (Key guides for effective teaching in higher education series). London: Routledge, Taylor and Francis.

Wright, C., Hogard, E., Ellis, R., Smith, D. and Kelly, C. (2008) Effect of PETTLEP imagery training on performance of nursing skills: Pilot study. *Journal of Advanced Nursing,* 63(3): 259–65.

Yuan, H., Williams, B.A. and Lin Fan (2008) A systematic review of selected evidence on developing nursing students' critical thinking through problem-based learning. *Nurse Education Today,* 28: 657–63.

AUTHOR INDEX

This index is in word-by-word order. Page references in *italics* indicate figures, those in **bold** indicate tables, and those in ***bold italic*** indicate boxes.

SUBJECT INDEX